Introduction to Audiology, 11e, Frederick N. Martin and John Greer Clark, © 2012, ISBN: 0132108216

A Research Primer for Communication Sciences and Disorders, Timothy Meline, © 2010, ISBN: 0137015976

The Auditory System: Anatomy, Physiology, and Clinical Correlates, Frank E. Musiek and Jane A. Baran, © 2007, ISBN: 0205335535

Language and Literacy Disorders: Infancy through Adolescence, Nickola W. Nelson, © 2010, ISBN: 0205501788

Introduction to Communication Disorders: A Lifespan Evidence-Based Perspective, 4e, Robert E. Owens, Jr., Dale E. Metz, Kimberly A. Farinella, © 2011, ISBN: 0137000081

Language Development: An Introduction, 8e, Robert E. Owens, Jr., © 2012, ISBN: 013258252X

Language Disorders: A Functional Approach to Assessment and Intervention, 6e, Robert E. Owens, Jr., © 2014, ISBN: 0132978725

Linguistics for Non-Linguists: A Primer with Exercises, 5e, Frank Parker and Kathryn Riley, © 2010, ISBN: 0137152043

Language Development from Theory to Practice, 2e, Khara L. Pence Turnbull and Laura M. Justice, © 2012, ISBN: 013707347X

Foundations of Audiology, Miles E. Peterson and Theodore S. Bell, © 2008, ISBN: 0131185683

Communication and Communication Disorders: A Clinical Introduction, 4e, Elena M. Plante and Pelagie M. Beeson, © 2013, ISBN: 0132658127

An Introduction to Children with Language Disorders, 4e, Vicki A. Reed, © 2012, ISBN: 0131390481

Building ASL Interpreting and Translation Skills: Narratives for Practice (with DVD), Nanci A. Scheetz, © 2009, ISBN: 0205470254

Deaf Education in the 21st Century: Topics and Trends, Nanci A. Scheetz, © 2012, ISBN: 0138154449

Evaluating Research in Communicative Disorders, 6e, Nicholas Schiavetti, Dale Evan Metz, and Robert F. Orlikoff, © 2011, ISBN: 0137151551

Introduction to Audiologic Rehabilitation, 6e, Ronald L Schow and Michael A. Nerbonne, © 2013, ISBN: 0132582570

A Primer on Communication and Communicative Disorders, Howard D. Schwartz, © 2012, ISBN: 0205496369

Clinical Phonetics, 4e, Lawrence D. Shriberg and Raymond D. Kent, © 2013, ISBN: 0137021062

Fundamentals of Phonetics: A Practical Guide for Students, 3e, Larry H. Small, © 2012, ISBN: 0132582104

Stuttering: Foundations and Clinical Applications, Ehud Yairi and Carol H. Seery, © 2011, ISBN: 0131573101

Introduction to Audiology Today, James W. Hall, III, © 2014, ISBN: 0205569234

Speech Science: An Integrated Approach to Theory and Clinical Practice, 3e, Carole T. Ferrand, © 2014, ISBN: 0132907119

Counseling-Infused Audiologic Care John Greer Clark and Kristina M. English, © 2014, 013315324X

For a full listing of the latest resources of interest, browse our online catalog at

www.pearsonhighered.com

ALWAYS LEARNING

PEARSON

Ninth Edition

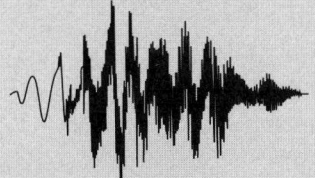

The Voice and Voice Therapy

DANIEL R. BOONE

University of Arizona

STEPHEN C. McFARLANE

University of Nevada Medical School

SHELLEY L. VON BERG

California State University, Chico

RICHARD I. ZRAICK

University of Arkansas for Medical Sciences/
University of Arkansas at Little Rock

PEARSON

Boston • Columbus • Indianapolis • New York • San Francisco • Upper Saddle River
Amsterdam • Cape Town • Dubai • London • Madrid • Milan • Munich • Paris • Montréal • Toronto
Delhi • Mexico City • São Paulo • Sydney • Hong Kong • Seoul • Singapore • Taipei • Tokyo

Executive Editor and Publisher: Stephen D. Dragin
Editorial Assistant: Michelle Hochberg
Marketing Manager: Joanna Sabella
Production Editor: Mary Beth Finch
Editorial Production Service: Jouve North America
Manufacturing Buyer: Megan Cochran
Electronic Composition: Jouve India
Interior Design: Jouve North America
Cover Designer: Laura Gardner

Library of Congress Cataloging-in-Publication Data
Boone, Daniel R.
  The voice and voice therapy/Daniel R. Boone, University of Arizona, Stephen C. McFarlane, University of Nevada Medical School, Shelley L. von Berg, California State University, Chico, Richard I. Zraick, University of Arkansas for Medical Sciences/ University of Arkansas at Little Rock. —Ninth edition.
    pages cm
  Includes bibliographical references and index.
  ISBN-13: 978-0-13-300702-2
  ISBN-10: 0-13-300702-2
  1. Voice disorders—Textbooks. I. McFarlane, Stephen C. II. Von Berg, Shelley L.
    III. Zraick, Richard I., 1962– IV. Title.
  RF540.B66 2013
  616.85'56—dc23

                                                            2012050999

10 9 8 7 6 5 4 3 2 1

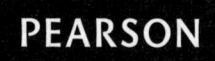

ISBN-10: 0-13-300702-2
ISBN-13: 978-0-13-300702-2

From Dan to his sister, Barbara Boone Brueggemann, who typed the raw manuscripts of the first two editions of this textbook.

From Stephen to his wife, Patty, and his family.

From Shelley to her mother, Sarah Von Berg, an extraordinary speech pathologist and mentor.

From Richard to his wife, Amanda, and his twin daughters, Kaitlyn and Brooklyn, whose voices fill his heart with joy.

About the Authors

Daniel R. Boone celebrates his 60th year as a speech-language pathologist with the publishing of this ninth edition of *The Voice and Voice Therapy*. Dr. Boone has held professorships over the years at Case Western Reserve University, University of Kansas Medical Center, University of Denver, and the University of Arizona (where he is now a professor emeritus). Dr. Boone is a former president of the American Speech-Language-Hearing Association and holds both a Fellowship and the Honors of that organization. He is the author of over 100 publications and is well known nationally and internationally for his many workshop presentations. Dr. Boone is perhaps best known for his love of his students and turning them on to the excitement of clinical voice practice.

Stephen C. McFarlane is a professor emeritus at the School of Medicine at the University of Nevada, Reno. He was awarded ASHA Fellowship in 1982 and ASHA Honors in 1999. He received both his B.S. and M.S. degrees from Portland State University and his Ph.D. degree from the University of Washington. Dr. McFarlane has a long history of research interests in the area of voice disorders. Study of the outcomes from voice therapy and the development of new treatment techniques is of particular interest. His scholarly work has been published in dozens of books and journals, among them *Seminars in Speech and Language*; *American Journal of Speech Language Pathology*; *Phonoscope*; and *Current Opinion in Otolaryngology & Head and Neck Surgery*.

Shelley L. Von Berg teaches, practices, and researches in the areas of voice, dysphagia, and motor speech disorders in adults and children in the Department of Communication Sciences and Disorders at California State University, Chico, where she holds the rank of Associate Professor. She earned her M.S. and Ph.D. degrees from the School of Medicine at the University of Nevada, Reno. She has presented on the assessment and intervention of neurogenic speech-language disorders nationally and abroad. She also teaches abroad on occasion. Dr. Von Berg has been published in the ASHA *Leader* Series; *Unmasking Voice Disorders*; *Language, Speech, and Hearing Services in Schools*; *Current Opinion in Otolaryngology & Head and Neck Surgery*; *Cleft Palate–Craniofacial Journal*; and *AAC Journal*. Areas of interest are intelligibility and comprehensibility of synthetic speech and speech produced by individuals with motor speech disorders.

Richard I. Zraick holds the rank of Professor in the Department of Audiology and Speech Pathology, a consortium program offered by the University of Arkansas for Medical Sciences (UAMS) and the University of Arkansas at Little Rock (UALR). He earned his doctorate at Arizona State University. Dr. Zraick is a clinician and teacher-scholar with over 25 years of experience in clinical practice and academia. His research grants, journal articles, and book chapters are in the areas of voice disorders, neurogenic speech-language disorders, speech and voice perception, clinical skills training, and health literacy. He regularly speaks about these topics at state, regional, and national scientific and professional conventions. He is a recipient of multiple Faculty Excellence in Research and Faculty Excellence in Teaching awards from both UALR and UAMS.

Contents

Chapter 3   Functional Voice Disorders   65

Chapter 4   Organic Voice Disorders   87

Chapter 7   Voice Facilitating Approaches   185

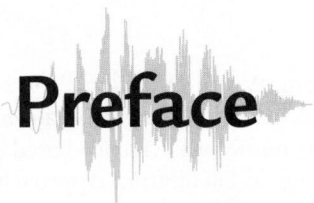

Preface

NEW TO THIS EDITION

The original edition of *The Voice and Voice Therapy* was published in 1971. The preface to the first edition concluded with a statement that has as much relevance today as it did some forty years ago:

> *The Voice and Voice Therapy* is an attempt to take some of the magic out of voice therapy. I hope there is something here not only for the student of voice therapy, but also for the clinical speech pathologist and the practicing laryngologist. I think there is.

In subsequent revisions, we have attempted to maintain the book's relevance to students and voice clinicians alike. Each edition has incorporated the most current scientific knowledge from a variety of disciplines, as well as information about the latest advances in technology. This current edition has some major updates to both the fundamental content of the book and to the pedagogical elements supporting its use in the classroom and clinic. Some chapter-by-chapter highlights include:

- Chapter 1, "An Introduction to Voice Disorders and Their Management," features current data on the incidence and prevalence of voice disorders in the general population and in specific populations. There are also expanded discussions of the classification of voice disorders and of the various approaches to managing the person with dysphonia.
- Chapter 2, "Normal Voice: Anatomy and Physiology Through the Lifespan," has been expanded considerably. It features a more comprehensive description of the anatomy and physiology of normal voice production. In addition, the chapter has all new anatomy illustrations. This chapter can stand alone, thus eliminating the need for students, instructors, or clinicians to refer to outside source material.
- Chapter 3, "Functional Voice Disorders," presents practical approaches to identifying and managing behaviorally based voice disorders. The chapter includes expanded discussions of excessive laryngeal muscle tension and the benign laryngeal pathology that may develop as a result, as well as voice disorders with a psycho-emotional basis or overlay. We also review evidence-based practice (EBP) studies supporting the value of our Voice Facilitating Approaches in treating persons with functional or psychogenic dysphonia.
- Chapter 4, "Organic Voice Disorders," presents practical approaches to identifying and managing organic voice disorders. We present current literature on the medical management of these disorders and on the role of the voice clinician in evaluation and therapy.

- Chapter 5, "Neurogenic Voice Disorders," presents the latest research in the behavioral, pharmacological, and surgical management of neurogenic voice disorders. We also review numerous evidence-based practice (EBP) studies supporting the value of our Voice Facilitating Approaches in treating the respiration, phonation, and resonance subsystems in persons with dysarthria.
- Chapter 6, "Evaluation of the Voice," has been expanded considerably. It features the latest approaches to the auditory-perceptual evaluation of the voice and to assessment of voice-related quality of life. Multiple case studies illustrate both instrumental and noninstrumental assessment of the voice across medical and educational settings. These case studies also provide a framework for report writing and special considerations for voice populations across the lifespan. New figures illustrate instrumental approaches to identifying and quantifying voice and resonance disorders. Over a dozen new tables present the student and clinician with normative data across the lifespan for a variety of acoustic, aerodynamic, and related voice measures. This chapter can stand alone, thus eliminating the need for students, instructors, or clinicians to refer to outside source material.
- Chapter 7, "Voice Facilitating Approaches," remains the bedrock of this textbook. We have retained our core set of 25 Voice Facilitating Approaches, and present the latest evidence-based practice (EBP) studies supporting their value in treating persons with dysphonia. Many of the cases illustrating the approaches have been updated to reflect the types of patients seen in current clinical practice, including applications for audiovisual feedback in therapy. We also discuss current literature on patient compliance and barriers to treatment.
- Chapter 8, "Therapy for Special Patient Populations," features expanded discussions of the identification and management of children, adolescents, and older adults with dysphonia. In particular, we discuss in greater detail the professional voice user and the management of dysphonia in this increasing population of patients. We also discuss in more detail the management of dysphonia in children and adults with hearing impairment, in those who are transgendered, and in those with a variety of respiratory-based conditions.
- Chapter 9, "Management and Therapy Following Laryngeal Cancer," is new and features expanded discussion of the medical management of patients with laryngeal cancer and the role of the voice clinician in evaluation and therapy. We have added new illustrations and photographs throughout the chapter.
- Chapter 10, "Resonance Disorders," features both the instrumental and noninstrumental assessment of persons with disorders of nasal or oral resonance. We have expanded the chapter's discussion of the team management of persons with cleft palate speech. Application of our Voice Facilitating Approaches to treatment of resonance disorders is illustrated.

Close to 1,000 references to other studies are included throughout the text. Cardinal literature from the past 40 years of voice science and care is included, as well as the most current literature from a variety of disciplines. Greater than half the references are new in this edition, with the majority representing advances in our field from the year 2000 to the present.

All new pedagogical elements supporting the use of the book for teaching include the following:

- The Learning Objectives at the beginning of each chapter have been expanded.
- Check Your Knowledge boxes within each chapter stimulate critical thinking.

- Clinical Sidebars reinforce clinical application of material.
- Clinical Concepts at the end of select chapters reflect many of the learning objectives.
- Guided Reading exercises at the end of select chapters reference key clinical articles.
- Multiple-choice questions (Preparing for the PRAXIS™) at the end of select chapters help readers master the type of content covered in the Praxis II™ examination in speech-language pathology.
- A companion website contains a wealth of supplemental materials.

Did you know this book is also available as an enhanced Pearson eText? The affordable, interactive version of this text includes 3–5 videos per chapter that exemplify, model, or expand upon chapter concepts. Look for the play button in the margins to see where video is available in the affordable enhanced eText version of this text. To learn more about the enhanced Pearson eText, go to www.pearsonhighered.com/etextbooks.

We are fascinated by the human voice and intrigued by the art and science of voice therapy. As the great American poet Henry Wadsworth Longfellow wrote,

"Oh, there is something in that voice that reaches the innermost recesses of my spirit!"

We invite you to join us as lifelong students of the human voice, and we hope that while you read this edition, you will share the passion we had for writing it.

DANIEL R. BOONE
STEPHEN C. MCFARLANE
SHELLEY L. VON BERG
RICHARD I. ZRAICK

Acknowledgments

We would like to thank our reviewers: Stephanie Hughes, Governors State University; Kathleen Fahey, University of Northern Colorado; Barbara R. Brindle, Western Kentucky University; and Nandhu Radhakrishnan, University of Missouri; we'd also like to thank Denise Stats-Caldwell, Arizona State University, for her suggestions regarding the book's features. This book contains material produced with our valued colleagues, as follows: (i) The Laryngeal Pathology Photo Gallery and Laryngeal Pathology Video Library are from the Voice and Swallowing Center in the Department of Otolaryngology—Head and Neck Surgery at the University of Arkansas for Medical Sciences (UAMS) (Little Rock, Arkansas). We are grateful to Dr. Ozlem Tulunay-Ugur and Dr. James Suen for allowing their inclusion. (ii) The Voice Facilitating Approaches videos would not have been possible without the expertise of Mark Gandolfo and his team in Media Design and Production at Teaching and Learning Technologies at the University of Nevada, Reno. The new medical illustrations were generated by the gifted hand of Maury Aaseng. Chapters 9 and 10 contain contributions from Leah Skladany, Ph.D. Bonnie Slavych, M.S., assisted with manuscript preparation. Douglas Kucera provided eagle-eyed manuscript scrutiny.

DANIEL R. BOONE
STEPHEN C. McFARLANE
SHELLEY L. VON BERG
RICHARD I. ZRAICK

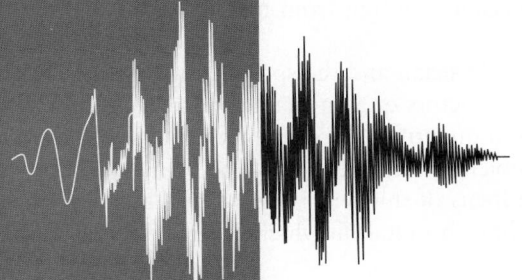

CHAPTER 1

An Introduction to Voice Disorders and Their Management

. . . . . ———————————— LEARNING OBJECTIVES ———————————— . . . .

After reading this chapter, one should be able to:

- List and describe the biological, emotional, and linguistic functions of the larynx.
- List and describe the kinds of voice disorders.
- Describe the incidence and prevalence of voice disorders in the general population.
- Describe the incidence and prevalence of voice disorders in specific populations.
- Describe the types of intervention for voice disorders.

When we hear the long-awaited cry of the newborn infant, we are hearing the infant's first coordination of the outgoing use of the breath stream passing between the vocal folds. More important, we are hearing the confirming evidence that a new life has been born. From that moment on, the mother and those nearby listen closely to the baby's vocalizations. The mood states of anger, loving, and hunger can be heard in the baby's vocal shadings. Similarly, for a lifetime, the sound of the voice often carries more meaning than the words that we say.

Speaking is a distinctive way of using the larynx. The act of singing is even more so. Both speaking and singing demand a combination and interaction of respiration, phonation, resonance, and speech articulation. The best speakers and singers are often those persons who, by natural gift or training, or by a studied blend of both, have mastered the art of optimally using these vocal mechanisms. For most of the population, however, we count on our voices being there when we speak, sing, cry, or laugh with very little conscious effort required.

The larynx sits at the top of the airway, and it appears that its primary function in mammals (including humans) is protecting the airway from any kind of obstruction. Production of the human voice is a secondary function. While the focus of this text is on voice habilitation and rehabilitation, whatever we do in therapy must be consistent with the primary demands of the respiratory system. We will also see that, beyond breathing problems, voicing difficulties can be the result of anatomic deviation and disease, or of emotions overriding normal vocal function, or of a change of vocal function resulting from misuse and overuse of vocal mechanisms.

The voice evaluation by both the physician and the speech-language pathologist (SLP) attempts to identify the causal factors of a particular voice disorder. This dual evaluation of voice documents and quantifies the elements for possible vocal change. If remediation of the voice problem is indicated, it will be by medical treatment and/or voice therapy alone. The focus of this text is on voice therapy by the SLP, regardless of the setting (school, clinic, hospital) in which he or she works with the patient with a voice disorder.

THE BIOLOGICAL FUNCTION OF THE LARYNX

As you watch this **video,** note how the clinician takes time to frame strategic questions to attempt to approach the voice disorder holistically. He is interested in the entire person, not just the pathology. Grand Rounds: What additional questions might you ask this patient? Explain why you would ask these questions.

A description of the biological aspects of laryngeal function provides us an early hint of how the biological demands of the airway and the larynx will always take precedence over artistic or communicative vocal production. When the brain signals the body's need for renewal of oxygen in the breath cycle, we automatically take in a breath. Oxygen-laden air flows through the passages of the upper airway into the lungs, followed by the outgoing carbon dioxide–loaded air flowing out of the body through the airway. This transportation of air into and out of the lungs is the primary function of the airway. Protecting the airway for an unobstructed passage of the air supply is the larynx. The primary biological function of the larynx is to keep fluids and foods from going into the airway (aspiration).

The larynx sits in a vital site at the front, bottom of the throat (pharynx), and at the top of the windpipe (trachea). As fluids and chewed food (bolus) come down the posterior throat, they are diverted from the lower throat (hypopharynx) into the open esophagus, where they continue their journey through the esophagus down into the stomach. As part of the swallowing act, the larynx raises high in the neck (elevating the esophagus and trachea with it). As swallowing progresses, the tongue comes back, and the epiglottis, which acts as a partial cover, closes over the open glottis (see Sidebar 1.1).

SIDEBAR 1.1

To appreciate this movement, put your right index finger on your Adam's apple and swallow repeatedly. You should feel the larynx rising and gliding forward, and then gliding back and lowering to its resting position.

Whenever the larynx plays this sphincteric role of closing off the airway to permit the posterior passage of liquids or food, the entire laryngeal body rises. Also, in fear situations, the larynx may reflexively elevate as part of its primary role in protecting the airway. Some voice patients, sometimes those with excessive fears, will attempt voice with the larynx in its elevated "protector" posture. Such excessive laryngeal elevation is not a good posture for producing a normal voice. This may be associated with the Polyvagal theory (see Porges, 2003).

Besides the elevating capability of the larynx, which helps prevent aspiration, airway closure is aided by three laryngeal muscle valves, described in Chapter 2 as the aryepiglottic folds, the ventricular folds (false folds), and the thyroarytenoid muscles (the true vocal folds). The most vertical of these valve pairs in the larynx are the aryepiglottic folds, which are considered part of the supralarynx. Under vigorous valving conditions, such as severe coughing, they begin to approximate (adduct). Below them are the ventricular folds; only during vigorous adductory activities, like the cough, do they approach each other. The lowest and more medial of the three laryngeal valves are the thyroarytenoid muscles, the true vocal folds. During swallowing, they always adduct to prevent possible aspiration. Also, the individual has fine control of the true vocal folds, with some capability of altering their shape, length, and tension, to produce various voicing changes.

When one breathes naturally, all three valve sites are open. The vocal folds separate further on inspiration, allowing a greater volume of air to pass through quickly; on expiration, they move slightly toward (adduct) one another. As further described in Chapter 2, voice is produced when the vocal folds adduct slightly together, allowing expired air to pass between them, setting the folds into vibration. This vibration produces voice (phonation). This phonation is then resonated through various sites of the vocal tract. The resonance of the voice begins with this vibratory sound in the larynx, traveling up through the pharynx and the oral and nasal cavities above. The voice we hear, then, is produced by a combination of respiratory activation, phonation, and amplifying resonance. Although the primary role of the larynx is to protect the airway, the larynx and voice in the human plays an important role in emotional and linguistic expression.

THE EMOTIONAL FUNCTION OF THE LARYNX

The infant seems to express emotions by making laryngeal sounds. Certainly, the caregiver can soon detect differences in the emotional state of the baby by changes in the sound of the baby's vocalizations: A cry from hunger may sound different from a cry of discomfort or the vocalization of anger. Contentment (after a full stomach or being held) can be heard in the relaxed cooing responses of the baby. From early infancy throughout the lifespan, the sound of one's vocalization often mirrors one's internal emotional state.

Our voice can sound happy or sad, contented or angry, secure or unsafe, placid or passionate (see Sidebar 1.2). How one feels affectively may be heard in the sound of the voice as well as in changes of the prosodic rhythm patterns of vocalization. Our emotional status plays a primary role in the control of respiration; for example, nervousness may be heard in one's shortness of breath. Our emotional state seems to dictate the vertical positioning of the larynx, the relative relaxation of the vocal folds, and the posturing and relaxation of the muscles of the pharynx and tongue.

One's emotionality can be heard in the voice, a fact that can be threatening to the professional singer, or harmful to sales for the nervous salesperson, or embarrassing to someone who sounds like he or she is crying when actually happy. Our mood state can be harmful to voice. Many voice disorders are the result of various affective excesses; for example, a young professional woman attempts to use normal conversational voice when her larynx is postured in a high, sphincter-like position, resulting in a tight, tense voice. Her problem may be more related to unchecked and unrealistic fear than it is to faulty use of the vocal mechanisms per se.

Because emotionality and vocal function are so closely intertwined, effective voice therapy often requires the treatment of the total person and not just remediation of voice symptoms. Therefore, as we will see in later chapters, getting to know the patient is an important prerequisite to taking a case history or making an instrumental-perceptual voice evaluation. Voice clinicians have long recognized that the patient in the office may not resemble the same person in play or stress settings; the patient's voice will change according to his or her mood state. To assess voice realistically, we often have to observe and listen to the patient in various life settings.

SIDEBAR 1.2

To appreciate this, try to express various emotional states using just your voice. See if the person who is listening to you can detect which emotional state you are trying to convey.

THE LINGUISTIC FUNCTION OF THE VOICE

Voice seems to hold spoken language together. From the primitive emotional vocalization that may color what we say to the skilled use of voice stress to emphasize a particular utterance, the voicing component of spoken language plays a primary role. It is not always what we say that carries the message, but how we say it.

New interest in infant vocalization is producing a fascinating literature. By the time typical one-year-old babies utter their first word, they have already used their voice in highly elaborate jargon communication. While human babies all seem to babble about the same way from four to six months of age, babbling becomes more language-differentiated beyond that age. That is, babies no longer sound alike after six months; rather, they begin to sound like the primary language they have been hearing. The melody of the parent language, or its prosody, begins to color the vocalizations of the baby. The vocalizations of Chinese babies begins to sound like the sweeping tonal patterns of the Chinese Mandarin language; the pharyngeal sounds of an Arab language begin to be heard in the vocalizations of Arab babies.

These prosodic vocal patterns exist far beyond the individual word or segment. Such voicing is known as suprasegmental phonation. In young babies, suprasegmental vocalization far exceeds the voicing of actual word segments. As infants speak new words, they often place them in the proper place of their ongoing voicing rhythm. If they want to say "milk," they are far more likely to say the word at the end of a jargon phrase, such as "gawa na ta milk," rather than say the word in isolation. The jargon leading up to the word is suprasegmental voicing. The jargon voice carries a noncoded message with no specific meaning but seems to convey some general meaning by the overall sound of it. The mood and need state of the baby influence the sound of the vocalization.

Although jargon speech appears to diminish after the first 18 months of life, we continue to use suprasegmental vocalization in all aspects of spoken communication. We may add vocal stress patterns to augment the meaning of what we say. The actual words we say are only part of the communication. The "how we say it" is conveyed by various vocal stress strategies, such as changing loudness, grouping words together on one breath, changing pitch level, changing vocal quality and resonance to match our mood. These stress changes of the suprasegmentals can be produced with or without intent. That is, if it serves our purpose, we can sound angry by talking louder, or we may sound angry despite our best efforts to hide our anger from our listener. Once again, the voice carries much of the message. The same words spoken or written may convey different messages (as any lawyer taking depositions will tell you) depending on the stress patterns given the words by the speaker, with or without intent.

Considering the role of the voice in both emotional and linguistic expression, it is no wonder that people with voice disorders may find themselves handicapped in their communication. A young girl with vocal nodules, for example, may have developed them in part from excessive emotional vocalization (such as constantly yelling). Once the nodules were developed, however, she may be unable to use the vocal suprasegmentals and stress patterns she had previously used with ease in communication. As anyone knows who has ever suffered a complete loss of voice from severe laryngitis, the lack of voice prevents you from being you. Whisper and gesture somehow do not carry the communication effectiveness that normal voice allows you to add to the words you say (see Sidebar 1.3).

SIDEBAR 1.3

To experience this restriction, whisper the phrase *Today is Tuesday* two different ways—once as a statement and once as a question. Repeat these phrase contrasts using a normal voice. Which is more effective: whisper or voice?

While a primary role of the human larynx appears to be biological (guarding the airway), laryngeal voicing plays a vital role in the expression of both emotional and linguistic communication. When we add the voicing dimensions of acting and singing as laryngeal functions, we can truly appreciate the amazing artistic capabilities of the vocal tract (that a few people are fortunate to have and sometimes use). The role of the human larynx is obviously more complex and more subtle than the way the larynx functions as an airway protector in most other mammals.

CHECK YOUR KNOWLEDGE

1. What is the primary biological function of the larynx?
2. List and describe three emotional or linguistic functions of the larynx.

PREVALENCE OF VOICE DISORDERS IN THE GENERAL POPULATION

It is difficult, for several reasons, to establish normative incidence and prevalence data on voice disorders (see Sidebars 1.4 and 1.5). For example, voice can become temporarily disordered from a common cold that changes laryngeal tissue vibration and may fill resonating sinuses with infected mucus; almost everyone has experienced some voice change (phonation or resonance) as a result of a cold. Or some people experience voice changes from allergies. Therefore, if we were to take a large segment of the population and determine the present and past incidence of a voice disorder, our incidence reporting would be near 100%. Such incidence data would be meaningless. Rather, if we took a segment of a population, such as airline pilots, and looked back at the occurrences of hoarseness in a certain time period, we would determine some prevalence data for that particular group. Even these data would have far more meaning if there were a comparison between the pilots' voices and the voices of matched controls (matched, for example, by gender and age).

There have been only a handful of epidemiologic studies of the prevalence and risk factors of voice disorders in the general population (see Cohen and colleagues, 2012a; Verdolini and Ramig, 2001; and Best and Fakhry, 2011, for reviews). There has been substantial variability in reported prevalence estimates across the studies (Roy and colleagues, 2005). Conflicting definitions of voice disorder and methodological differences in procedures, and patient populations and sizes, are some of the causes of variations in the overall reported prevalence (Van Houtte and colleagues, 2010). The absence of acceptable epidemiologic data makes it difficult to precisely identify specific populations at risk, delineate the causes and effects of voice disorders, develop early screening procedures to identify those at risk, estimate societal costs related to voice disorders, and plan healthcare services designed to prevent or treat such problems (Roy and colleagues, 2005, p. 1988).

Roy and colleagues (2005) conducted a cross-sectional telephone interview survey of over 1,300 adults chosen at random. They discovered that nearly 7% of respondents had a voice disorder at the time of the interview and that nearly 30% had experienced a voice disorder at least once in their lifetime. About 7% of adults had missed work for more than one day because of their voice disorder. These findings are remarkably similar to those reported by Cohen (2010), who surveyed over 850 adults seeking medical care by their primary care physician for a variety of

---

SIDEBAR 1.4

Incidence is a frequently used epidemiological measure of rate of occurrence of new cases of a disease or condition. Incidence is calculated as the number of *new cases* of a disease or condition in a specified time period (usually a year) divided by the size of the population under consideration who are initially disease-free (Le and Boen, 1995).

SIDEBAR 1.5

Prevalence is a frequently used epidemiological measure of how commonly a disease or condition occurs in a population. Prevalence measures *how much of some disease or condition occurs in a population at a particular point in time*. The prevalence is calculated by dividing the number of persons with the disease or condition at a particular point in time by the number of individuals examined (Le and Boen, 1995).

reasons. Cohen discovered that the lifetime prevalence of dysphonia in this population was 29%, and that the point prevalence (number of persons with dysphonia at the time) was just over 7%. Four percent of patients had experienced dysphonia for more than 4 weeks, and 73% had experienced dysphonia more than once. With over 300 million people in the United States, a 7% point prevalence rate means that approximately 20 million people have a voice disorder at any given time.

Cohen and colleagues (2012a) recently examined the prevalence and common causes of dysphonia as diagnosed by primary care physicians (PCPs) and otolaryngologists (ENTs) and evaluated differences in etiologies offered by these care providers. A retrospective analysis of data from a nationally representative administrative U.S. claims database of 55 million individuals revealed that about 1% of patients received a diagnosis of dysphonia. It was further discovered that females were almost twice as likely as males to be diagnosed with dysphonia, and that adults over the age of 70 years were two-and-a-half times more likely than those under age 70 years to be diagnosed with a voice disorder. The most frequent diagnoses overall were acute laryngitis, nonspecific dysphonia, benign vocal fold lesions, and chronic laryngitis. Some trends noted by Cohen were that prevalence decreased slightly after age nine years, and increased after the age of 30 years, peaking among those greater than 70 years old (p. 344). Also, within age categories, males had a higher prevalence rate in zero- to nine-year-olds, and females had a higher prevalence beginning with puberty and persisting until age 70 years or older (p. 345).

In a similar study using the same database, Cohen and colleagues (2012b) reported that nearly three-fourths of patients who received a diagnosis of dysphonia received medical treatment for 12 months or more. More women than men required follow-up treatment. These clinical researchers estimated that the total annual direct costs of caring for such persons ran into the hundreds of millions of dollars, which is comparable to other chronic disease states. The mean cost per patient over 12 months was between approximately $500 and $1,000. In an effort to identify how ENTs manage such patients, Cohen, Pittman, and colleagues (2012) surveyed 1,000 ENTs about their practice patterns. Approximately 300 physicians responded, and they reported that prescribing medication to control laryngopharyngeal reflux disease was their most common approach, followed closely by referral to speech-language pathology for voice therapy. The most common laryngeal conditions leading to voice therapy referral were vocal fold nodules and muscle tension dysphonia.

CHECK YOUR KNOWLEDGE

1. Define the terms *incidence* and *prevalence*.
2. What is the prevalence of voice disorders in the general population?

PREVALENCE OF VOICE DISORDERS IN SPECIAL POPULATIONS

While the information already summarized in this chapter is helpful, a look at the prevalence of voice disorders in particular segments of the population may be more meaningful than looking at the population as a whole. Doing so may help clinicians focus their prevention, screening, and intervention efforts. In the following sections, we summarize the prevalence data on voice disorders in children and older adults, and across occupations (see also Chapter 8).

Prevalence of Voice Disorders in Children

The actual prevalence of voice disorders in children is difficult to determine. As summarized in McKinnon and colleagues (2007), a variety of different methods have been used to establish the presence of a communication disorder. The methods depend on both the age of the individual and the setting. Both direct (face-to-face assessment including screening and diagnostic techniques) and indirect (parent or teacher report) methods have been used extensively. Parent report measures are commonly used with preschool-age children while teacher report measures are commonly used with school-age children. Lower prevalence rates are typically derived from indirect methods in comparison to direct methods. Methodological challenges notwithstanding, it is very important that children be identified because it has been shown that a communication disorder such as dysphonia can negatively affect academic achievement and affect vocational choices later in adulthood (Pack, 2008; Ruben, 2000).

A number of researchers have concluded conservatively that between 6 and 9% of school-age children may have a voice disorder (Andrews, 2002; Carding and colleagues, 2006; Cornut and Troillet-Cornut, 1995). Some studies, such as the one conducted by Duff and colleagues (2004), have reported a slightly lower prevalence rate of 4%. Other studies have reported that the prevalence rate may actually be as high as 20 to 30% (Angilillo and colleagues, 2008; Boyle, 2000; Faust, 2003; Silverman and Zimmer, 1975). According to the U.S. Census Bureau (2010), there are approximately 74 million persons between the ages of 0 and 18 years; this is approximately 25% of the total U.S. population. Using a conservative prevalence rate of 6 to 9% suggests that there are between 4.5 and 6.6 million children who may have a voice disorder (for information about voice-disorder prevalence rates for other countries, see Akif Kilic and colleagues, 2004; Milutinovic, 1994). Perhaps even more alarming than this actual number is the fact that most of these children are not receiving voice therapy (Andrews and Summers, 2002). This is consistent with school SLPs who report a much higher incidence. Very little data are available on the incidence or prevalence of voice disorders among students in middle school (where among the students most normal voice changes occur) or in high school.

Prevalence of Voice Disorders in the Elderly

According to the U.S. Census Bureau (2010), there are approximately 40 million persons age 65 years or older, comprising about 13% of the total U.S. population. In spite of this large number (which is expected to grow), there are very few studies of the prevalence, risk factors, and psychosocial impact of dysphonia in the elderly. Studies of the incidence and prevalence of dysphonia in this population have been restricted solely to investigations of those seeking treatment; thus, the true prevalence of voice disorders in the general elderly population remains largely unknown. Three separate studies examining the prevalence of voice disorders in a non-treatment-seeking population over age 65 years (Cohen and Turley, 2009; Golub and colleagues, 2006; Roy and colleagues, 2007) discovered that between 20 and 30% of persons completing a survey about their voices reported having a current voice disorder, and that more than half these persons experienced significant quality-of-life impairment resulting from their dysphonia. The prevalence data reported by Roy and colleagues and Golub and colleagues are supported by the finding reported by Cohen and colleagues (2012a) that adults over the age of 70 years were two-and-a-half times more likely than those under the age of 70 years to be diagnosed with a voice disorder; in fact, adult males over the age of 70 years were the most likely persons to experience a voice disorder. The risk of an elderly person having a voice disorder is greater if the person also has a hearing loss, and having either disorder is more likely to lead to depression (Cohen and Turley, 2009).

Prevalence of Voice Disorders in Teachers and Student Teachers

It has been estimated that 5 to 10% of the U.S. workforce are "heavy occupational voice users" (Titze and colleagues, 1997). Within this group are over 3 million primary and secondary school teachers—the largest group of professionals who use their voice as a primary tool of their trade (U.S. Department of Labor, Bureau of Labor Statistics, 2006; U.S. Census Bureau, 2010). As described in VanHoudt and colleagues (2008, p. 371), these teachers are at risk for having a voice disorder due to vocal load (hours of voice use, number of communication partners), physical factors (physical condition, mucosal problems), psycho-emotional factors (stress, emotions, work pressure), and environmental factors (acoustics, humidity, environmental pollutants) (see also Da Costa and colleagues, 2012; Ferrand, 2012).

The prevalence of voice disorders in U.S. teachers has been studied quite extensively, yielding prevalence rates ranging from 4 to 50% or higher (Munier and Kinsella, 2008; Roy and colleagues, 2004a, 2004b), with most studies indicating a prevalence rate higher than that for comparable persons from the general population. For example, Roy and colleagues (2004a) surveyed about 1,200 teachers and 1,300 nonteachers and reported a prevalence rate for teachers of 11% compared to 6% for nonteachers; furthermore, 57% of these teachers had experienced a voice disorder at some point in their lives, compared to 26% for the nonteachers. Of those teachers who had experienced a voice disorder at some point in their lives, only 14% sought help from physicians and/or SLPs. Roy and colleagues also examined risk factors, and discovered that being a teacher, being a woman, being between 40 and 59 years of age, having 16 or more years of education, and having a family history of voice disorders were each positively associated with having experienced a voice disorder. In a related survey study of the same two groups, Roy and colleagues (2004b) discovered that teachers, compared with nonteachers, had missed more workdays over the preceding year because of voice problems and were more likely to consider changing occupations because of their voice (p. 542). To address this issue, vocal training programs targeting vocal health in teachers have been developed (see Roy and colleagues, 2001, for an example). The problem of voice disorders in teachers is not limited to those working in the United States; similar problems have been reported by teachers working in other developed countries (see Medeiros and colleagues, 2011, for a review).

Student teachers are also at risk for developing a voice disorder. Thomas and colleagues (2007) compared the incidence of voice complaints in student teachers versus students from nonteaching disciplines, and reported an incidence rate of 17% for student teachers compared to slightly less than 10% for their peers. Timmermans and colleagues (2005) reported that student teachers experience significantly more symptoms of dysphonia than their peers, including throat clearing, coughing, hoarseness, pain in the throat, fatigue, and difficulty being heard. One study reported that 90% of future teachers who experienced voice problems during their education experienced voice problems later in their teaching career (deJong and colleagues, 2006). To address this issue, individual and group training programs have been developed to address vocal health in student teachers (see Simberg and colleagues, 2006, and Timmermans and colleagues, 2011, for examples). In Chapter 8, we discuss the issue of voice disorders in teachers and student teachers in greater detail.

Prevalence of Voice Disorders in SLPs and Future SLPs

SLPs are professionals who also rely on healthy voices. SLPs and those in training to be SLPs have high vocal loads and often use their voices in emotional or stressful contexts, such as therapy, counseling, conferencing, and public speaking. They must also demonstrate and model appropriate voice use. Gottliebson and colleagues (2007) investigated the prevalence of voice disorder in 104 U.S. student SLPs (94% female) and reported that 12% had perceptual features of dysphonia in their habitual voice—a higher prevalence rate than that of the general population of students, and one that is similar to that of student teachers (see Thomas and colleagues, 2007). Because of the risk to this population, intervention programs have been developed to address vocal health and performance (see Van Lierde and colleagues, 2011, 2012, for examples).

 The identification of causes of vocal fatigue is a journey made by the patient with guidance from the clinician. In this **video,** the clinician actively listens to the SLP patient and then reiterates the patient's observations to ensure that both are "on the same page." Grand Rounds: Describe how the Voice Facilitating Approaches of focus, open mouth and yawn-sigh reduce vocal hyperfunction and increase use of the resonating chambers.

CHECK YOUR KNOWLEDGE

1. Describe the direct and indirect methods for determining prevalence of a disorder.
2. Which specific populations are at higher risk for having a voice disorder?

KINDS OF VOICE DISORDERS

When we talk about "kinds of voice disorders," we are usually talking about classifying the cause of voice disorders. This kind of classification over time has led to the historic causal simplification: the organic and functional dichotomy. In most classification systems, there is a mixture of etiologic causations and descriptive names of conditions, such as *cancer* as a causative form of an organic disorder, and *dysphonia* as the name of a condition that may have organic or functional origins.

Let us look at a few literature presentations of voice disorder classifications. The Classification Manual for Voice Disorders–I (Verdolini and colleagues, 2006) describes seven distinct causal classifications: laryngeal problems related to structural (1) pathologies, (2) inflammatory conditions, and (3) trauma or injury; (4) systemic conditions; (5) nonlaryngeal aero digestive disorders; (6) psychiatric-psychological disorders; and (7) neurological disorders. The manual also offers two other categories ("other disorders" and "undiagnosed"). Under each of the causative categories is specific information about etiology, behavioral description of the voice disorder, severity criteria, and so on, all of which can be most helpful to the SLP. Such diversity of nomenclature generates many categories of voice patient groups, however, complicating the task for generating evidence-based data.

Addressing the need to develop useful outcome data, an Australian diagnostic system (Baker and colleagues, 2007) presents a modified classification system as part of an inter-rater reliability study. Baker and colleagues basically modify the historic two broad categories of voice disorders, organic and functional. The organic classification of voice disorder causation combines structural changes of the vocal folds or cartilages or by "interruption of neurological innervations of the laryngeal mechanism." Such a combination of organic problems under one heading may present a real hindrance in evaluating treatment outcome effectiveness. Study of clinical effectiveness would probably be simpler if the organic causations and neurogenic categories were separated. Similarly, the functional voice disorder categories might be separated into two separate classifications: psychogenic voice disorders (PVD) and muscle tension voice disorder (MTVD, otherwise known as muscle tension dysphonia). While both PVD and MTVD are both functional voice disorders, they have distinctly different origins.

A different etiologic classification for causes of voice disorders was introduced by Stemple (2007) who presented these four pathology classifications: congenital laryngeal pathologies, pathologies of the vocal fold cover, neurogenic laryngeal pathologies, and pathologies of muscular dysfunction. The first category, congenital, includes only five relatively rare congenital conditions, such as congenital web or congenital cyst. The vocal cover category lists 15 various laryngeal conditions, from nodules to papilloma to sulcus vocalis. The neurogenic category does not include degenerative diseases and their possible influence on vocal fold function.

In this text, we have made an effort to use a classification system that allows easy identification of a voice disorder population—one that will promote valid and reliable clinical research. There appear to be three distinct categories of voice problems, one of them functional in causation and two of them organic in origin. Under the first category, functional voice disorders, there appears to be two subcategories: muscle tension voice disorders, which can develop from excessive muscle tension and use, and psychogenic voice disorders, which are caused by psychosocial factors. The second category, organic voice disorders, includes any organic structural deviation that affects vocal fold function. The third category, neurogenic voice disorders, relates to neurological conditions that cause faulty vocal fold closure from either paralysis (or weakness) or from neurological disease. In summary, these three categories—functional voice disorders, organic voice disorders, and neurogenic voice disorders—appear clear and distinct.

Functional Voice Disorders

There are basically two types of functional voice disorders: muscle tension dysphonia and psychogenic voice disorders. Each has a different etiology requiring different management and therapy approaches.

Muscle Tension Dysphonia. Muscle tension dysphonia (MTD) is the most common voice disorder seen in both children and adults. MTD is the most common manifestation of vocal hypertension—using too much muscular effort to phonate. This overuse of the respiratory, laryngeal, and supralaryngeal systems when voicing usually begins gradually. After talking awhile, the individual may begin to experience some pain and discomfort in the throat area. Before any dysphonia can be heard in the voice, the patient may experience fatigue and effort that increases with voice use. Children's loud voices and yelling over time seems to produce some hoarseness of voice. Also, adults may experience more hoarseness after prolonged voice use. Physical examination of the larynx shows no organic pathologies, and the voice problem is considered functional in origin. Baker and colleagues (2007) classify the patient's discomfort coupled with hoarseness (and normal laryngeal structures) as representing primary muscle tension dysphonia. With continued misuse of the voice over time, however, children and adults may develop secondary tissue changes related to this vocal hyperfunction, such as vocal fold changes (swelling, thickening, nodules, polyps, etc.). Both primary and secondary forms of MTD can usually be minimized with voice therapy that is designed to reduce excessive tension by restoring the normal balance among the respiratory, phonatory, and resonance systems.

Psychogenic Voice Disorders. Some children and adults experience severe emotional trauma or conflict that shows itself in some kind of physical alteration. Reaction to the trauma may manifest itself in a complete loss of voice, often labeled as a conversion aphonia. More commonly, the emotional reaction may show itself in a functional dysphonia—a hoarseness that has no physical cause. Or excessive emotionality may cause an alteration of voice pitch or speaking style that has no physical cause. In aphonia, the patient usually continues to whisper and attempts to speak. The complete lack of voice prevents the patient from having normal conversational interactions and may have devastating effects vocationally. Clinically, we have seen aphonic teachers unable to teach, an airline pilot unable to fly, a politician unable to continue a political campaign. Similarly, patients with a psychogenic dysphonia may suffer severe social and vocational limitations. Conversion-type voice problems vary dramatically, perhaps showing only in particular emotional or physical situations. For example, a Jesuit priest could interact with a normal voice with his Jesuit teaching peers, but he may lose his voice completely when he enters the classroom. In psychogenic aphonia or dysphonia, the patients are not willfully experiencing voice limitation. Rather, their vocal symptoms are often the result of long-term or recent psychologically damaging circumstances, such as a loss of a loved one or from continued sexual abuse. Although the patient with a psychogenic voice disorder may experience some voice improvement from direct voice therapy, in most cases, the voice disorder will not resolve unless there is some concomitant counseling or psychotherapy to address the underlying emotional problem.

Organic Voice Disorders

Organic voice disorders are related to structural deviations of the vocal tract (lungs, muscles of respiration, larynx, pharynx, and oral cavity) or to diseases of specific structures of the vocal tract. An example of a structural deviation is cleft palate, where there is abnormal coupling of the oral and nasal cavities, producing hypernasality during voicing attempts. An example of a vocal tract disease is viral papilloma of the larynx, where the child or adult experiences additive growths in the larynx, which might compromise the airway and interfere with vocal fold vibration. In Chapters 3 to 5 and Chapters 8 to 10, we will consider various organic diseases that may affect voice. Although the SLP may play an active role in the identification and evaluation of the patient with an organic voice disorder, the primary treatment of the disorder is often medical, dental, or surgical. Treatment by the SLP may have several goals, such as helping to improve the physiologic function of a damaged larynx. When the structural problem is controlled or stabilized, the SLP works with the patient to develop the best voice possible using various therapy methods.

Neurogenic Voice Disorders

The muscle control and innervation of the muscles of respiration, phonation, resonance, and articulation may be impaired from birth or from injury or disease of the peripheral or central nervous systems occurring at any age. For example, the SLP may work closely with a young child with cerebral palsy, perhaps working on both respiratory–voice control and helping the child to develop language. Or the SLP may work with the adult patient with a motor speech disorder acquired after a stroke, not only to improve respiration, voice, and articulation, but also to address concomitant swallowing problems. The tight, spasmodic voices of patients diagnosed with adductor spasmodic dysphonia appear to have unspecified neurogenic origins. Most of the neurological diseases presented in Chapter 4 alter normal voice in some way. The SLP plays a vital role in the assessment and management of the patient with a neurological voice disorder, such as assessing the patient's respiratory volumes and expiratory control, or visualizing through endoscopy a paralyzed vocal fold, or applying diagnostic probes to the Parkinson's disease patient to determine which therapy approaches produce a better voice.

While the majority of neurological impairments and diseases that impair swallowing, breathing, voice, and resonance cannot be cured or eradicated, the SLP frequently plays a vital role in maximizing function to as near normal levels as possible. For many neurologically impaired patients, there is a functional margin of disability that can be minimized by improved patient management and direct therapy intervention.

CHECK YOUR KNOWLEDGE

1. Describe the three categories of voice disorders presented in this text.
2. Why is it important to use a classification system?

MANAGEMENT AND THERAPY FOR VOICE DISORDERS

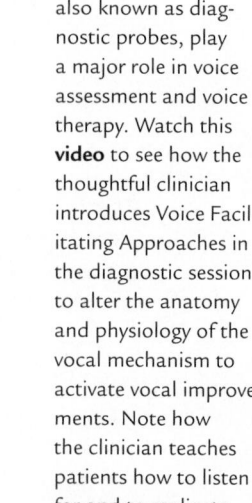

Stimulability probes, also known as diagnostic probes, play a major role in voice assessment and voice therapy. Watch this **video** to see how the thoughtful clinician introduces Voice Facilitating Approaches in the diagnostic session to alter the anatomy and physiology of the vocal mechanism to activate vocal improvements. Note how the clinician teaches patients how to listen for and to replicate these improvements using the open mouth approach. Grand Rounds: Describe elements of the close working relationship among the speech language pathologist and the otolaryngologist.

Probably no client/patient groups seen by the SLP are more responsive to management and therapy than children and adults with voice disorders. Successful intervention for a voice disorder first requires the identification of the cause of the disorder. We have grouped causal factors of voice disorders into three etiologic categories: functional, organic, and neurogenic. The typical history shows the patient experiencing some problem in respiration, voice, and/or resonance. Breathing and resonance problems are often long-standing, perhaps experienced by the patient over time. Voice or phonation problems, such as hoarseness, are more likely to develop more recently. The SLP often counsels patients that, unless they are experiencing hoarseness (dysphonia) as part of an allergy or upper respiratory infection (URI), they should wait no more than seven days to have a medical evaluation of the hoarseness. The SLP and otolaryngologist (ear-nose-throat physician, or ENT) have a close working relationship (Thibeault, 2007), and the SLP would refer the hoarse patient to the ENT for identification of the problem and possible medical treatment.

The ENT often refers the patient to the SLP who, by training is able to evaluate and diagnose the voice problem. The SLP takes a detailed history, observes the patient closely, and uses instrumental and noninstrumental assessment approaches. The SLP collects measurement values related to respiratory volumes and performance; performs acoustic measurement of vocal function; visualizes the larynx; and determines resonance function, particularly as related to velopharyngeal closure. Added to these observations and measurements of structure and function, the SLP determines how the patient feels about his or her voice problem, its effect on personality and interaction with others, and the influence of the voice problem on vocational performance. For many voice problems at the time of the evaluation, the SLP tests voice stimulability by introducing a few voice therapy approaches, often called diagnostic probes, with the patient. The SLP determines the outcome from using a particular technique, such as opening one's mouth more or speaking in a louder voice. If such an approach facilitates the production of a target voice, it might well be among the first used in therapy.

Many forms of voice therapy are available for the SLP to use with different kinds of voice problems. The client's response to the diagnostic probe may indicate the general direction of the therapy to be provided. For example, changing the loudness of the patient's voice may be an option. Perhaps with two young boys with vocal nodules, the SLP would recommend using a softer voice, such as "the voice to use when not wanting to awaken a sleeping person, a quiet voice" (Boone and colleagues, 2009, p. 190). Such a quiet voice is also presented by Casper (2000) as the "confidential voice." Or increasing loudness with an aging patient with Parkinson's disease may improve both articulation and voice, achieved by using a voice loud enough to be heard "20 or 30 feet away" (Boone and Wiley, 2000). Working on loudness changes—developing a softer voice or a louder voice—may go either way.

We have a professional need to develop scientific evidence to support what we do in therapy, but group data are difficult to gather because voice therapy is so individualized. Two patients with the same causative voice problem may require a distinctively different combination of therapy procedures. It is possible, however, to look at therapy effectiveness using different levels of evidence, as suggested by Butler and Darrah (2001) in their determination of treatment outcomes with patients with cerebral palsy. Their five levels of evidence range from Type I (clinic versus control group study) to Type V (descriptive case series/case reports.) The construct validity of each level of typing may have to be questioned. The effectiveness of "Voice Facilitating Approaches" presented in Chapter 7 can probably best be determined by comparing pre-therapy evaluation measurement with post-therapy evaluation by the same measurements. As we shall see when we discuss evaluating the outcome of therapy techniques in Chapter 7, validity of outcome data are often compromised by limitations in the number of voice patients available, SLP fiscal requirements, patient fee difficulties, and the demand for rapid progress.

For organic voice problems, the SLP may work closely with other specialists, such as in physical medicine or respiratory therapy, depending on the particular problem. For example, a preschool youngster with a growth in the airway called papilloma (caused by a virus) may require the clinical services of a surgeon; a respiratory therapist; extra nursing care; and the close watching by the SLP, who may need to work with the child to address breath support and voice. The voice therapy goal with such a child may be solely to develop the best voice possible with a vocal mechanism heavily laden with multiple papilloma growths. When such papillomas become large enough to impinge on the airway, the surgeon excises or reduces them, as needed, to improve breathing function.

Neurogenic voice problems come in many different forms, as we will see in Chapter 5. The SLP may be the first healthcare professional to see a patient who is just beginning to experience voice symptoms. For example, a recent patient was seen in our clinics because he felt he was experiencing a new problem pronouncing occasional words. A subsequent evaluation by the SLP found evidence of tongue tremor (fasciculations) and a problem in tongue diadochokinesis (he could not move his tongue rapidly when making alternating movements, such as saying "ta-ka" in a rapid series). A subsequent referral by the SLP to a neurologist confirmed that the patient was showing beginning signs of amyotrophic lateral sclerosis. Or the neurologist may be the first professional to see the patient with a neurogenic disorder and then refer the patient to the SLP for detailed assessment of breathing, phonation, and speech. The SLP sends his or her evaluation back to the neurologist, and together they may develop a management plan for the patient. Such a plan frequently includes medications for improving the patient's motor functions, with specific goals for the patient to achieve with the SLP in voice resonance and articulation therapy.

The SLP often works with actors, singers, and teachers who want to improve their speaking voices. The role of the SLP in improving the speaking voice of the professional user of voice was defined in a joint statement published by ASHA, the National Association of Teachers of Singing (NATS), and the Voice and Speech Trainers Association (VASTA) (ASHA/NATS/ASTA, 2005). This joint statement defines how the SLP would work collaboratively with members of NATS and VASTA. Since the establishment of roles for each voice specialist, there has been an increase in cross-referrals among the three voice specialties. For the actor and singer, the SLP can often offer vocal hygiene and voice therapy techniques that the professional can use in a normal day of voice usage when not acting or singing.

The SLP often works closely with the counselor, psychologist, or psychiatrist with patients with psychogenic voice problems. Working on voice symptoms alone often needs to be supplemented with psychological therapy to deal with underlying emotional problems that may be driving the voice problem. While loss of voice (aphonia) can often be treated successfully by symptomatic voice therapy, the vocal gains may only be temporary or they may recur in particular environmental situations. Similarly, long-term dysphonias without identifiable physical causes often resist successful resolution because the voice symptoms serve the patient in some way. Mutational falsetto, or continuing to use a higher-sounding voice after puberty (puberphonia), is often thought to be a psychogenic voice disorder among our psychology colleagues. The experience of most SLPs, however, is that the higher voice in the postpubertal male is usually changed in one or two voice therapy visits. Most young men seem to be trapped by habit in using the higher voice and are dramatically relieved with the discovery of the adult male voice. On occasion, the SLP may still refer these adolescents for some counseling or psychological therapy.

Most functional voice disorders result from the patient using excessive effort and are classified as muscle tension dysphonia (MTD). Both children and adults with MTD often abuse, overuse, or misuse their voices. The primary focus of the SLP with these patients is to identify their vocal excesses; once identified, vocal misuse can be reduced and often eliminated by voice therapy alone (Cohen and Garret, 2007). In Chapters 7 and 8, we will cite numerous other successful voice therapy outcome studies, similar to the seminal study of Benninger and Jacobson (1995). These clinical researchers followed 115 MTD patients who eventually developed vocal nodules or polyps from continued vocal excesses. After receiving appropriate voice therapy to reduce their vocal excesses, 94% of the patients experienced resolution of their problem. The authors concluded that, with appropriate voice modification and therapy provided by the SLP, "nodules will generally resolve with return of normal vocal function" (p. 326). Voice therapy for patients with MTD is usually a collection of Voice Facilitating Approaches that result in the proper balance of respiratory, voice, and resonance behaviors.

Progress in voice therapy can be determined from pre- and post-treatment measures of respiratory function, acoustic comparisons, and voice quality and resonance changes. The voice patient's self-perception (Bogaardt and colleagues, 2007) of any change in voice and its impact on quality of life adds needed outcome data. Useful outcome data also come from follow-up contacts and measures by the SLP over a specified period of time.

SUMMARY

In this chapter, we looked at voice and the larynx in the biologic viability of the individual as a tool in emotional expression, and in its complicated and extensive role in spoken human communication. We reviewed the prevalence of voice disorders in the general population and in specific subpopulations. We saw that there appear to be three causal factors in the development and maintenance of voice disorders: functional, organic, and neurogenic. The child or adult with a voice problem is evaluated by the SLP who uses instrumental and noninstrumental approaches for various respiratory and acoustic measures in the attempt to identify causal factors and define aspects of voice production. Diagnostic probes, the application of trial therapy approaches, are then used to determine the efficacy of a particular therapy technique for improving the patient's voice productions. The patient's self-perception of the handicaps presented by the voice disorder in his or her life is then recorded. If evaluation measures indicate that the patient can profit from therapy, the SLP then provides needed voice therapy. At the conclusion of voice therapy, therapy success is determined by comparing pre- and post-therapy measures, providing needed outcome data.

CLINICAL CONCEPTS

The following clinical concepts correspond with many of the objectives at the beginning of this chapter:

1. Some voice-disordered patients will come to you because they have a larynx that cannot adequately protect their upper airway from aspiration of food or liquids, or the larynx cannot adequately regulate the flow of air through the glottis in order to produce normal voice. Some examples include a speaker with a paralyzed vocal fold (see Chapter 5), a patient with dysarthria (see Chapter 5), a speaker with adductor spasmodic dysphonia (see Chapter 5), a speaker who has a mass on his or her vocal fold (see Chapters 4 and 9), a speaker with paradoxical vocal fold movement (see Chapter 8), and a patient who has undergone a partial laryngectomy (see Chapter 9).
2. Some voice-disordered patients will come to you because they cannot use their voice to express emotion or linguistic subtlety. Some examples include a speaker with muscle tension dysphonia (see Chapter 3), a speaker with psychogenic dysphonia (see Chapter 3), a speaker with a paralyzed vocal fold (see Chapter 5), a patient with dysarthria (see Chapter 5), a speaker with vocal fold nodules (see Chapter 3); a speaker with adductor spasmodic dysphonia (see Chapter 5), and a speaker with hearing loss (see Chapter 8).
3. Obtaining valid data about the incidence and prevalence of voice disorders entails theoretical considerations and practical challenges. It is probable that many persons with voice disorders are underserved because they are either not identified or not referred for voice therapy.

4. There is no universally accepted classification of voice disorders. Regardless of whether or not one adopts the classification system put forth in this text, the voice clinician must have a thorough understanding, not only of the cause of an individual's voice disorder, but also of the personal and environmental factors that may perpetuate the voice disorder. This requisite knowledge is needed in order to plan and deliver effective treatment.

GUIDED READING

Read the following article:

Baker, J., Ben-Tovim, D. I., Butcher, A., Esterman, A., & McLaughlin, K. (2007). Development of a modified diagnostic classification system for voice disorders with inter-rater reliability study. *Logopedics Phoniatrics Vocology, 32,* 99–112.

What are the pros and cons of using Baker's classification system compared to the one proposed in this text?

Read the following article:

Cohen, S. M., Kim, J., Roy, N., Asche, C., & Courey, M. (2012a). Prevalence and causes of dysphonia in a large treatment-seeking population. *Laryngoscope, 122,* 343–348.

What voice disorder incidence and prevalence data are still lacking? Explain.

PREPARING FOR THE PRAXIS™

Directions: Please read the case study and answer the five questions that follow. (Please see page 319 for the answer key.)

Michelle is a 32-year-old kindergarten teacher. Her chief voice complaints are a hoarse voice, vocal fatigue, and pain when using her voice. She has not yet been seen by an otolaryngologist.

1. This patient asks you how common it is for teachers to have voice problems. You tell her that the prevalence of voice disorders in this population is:
   A. Less than 5%
   B. 5 to 10%
   C. 11 to 15%
   D. 16 to 20%
   E. More than 20%

2. This patient then asks you how common it is for people in the general population to have voice problems. You tell her that the prevalence of voice disorders in the general population is:
   A. Less than 5%
   B. 5 to 10%
   C. 11 to 15%
   D. 16 to 20%
   E. More than 20%

3. This patient then asks you how common it is for her kindergarten students to have voice problems. You tell her that the prevalence of voice disorders in this population is:
   A. Less than 5%
   B. 5 to 10%
   C. 11 to 15%
   D. 16 to 20%
   E. More than 20%

4. This patient has a student teacher this semester, so she asks you how common it is for student teachers to have voice problems. You tell her that the prevalence of voice disorders in this population is:
   A. Less than 5%
   B. 5 to 10%
   C. 11 to 15%
   D. 16 to 20%
   E. More than 20%

5. This patient is concerned about her grandfather's voice, so she asks you how common it is for senior citizens to have voice problems. You tell her that the prevalence of voice disorders in this population is:
   A. Less than 5%
   B. 5 to 10%
   C. 11 to 15%
   D. 16 to 20%
   E. More than 20%

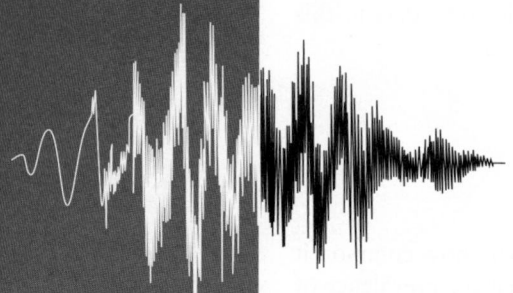

CHAPTER 2

Normal Voice
Anatomy and Physiology
Throughout the Lifespan

This chapter describes the normal voice and how it is produced. It is important to understand the normal voice in order to be able to diagnose and treat the abnormal voice. Few things are so difficult to define or understand as "What is normal and what constitutes normal limits?" Because of maladaptive vocal behaviors and/or disease, many patients present to the clinician with overworked voice production systems. To help the patient to abandon the abnormal functions, the clinician must know how normal voice is produced, and be able to communicate this information appropriately to the patient. Modern-day voice evaluation often involves consultation with medical professionals who are well-grounded in human anatomy and physiology. For these reasons and more, voice clinicians must have a good working knowledge of the structures and functions serving normal and abnormal voice production throughout the lifespan.

NORMAL ASPECTS OF VOICE

Normal voice may be characterized by five aspects, each related to function. First, the voice must be loud enough to be heard. We may refer to this as adequate carrying power. This means that the voice can be heard and speech can be understood over the noise of most everyday environmental sounds such as the television, air conditioning, keyboard typing, transportation noises, and so on. Second, the voice must be produced in a manner that is hygienic and safe, that is, without vocal trauma and resulting laryngeal lesions. Third, the voice should have a pleasant quality, one that is not distracting and thus interferes with verbal communication. Fourth, the normal voice should be flexible enough to accurately express emotion. The human voice can be thought of as a "window into the soul" in that we sometimes judge how a loved one or close friend feels based on the sound of his or her voice. We often think we know if the person is happy, sad, sick, excited, or nervous. Likewise, we sometimes find it hard to mask our own emotional state with our voice. We can also change the meaning of a verbal message by changing the emotional tone of our voice. The sentence, "I am so happy for you," can be said in such a manner as to be sincere or sarcastic just by the tone of voice, even while the words remain the same. The expression, "Oh wonderful," can be said with excitement or with scorn. Last, the voice should represent the speaker well in terms of age and gender. We should not be surprised to meet someone for the first time after speaking to him or her on the phone. Our voice should not portray us as either older, younger, or as less mature than we are. Nor will we likely be pleased if we are mistaken for the opposite gender. The normal voice should represent the speaker faithfully.

Keep the five aspects of loudness, hygiene, pleasantness, flexibility, and representation in mind as we explain in the next section how the normal voice is produced. That the voice can serve us so well through our lifespan is a true testament to the uniquely human aspects of voice we just described.

CHECK YOUR KNOWLEDGE

1. What are the five key aspects of the normal voice?
2. Give an example of how each of these aspects can be abnormal.

NORMAL PROCESSES OF VOICE PRODUCTION

Separating the normal speaking voice into three individual processes (respiration, phonation, and resonance) for purposes of study is helpful, but we must remember that these three components of voice production are highly interdependent. For example, without the expiratory phase of respiration, there would be no phonation or resonance. Without adequate functioning of the velopharyngeal mechanism, there would be an imbalance of oral-nasal resonance. Also, these three processes are constantly changing simultaneously. Let us first consider the structures and function of respiration, particularly as they relate to production of voice.

THE RESPIRATORY SYSTEM

For speech to be possible, humans have learned to use respiration for the purpose of phonation. Both speaking and singing require an exhalation (outgoing air stream) capable of activating vocal fold vibration. When training their voice, speakers or singers frequently focus on developing conscious control of the breathing mechanism. This conscious control must not conflict, however, with the physiological air requirements of the individual. When a problem occurs with respiration, it is often the conflict between the physiological needs and the speaking-singing demands for air that causes faulty usage of the vocal mechanism. Our dependence on the constant renewal of oxygen supply imposes certain limitations on how many words we can say, how many phrases we can sing, or how much loud emphasis we can use on one expiration.

STRUCTURES OF RESPIRATION

Respiration is a vital life-sustaining and voice-enabling process that results from the movement of support structures within the musculoskeletal system. While a complete review of the musculoskeletal components for speech and voice is beyond the scope of this text, an overview is presented here that will provide the student or clinician with core information that can be applied to the diagnosis and management of persons with respiratory-based voice disorders.

The Bony Thorax

The bony thorax includes the vertebrae and vertebral column, the thoracic cage (ribs and sternum, and associated muscles), the pectoral girdle, and the pelvic girdle. The thorax is suspended from the vertebral (spinal) column, a strong but flexible structure that serves many purposes. The vertebral column consists of 33 individual vertebrae stacked loosely on top of each other, forming a strong pillar for the support of the head and trunk. The vertebrae can be grouped into five regions. The 31 pairs of spinal nerves emerge and enter the spinal cord through spaces between each pair of vertebrae, beginning at the thoracic level.

The seven cervical vertebrae are smaller and more delicate than the remaining vertebrae, and within these vertebrae the left and right vertebral arteries course superiorly on their way to joining the basilar artery at the base of the brain. Two of the cervical vertebrae (C1—Atlas, C2—Axis) are unique because they connect the skull to the spinal column and also allow for diverse head movement (e.g., rotate side to side, bend forward and backward). The C7 vertebra—the cervical prominence—can be felt if you pass your fingers down the back of your neck, in between the base of your skull and the top of your spine. In terms of adult landmarks, the base of the nose and the hard palate corresponds to C1, the teeth (when mouth remains closed) correspond to C2, the mandible and hyoid bone corresponds to C3, the thyroid cartilage spans from C4 to C5, and the cricoid cartilage spans from C6 to C7. In infants and children, the laryngeal landmarks are situated higher, at the level of C1 to C3.

The 12 thoracic vertebrae are intermediate in size between those of the cervical and lumbar regions; they increase in size as one proceeds down the spine, the upper vertebrae being much smaller than those in the lower part of the region. The first 12 pairs of spinal nerves emerge from between the thoracic vertebrae.

The thoracic vertebrae provide the basis for the respiratory framework because they form the posterior point of attachment for the ribs (Seikel and colleagues, 2010). The thoracic spine's range of motion is limited due to the many rib/vertebrae connections

The five lumbar vertebrae graduate in size from L1 through L5. These vertebrae bear much of the body's weight and related biomechanical stress. They provide direct or indirect attachment for a number of back and abdominal muscles, as well as for the posterior fibers of the diaphragm (Seikel and colleagues, 2010). The lumbar vertebrae allow significant forward and backward bending at the waist, moderate side bending, and a small degree of rotation.

The sacrum is a large, triangular bone at the base of the spine and at the upper and back part of the pelvic cavity, where it is inserted like a wedge between the two hip bones. Its upper part connects with the last lumbar vertebra, and the bottom part connects with the coccyx (tailbone). It consists of usually five initially non-fused vertebrae that begin to fuse between the ages of 16 and 18 years and are usually completely fused into a single bone by age 34.

The coccyx, commonly referred to as the tailbone, is the final segment of the vertebral column. Comprising three to five separate or fused vertebrae (the coccygeal vertebrae) below the sacrum, it is attached to the sacrum by a joint that permits limited movement between the sacrum and the coccyx.

The thoracic (rib) cage is formed by the thoracic vertebral column, 12 pairs of ribs and their costal cartilages, the sternum, and the internal and external intercostal muscles. Each of the ribs is made up of bone and cartilage, allowing for both strength and mobility. The 12 pairs of ribs can be subdivided into three general classes: true ribs (the first seven pairs), false ribs (the next three pairs) and floating ribs (the last two pairs). The true and false attach to the vertebral column and the sternum, while the floating ribs attach only to the vertebral column. The ribs connected to the thoracic vertebral column and their connecting muscles play an important role in respiration, as we shall see when we discuss respiratory function.

The pectoral girdle is formed by the clavicle and scapula. It supports the upper limbs. It is suspended from the head and neck by the support fibers of the trapezius muscles, which descend from the cervical vertebrae and the skull and are attached to both the clavicle and the scapula (shoulder blade).

The pelvic girdle is formed by the ilium, sacrum, pubic bone, and ischium. The pelvic girdle provides a strong structure for attaching the legs to the vertebral column. By means of this structure, forces generated through movement of the legs are distributed across a mass of bone which, in turn, is attached to the vertebral column (Seikel and colleagues, 2010).

CHECK YOUR KNOWLEDGE

1. List the structures of the bony thorax.
2. List the five vertebral regions and the number of vertebrae in each.

The Muscles of Respiration

We now need to consider the muscles of respiration (see Figures 2.1 and 2.2). When discussing these muscles, it is helpful to think of three major categories: (1) the muscles of the rib cage, (2) the diaphragm, and (3) the muscles of the abdominal wall. Thinking of the muscles of respiration in this way makes it easier to discuss

FIGURE 2.1 A List of Muscles of Respiration

Muscles of the Rib Cage Wall
Sternocleidomastoid
Scalenus group (anterior, medial, posterior)
Pectoralis major
Pectoralis minor
Subclavius
Serratus anterior
External intercostals
Internal intercostals
Transversus thoracis
Lattisimus dorsi
Serratus posterior superior
Serratus posterior inferior
Lateral iliocostals
Levatores costarum
Quadratus lumborum
Subcostals

Muscles of the Diaphragm
Diaphragm

Muscles of the Abdominal Wall
Rectus abdominus
External oblique
Internal oblique
Transversus abdominis

the movements that occur due to the passive and active forces to be discussed later in this chapter, and the adjustment capabilities of the respiratory system for speech. Keep in mind now that the action of the respiratory muscles changes the dimensions of the thoracic cavity, which in turn changes the pressure within the thoracic cavity. The resulting changes in pressure result in the inspiratory-expiratory cycle with which we are all familiar.

The Inspiratory Muscles

The inspiratory muscles can be found within the thorax, back, neck, and upper limbs. The primary inspiratory muscles of the thorax are the diaphragm and external intercostal muscles. These muscles are assisted by accessory muscles in the neck, back, and upper limbs.

The Diaphragm. The diaphragm is a large (about 250 cm^2 in surface area) dome-shaped muscle that separates the thorax from the abdominal cavity, with openings for the esophagus and assorted arteries (see Figure 2.3 on page 24). The muscle fibers of the diaphragm insert into the sternum and the six lower ribs and their cartilages and into the first three of four lumbar vertebrae. The other ends of these muscle fibers converge to attach to the fibrous central tendon, which is also attached to the pericardium on its upper surface. At rest, the diaphragm is shaped like an inverted bowl. When you are standing and in the mid-phase of respiration, the dome of the diaphragm is at about the same level as the sixth rib. As described in

FIGURE 2.2 Muscles of Respiration

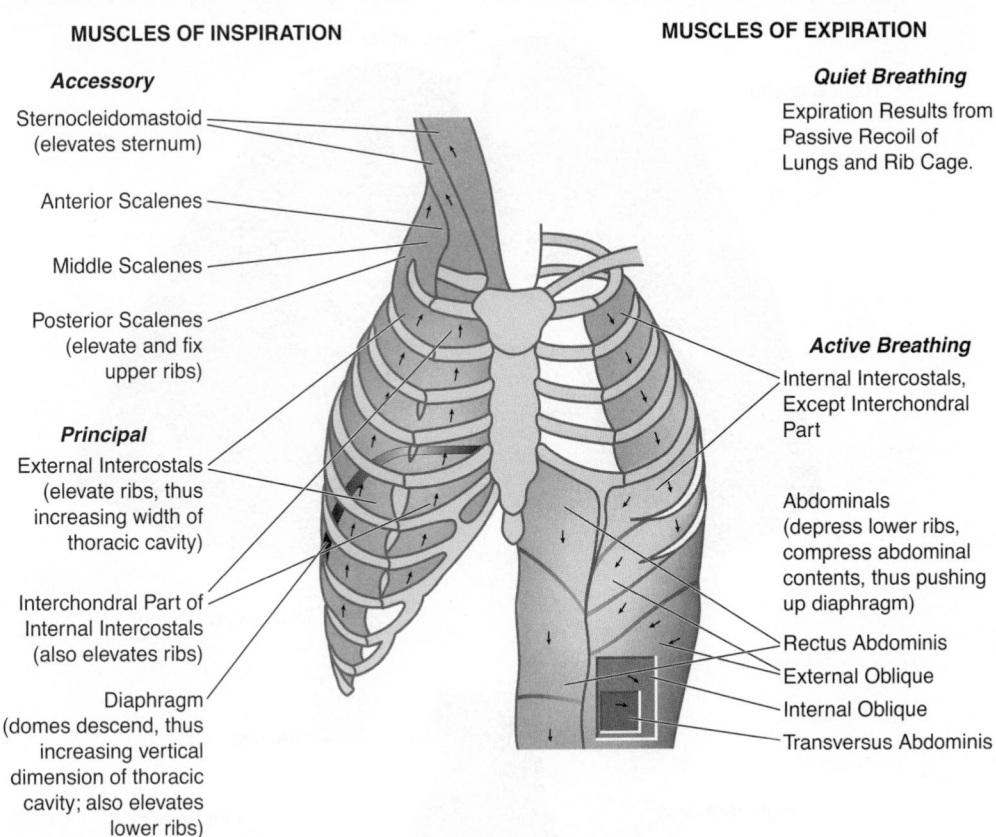

MUSCLES OF INSPIRATION

Accessory

Sternocleidomastoid
(elevates sternum)

Anterior Scalenes

Middle Scalenes

Posterior Scalenes
(elevate and fix
upper ribs)

Principal

External Intercostals
(elevate ribs, thus
increasing width of
thoracic cavity)

Interchondral Part of
Internal Intercostals
(also elevates ribs)

Diaphragm
(domes descend, thus
increasing vertical
dimension of thoracic
cavity; also elevates
lower ribs)

MUSCLES OF EXPIRATION

Quiet Breathing

Expiration Results from
Passive Recoil of
Lungs and Rib Cage.

Active Breathing

Internal Intercostals,
Except Interchondral
Part

Abdominals
(depress lower ribs,
compress abdominal
contents, thus pushing
up diaphragm)

Rectus Abdominis
External Oblique
Internal Oblique
Transversus Abdominis

Levitzy (2007), during normal quiet breathing, contraction of the diaphragm causes its dome to descend 1 to 2 cm into the abdominal cavity, with little change in its shape. This elongates the thorax in the cephalacaudal (top to bottom) dimension and increases its volume. These small downward movements of the diaphragm are possible because the abdominal viscera can push out against the relatively compliant abdominal wall. During a deep inspiration, the diaphragm can descend as much as 10 cm. With such a deep inspiration, the limit of the compliance of the abdominal wall is reached, abdominal pressure increases, and the central tendon becomes fixed against the abdominal contents. After this point, contraction of the diaphragm against the fixed central tendon elevates the lower ribs. When a person is in the supine position, the diaphragm is responsible for about two-thirds of the air that enters the lungs during normal quiet breathing. When a person is standing or seated in an upright posture, the diaphragm is responsible for only about one-third to one-half of the tidal volume. Motor and sensory innervation for the diaphragm comes primarily from the two phrenic nerves. These nerves originate in the cervical plexus (grouping) of spinal nerves C3 through C5 of both sides of the spinal cord (Seikel and colleagues, 2010). Thus, innervation to the diaphragm is bilateral, an indication of its biological importance. The diaphragm is under primary control of the autonomic nervous system, although one can place the diaphragm under voluntary control, albeit only temporarily (such as when holding one's breath).

FIGURE 2.3 Lungs and Tracheal Bifurcation

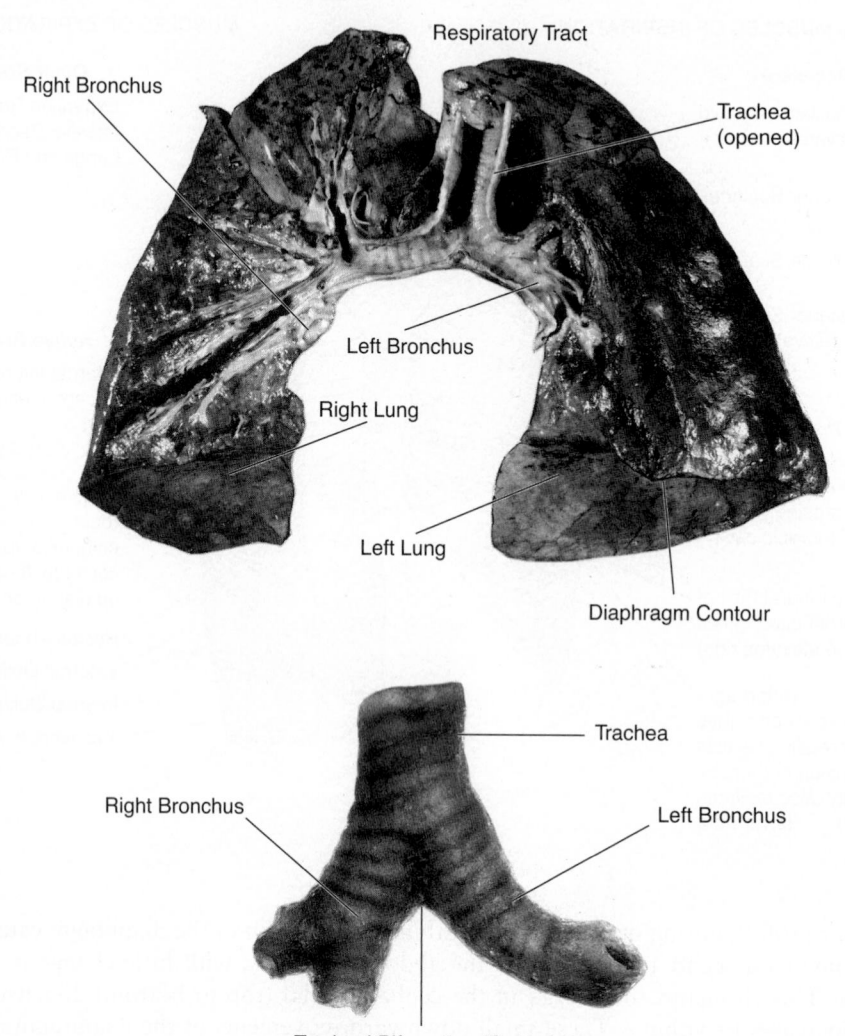

The External Intercostal Muscles. The eleven external intercostal muscles run downward and forward from the lower border of the rib cage above to the upper border of the rib cage below (see Sidebar 2.1). Together, these muscles form a large sheet of muscle that attaches the ribs to one another (Hixon and colleagues, 2008). The external intercostal muscles are positioned so that, when they contract, the entire rib cage elevates and expands (Seikel and colleagues, 2010). As can be seen in Figure 2.4, the true/upper ribs move with a pump-handle motion about the vertebrae. This motion increases the anterior-posterior dimension of the thoracic cavity. That is, it increases the distance between the sternum and the vertebral column (see Sidebar 2.2 on page 26). The distance front to back is increased, leading to an overall increase in volume. The false/middle ribs move with a bucket-handle motion about the vertebrae. This motion increases the horizontal dimension of the thoracic cavity; that is, it makes the chest

SIDEBAR 2.1

These muscles are sometimes referred to as the *front pocket muscles* because the fibers mimic the direction a hand would enter a front pocket.

FIGURE 2.4 Movements of the Thoracic Cavity

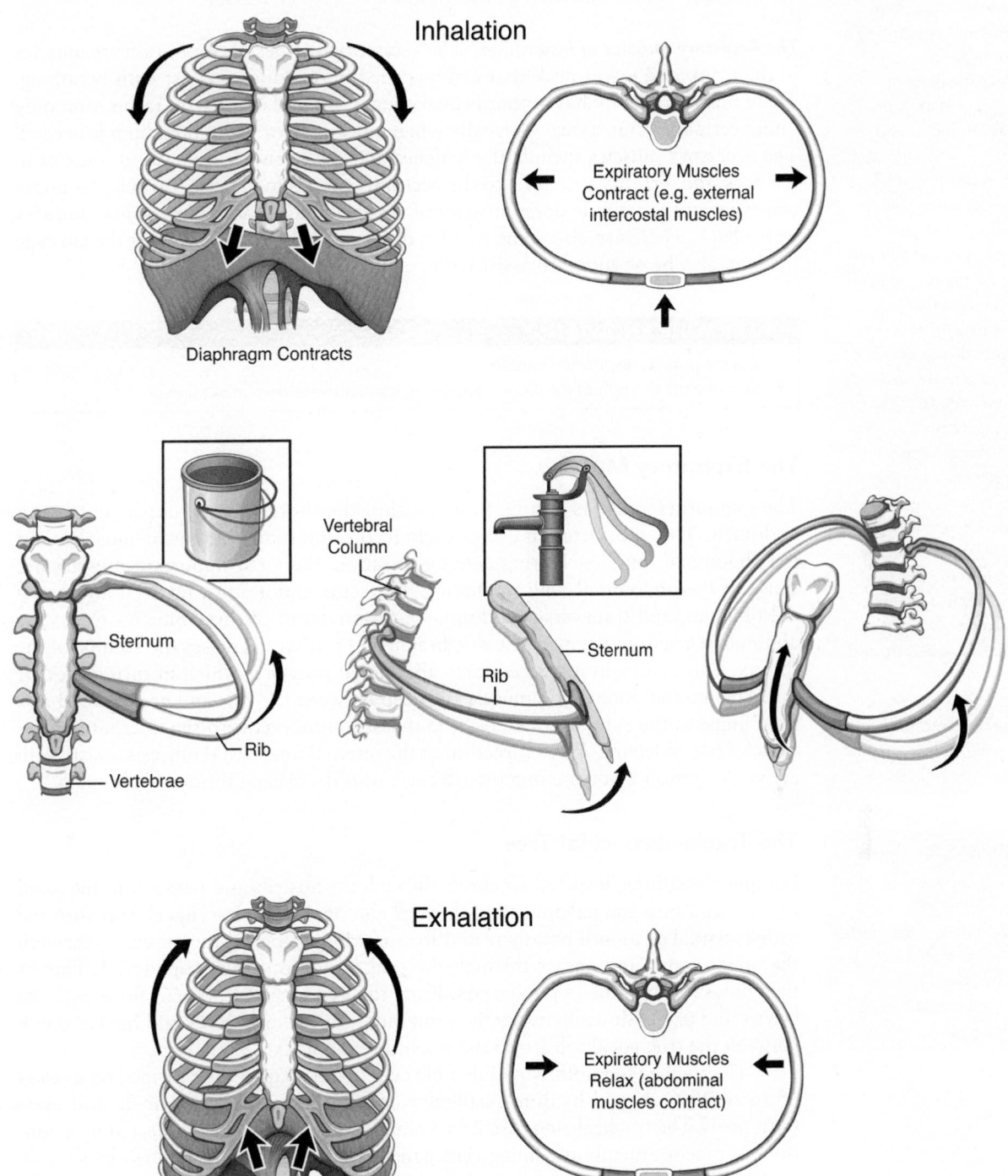

Inhalation

Diaphragm Contracts

Expiratory Muscles Contract (e.g. external intercostal muscles)

Sternum

Rib

Vertebrae

Vertebral Column

Sternum

Rib

Exhalation

Diaphragm Relaxes

Expiratory Muscles Relax (abdominal muscles contract)

SIDEBAR 2.2

To appreciate these movement dynamics, do the following: (1) Place the palm of your right hand on your sternum/chest and the back of your left hand on your spine at the level of your shoulder blades. Look down at your right hand as you take a breath, and you will notice that the distance between your hands increases. That is, your thorax expands from front to back. (2) Place the thumb of your right hand on the top of the uppermost rib on your right. Then, put the middle finger of your left hand on the bottom-most rib on your right. Look down at your right hand as you take a breath, and you will notice that the distance between your hands increases. That is, your thorax expands from top to bottom.

slightly wider, increasing the volume within, enabling breathing (see Sidebar 2.2). The floating ribs move with a caliper motion.

The Accessory Muscles of Inspiration. The accessory muscles of respiration are muscles in the trunk and lower neck that can be called into action to assist with breathing. These muscles usually have other primary functions and assist with respiration only under certain circumstances—usually when more deep or rapid breathing is needed. The accessory muscles include the scalenes and the sternocleidomastoid muscles in the neck, the serratus anterior and the pectoral muscles in the upper trunk, the upper trapezius and latissimus dorsi muscles of the trunk, and the erector spinae muscles of the back. There are also some smaller, deeper muscles that lie against the rib cage that can also be recruited to assist with respiration.

CHECK YOUR KNOWLEDGE

1. List the primary inspiratory muscles.
2. Describe the position of the diaphragm during normal versus deep inhalation.

The Expiratory Muscles

The expiratory muscles can be found within the thorax, back, upper limbs, and abdomen. The expiratory muscles include the internal intercostal muscles and the abdominal muscles. During active expiration, the most important muscles are those of the abdominal wall (including the rectus abdominus, internal and external obliques, and transversus abdominus). Contraction of these muscles forces the abdominal organs up against the diaphragm and further decreases the volume of the thorax. This results in increased intra-abdominal pressure, which in turn drives air out. The internal intercostal muscles lie deep between the ribs and are oriented at a right angle to the external intercostal muscles, continuous with the internal oblique muscles (see Sidebar 2.3). Contraction of the internal intercostal muscles assists with active expiration by depressing the rib cage, thus decreasing thoracic volume.

SIDEBAR 2.3

These muscles are sometimes referred to as the *back pocket muscles* because the fibers mimic the direction a hand would enter a back pocket.

The Tracheobronchial Tree

For quiet breathing, inspired air enters through the nostrils and passes into the nasal cavities and into the nasopharynx through the open velopharyngeal port into the oropharynx. For mouth breathers and for speaking purposes, the air enters through the open mouth and passes through the oral cavity into the oropharynx. The air then flows through the hypopharynx. From the hypopharynx, the air flows into the larynx and passes down between the ventricular (false) vocal folds and further down between the true vocal folds into the trachea (windpipe).

The trachea is a hollow and flexible cylindrical-shaped tube formed by a series of 16 to 20 C-shaped hyaline cartilage rings that are closed anteriorly and open posteriorly. The tracheal rings are 2 to 3 cm in diameter and are connected by a continuous mucous membrane lining. The gap between the rings is spanned by smooth muscle. The trachea runs from the inferior border of the larynx for about 11 to 12 cm, and then it bifurcates (divides) into two main-stem or primary bronchi at a point known as the carina, which is near the level of the fifth thoracic vertebra (see Figure 2.3). Each main-stem bronchus divides into smaller divisions known as the secondary (lobar) and tertiary (segmental) bronchi. The tertiary bronchi continue to branch and divide into smaller and smaller tubes and eventually branch into terminal (end) respiratory bronchioles. The respiratory bronchioles open into alveolar ducts. These ducts lead to outpouchings called alveolar sacs, which lead to microscopic alveoli (air sacs) inside capillary networks. In the alveolar sacs, gas exchange between oxygen and carbon dioxide occurs. Some of the bronchioli are visible in the upper picture of Figure 2.3, but most of the bronchioli and all the alveoli are covered by the pleural membrane that covers the lungs.

CONTROL OF BREATHING

As described in Moini (2012, p. 255), respiratory control has both involuntary and voluntary components. The involuntary centers of the brain regulate respiratory muscles, and control the depth and frequency of pulmonary ventilation. This occurs in response to sensory information that arrives from the lungs, the respiratory tract, and other sites. The voluntary control of respiration reflects activity in the cerebral cortex that affects either the output of the respiratory center in parts of the brainstem or the output of motor neurons in the spinal cord that control respiratory muscles (see Sidebar 2.4). Control of breathing for vocalization and speech has been associated with the primary motor and sensory cortex, supplemental motor area, cerebellum, thalamus, and limbic system.

THE RESPIRATORY CYCLE (INHALATION AND EXHALATION)

The respiratory tract functions much like a bellows. When we move the handles on the bellows apart, the bellows becomes larger and the air within it becomes less dense than the air outside it. The outside air rushes in due to the lower pressure of the less-dense air in the bellows and the greater pressure in the more-dense outside air. The inspiration of air into the bellows is achieved by active enlargement of the bellows' body. Similarly, in human respiration, the inspiration of air is achieved by active movement of muscles that enlarge the thoracic cavity. When the thorax enlarges, the lungs within the thorax enlarge. The air within the lungs becomes less dense than atmospheric air, and inspiration begins. The air is expired from the lungs by decreasing the size of the chest, thus compressing the air and forcing it to rush out. In human respiration, however, much of expiration is achieved by passive collapse of the thorax and not by active muscle contraction. This is an extremely important fact and can be valuable information for voice clinicians. Much of expiration is passive. Hixon and Hoit (2005) have described human respiration as having two types of forces that are always present: passive, nonvolitional forces and active, volitional forces.

Passive Forces

Much of the power required for normal speech can be supplied by the passive forces of respiration (passive exhalation). These forces include the natural recoil of muscles, cartilages, ligaments and lung tissue, the surface tension of a special film that lines the alveoli, and the pull of gravity. These forces reduce the size of the thorax during expiration (in a manner analogous to the recoil of a stretched spring) and thus contribute to outward airflow from the lungs, which may be used in speech. The mechanism of passive force can be understood by examining the concept of relaxation pressure.

Relaxation Pressure. Vocal quality is affected by extremely high or low air pressure at high or low lung volume (see Figure 2.5). The most efficient and most pleasing voice is produced at mid-air-pressure levels and mid-lung-volume levels of air (see Sidebar 2.5). Knowledge of this translates into an excellent clinical stimulation technique. We can often change the vocal quality of our dysphonic patients by instructing them to use the midrange of air pressure and lung volume. Teaching a shortened phrasing pattern may be important to teaching breath-stream management. Except in singers or actors, this generally is all the respiration training that needs to be given by the speech-language pathologist (SLP). All the emphasis placed on breathing exercises and respiration training in the past seems unproductive and unnecessary for nearly all of our patients with dysphonia. The clinical facilitation technique of glottal fry (discussed in Chapter 7) makes use of this information because glottal fry is produced with little air pressure and little airflow.

FIGURE 2.5 The Relaxation Pressure Curve

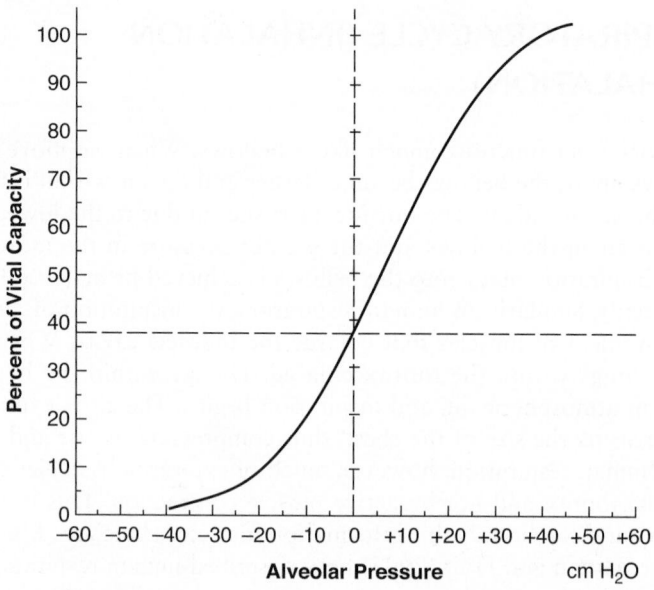

The passive forces of exhalation tend to generate force during inhalation that works to restore the lung and rib cage system to the normal resting state or equilibrium. After active inhalation, these passive forces of exhalation rebound to provide some of the expiratory force needed for speech. There is a nearly linear relationship between relaxation pressure and lung volume in the range between 20% and 70% of the vital capacity. This curve represents the pressure generated by the passive factors of the respiratory system.

Active Forces

Additional power required for normal speech can be supplied by the active forces of respiration (active exhalation). These forces include the strength of the muscles within the chest wall, their patterns of movement, and the amount of air contained in the lungs. As described by Hixon and Hoit (2005, p. 18), the more air the lungs contain, the greater the force that can be produced to decrease the size of the thorax (i.e., the greater the expiratory force that can be generated). By contrast, the less air the lungs contain, the greater the force that can be produced to increase the size of the thorax (i.e., the greater the inspiratory force that can be generated).

A key problem for many voice-disordered patients is the tendency to squeeze the glottis closed in order to produce the needed power, rather than to increase air pressure and airflow by contracting the abdominal muscles. We can better understand this poor technique by a simple analogy. If we are watering flowers in a garden and we want to reach the far row of plants, we can either place a thumb over the end of the hose and squirt the water further (increase the power), or we can increase the water power by turning the faucet on further. When we squeeze the glottis closed, we are "putting a thumb over the end of the hose." When we contract the abdominal muscles, we are "turning the faucet further on" and increasing the airflow. Even though squeezing the glottis tends to increase the vocal power, vocal quality is diminished because the voice sounds strained. If this method is habitual, the excessive effort becomes the basis of a hyperfunctional voice disorder. Such effort may lead to laryngeal changes that can result in abnormal voice. When we need increased power to speak louder, to stress words, or to extend a phrase when singing or speaking, we should use the larger muscles of the abdomen and "turn on the faucet" controlling the source of air. Thus, the pressure at the valve (the larynx) is not excessive, and vocal quality is improved with delicate laryngeal tissue not subjected to stress and strain, which produces laryngeal edema and laryngitis. Vocal quality is not diminished, and adverse tissue change is avoided. Voice clinicians can use this water analogy to teach patients how to monitor breath control by properly using expiratory reserve volume (see definition of terms in Table 2.1) via the abdominal muscles, rather than using excessive glottal valving in the larynx.

Figure 2.6, the simple tracings of a pneumotachometer, shows the relative time for inspiration-expiration for a passive, tidal breath, for saying the numbers "1, 2, 3, 4, 5," and for singing the musical passage, "I don't want to walk without you, baby," from the old song by that title. Note that the inspiratory time during normal tidal breathing is much longer than the quick inspiration for speech and singing. This is indicated by the rapid rise of the tracing from a resting baseline in an almost vertical move. In the tidal breath, the rise from the baseline is gradual and sloped rather than vertical.

 In this **video,** the clinician encourages the patient with Parkinson's disease to increase breath support, think about breath-phrase coordination, and to speak with intent to increase her comprehensibility. Grand Rounds: Describe the water analogy so that it would be clear to a patient unfamiliar with the four subsystems of speech.

CHECK YOUR KNOWLEDGE

1. List the passive and active forces of exhalation.
2. Describe in your own words how increasing expiratory pressure at the larynx can lead to muscle tension dysphonia and laryngeal tissue changes.

We will now define the terms we will use in following discussions to describe aspects of respiration. Methods for evaluating respiratory volumes and capacities will be discussed in Chapter 6.

FIGURE 2.6 Pneumotachometer Tracings

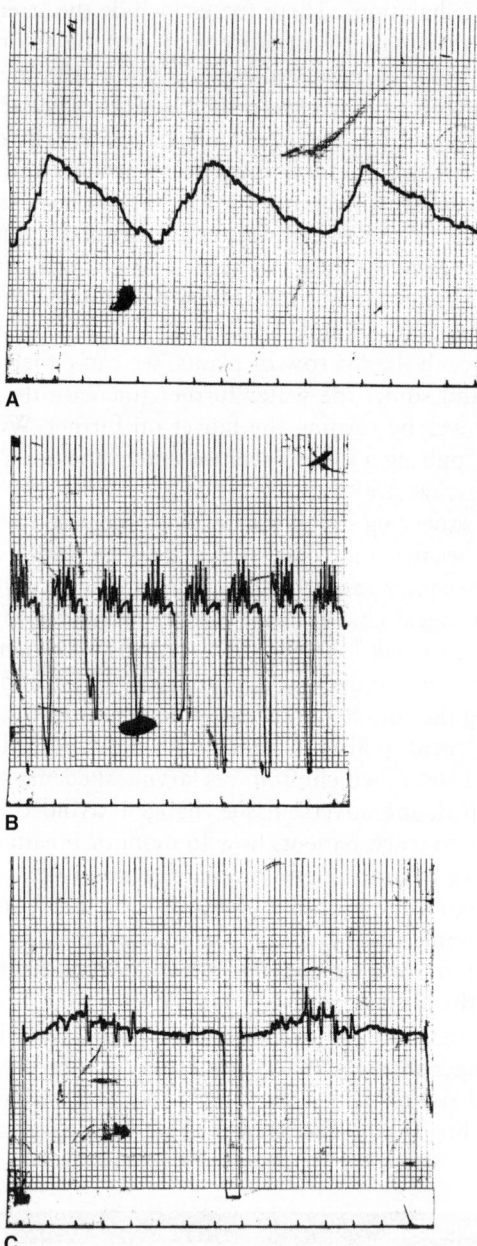

Note the relative time for inspiration as opposed to expiration for three conditions: tracing A (three tidal breaths) produces an inspiration–expiration time ratio of about 1:2; tracing B (counting from one to five on eight trials) produces a ratio of about 1:3; tracing C (singing twice, "I don't want to walk without you, baby") yielded an inspiration–expiration ratio of approximately 1:10.

RESPIRATORY VOLUMES AND CAPACITIES

Only a small amount of the air in the lungs is exchanged during a single quiet respiratory cycle. The total volume of the lungs can be divided into *volumes* and *capacities* (see Table 2.1). Respiratory volumes refer to the amount of air in the lungs at a given time and how much of that air is used for various purposes, including speech (Solomon and Charron, 1998). Respiratory volumes include *tidal volume, inspiratory reserve volume, expiratory reserve volume* and *residual volume.* Lung capacities combine two or more of the respiratory volumes and include *inspiratory capacity, vital capacity, functional residual capacity* and *total lung capacity.* These volumes and capacities are useful for diagnosing problems with pulmonary ventilation (Moini, 2012). Respiratory volumes and capacities vary depending on the patient's age, gender, level of physical exertion, and vocal training. Data reported by Hoit and Hixon (1987) and Hoit and colleagues (1989, 1990) indicate that, in general, lung volumes and capacities increase from infancy through puberty and then remain stable until advancing age, when they decrease slightly (see Table 2.2).

CHECK YOUR KNOWLEDGE

1. List and describe the respiratory volumes.
2. List and describe the respiratory capacities.

TABLE 2.1 Respiratory Volumes and Capacities

Type	Description	Calculation	Volume
Tidal volume (TV)	The amount of air inspired and expired during a single respiratory cycle.	Measured	500 mL
Inspiratory reserve volume (IRV)	The maximum volume of air that can be inspired beyond the end of a tidal inspiration.	Measured, or VC − (TV + ERV)	3,000 mL
Expiratory reserve volume (ERV)	The maximum volume of air that can be expired beyond the end of a tidal expiration.	Measured	1,100 mL
Residual volume (RV)	The volume of air that remains in the lungs after a maximum expiration.	Measured	1,200 mL
Inspiratory capacity (IC)	The maximum volume of air that can be inspired.	TV + IRV	3,500 mL
Functional residual capacity (FRC)	The volume of air remaining in the lungs and airways at the end of a resting tidal exhalation.	ERV + RV.	2,300 mL
Vital capacity (VC)	The maximum volume of air that can be expired following a maximum inspiration.	TV + IRV + ERV	4,600 mL
Total lung capacity (TLC)	The total volume of air contained in the lungs and airways after a maximum inspiration	TV + IRV + ERV + RV	5,800 mL

TABLE 2.2 Group Means of Seven Age Groups of Subjects for Some Lung Volumes and Capacities (in Cubic Centimeters)

Age Group	7	10	13	16	25	50	75
Males							
TLC	2120	3140	4330	6200	6740	7050	6630
VC	1670	2510	3550	5080	5350	5090	4470
FRC	980	1400	1970	2940	3120	3460	3440
ERV	530	770	1180	1810	1730	1500	1280
Females							
TLC	2070	2980	3740	4980	5030	5310	4860
VC	1580	2340	2999	3780	3930	3600	2940
FRC	970	1430	1690	2560	2420	2930	2590
ERV	480	780	940	1350	1320	1220	670

Source: Adapted from Hoit and Hixon (1987); Hoit, Hixon, Altman, and Morgan (1989); and Hoit, Hixon, Watson, and Morgan (1990).

THE EFFECTS OF AGING ON THE RESPIRATORY SYSTEM

It has been reported that changes in general pulmonary functioning with aging become measurable at around age 40 years (Rochet, 1991). As reported by Weismer and Liss (1991), there is increased stiffness of respiratory structures, resulting in increased relaxation pressure at corresponding lung volumes. Muscle weakness, muscle atrophy, and increased fibrotic content of muscle result in diminished pressure-generating capability at a given lung volume. Degeneration of nerve fibers and sensory receptors result in a loss of appreciation of absolute lung volumes, lung volume changes, and precision of motor commands for breathing. Less efficient gas exchange results in higher breathing frequency.

The first comprehensive studies reporting age-related changes in speech breathing were conducted in the late 1980s by Hoit and colleagues (1987, 1989, 1990). The major findings of the 1987 study were that elderly males demonstrated larger rib cage volume initiations, larger lung volume excursions, and larger lung volume expenditures per syllable than younger men, particularly during extemporaneous speaking. The major findings of the 1989 study were that, compared to younger women, elderly females demonstrated larger rib cage excursions during reading out loud, increased frequency of inhalation during reading out loud, increased air expenditure during non-phonated intervals during reading out loud, and larger lung volume initiations during extemporaneous speaking. (For a complete review of the speech and voice changes of geriatric speakers, see Zraick and colleagues, 2006).

CHECK YOUR KNOWLEDGE

1. Describe the effects of aging on the respiratory system.
2. How does aging affect voice?

BREATHING FOR LIFE VERSUS BREATHING FOR SPEECH

In breathing for life (that is, quiet breathing), the ratio of time for inhalation versus exhalation is nearly equal, with exhalation time just slightly longer than inhalation time. During breathing for speech, we have a bias toward longer exhalations, which is quite compatible with the need to extend expiration for purposes of speech (see Sidebar 2.6). Influences on speech breathing include the speaker's body position, body type, and age, as well as the type of utterance being produced, interactions between the speaker and the listener, the background noise in the setting, and so forth. As summarized by Hixon and Hoit (2005, pp. 105–106): (1) speech breathing while upright is different than speech breathing while lying down due to the effect of gravity on relaxation pressure and chest wall movements (see Sidebar 2.7); (2) body type influences speech breathing because of the effect of body fat on the movements of the abdominal wall and rib cage wall; (3) advanced age (seventh or eighth decade of life) brings changes in valving of the larynx, which result in larger lung volumes and rib cage wall excursions and greater average expenditures of air per syllable; (4) speech breathing patterns are highly variable until age 3 years and undergo refinement throughout childhood and adolescence; and (5) cognitive-linguistic factors affect when an inspiration occurs and how long it will be, how long the following expiration will be, how often silent pauses will occur, and how much speech is produced per breath group (see Sidebar 2.8). In addition to a change in the ratio times of inhalation/exhalation, there are changes in the volume of air inhaled/exhaled. During quiet breathing, the volume of air is approximately 10% of vital capacity, while during speech breathing it can be as high as 25% of vital capacity, depending on the length and loudness of the utterance. As described earlier in this chapter, muscle activity for exhalation is passive during quiet breathing, while it is active during speech breathing. Last, the abdomen is displaced outward relative to the rib cage during quiet breathing, while during speech breathing, it is displaced inward relative to the rib cage (see Sidebar 2.9).

SIDEBAR 2.6

To appreciate these timing differences, do the following: (1) Place the tip of your right index finger just in front of, but not touching, your lips and breathe quietly through your mouth. Close your eyes and pay attention to how long it takes you to inhale and how long you feel the exhaled air on your fingertip. (2) Keeping your fingertip in place, close your eyes and talk out loud for about 30 seconds. Pay attention to how short the inhalation time is and how you feel the exhaled air on your fingertip throughout your utterance.

SIDEBAR 2.7

To appreciate the effect of gravity, do the following: Say the Pledge of Allegiance out loud while sitting in a chair versus lying flat on your back. What are the differences you note?

SIDEBAR 2.8

To appreciate these influences, do the following: (1) Determine the number of quiet breaths you take per minute, then (2) silently read a passage for one minute and note the number of breaths you take. (3) Repeat the reading, this time aloud, and note the number of breaths you take. Was there a difference across conditions?

SIDEBAR 2.9

To appreciate these movement dynamics, do the following: (1) Put the palm of your right hand on your sternum/chest and the palm of your left hand on your belly. Look down at your hands as you take a quiet breath, and you will notice that your belly expands front to back to a greater degree than your chest. (2) Keeping your hands in the same locations, look down as you are talking out loud for about 30 seconds. Notice that each time you take a breath during speaking, your belly moves inward relative to your chest.

The SLP must take the aforementioned factors into consideration when conducting a speech breathing evaluation (more on this topic in Chapter 6). For example, when breath support or perhaps breath control is a problem in a voice-disordered patient, it is often related to failure to take breaths at appropriate places. At other times, the tendency to push too hard in extending the expiratory reserve volume results in a strained vocal quality. Understanding lung volumes and capacities, and the difference between breathing for life versus breathing for speech, is the foundation for identifying voice-disordered patients whose dysphonia is due in part to abnormal respiratory function.

CHECK YOUR KNOWLEDGE

1. Describe the difference between breathing for life versus breathing for speech.
2. Describe one sign or symptom of abnormal breathing for speech.

THE PHONATORY SYSTEM

The phonatory system is the source of voiced sound. Normal phonation (voice production) results from normal expiratory airflow, normal vocal fold structure and function, normal supraglottic structure and function, and normal nervous system control. One's voice can be heard while one is talking, singing, laughing, crying, or screaming. To quote Lord Byron in his poetic masterpiece *Don Juan* (1824), "The devil hath not, in all his quiver's choice, an arrow for the heart like a sweet voice" (Canto XV, Stanza 13).

ANATOMY OF PHONATION

The larynx, positioned atop the trachea, is a gateway to the respiratory tract. The larynx serves important biological functions, which include allowing air into and out of the lungs for life-sustaining breathing, protecting the airway from infiltration of food or liquid during swallowing, protecting the airway from infiltration of foreign bodies, and fixing the thorax during activities demanding highly elevated abdominal pressures (such as forced bowel and bladder evacuation, childbirth, and heavy lifting). Central to these functions is the ability of the vocal folds to *abduct* (move away from each other, starting together at midline) or *adduct* (move toward each other, ending together at midline), essentially serving as a valve between the speech tract and the respiratory tract. Using this valve to generate voice (to phonate) has required the development of intricate neural controls that permit humans to set the vocal folds into precise vibration for speaking and singing. Vocal fold vibration is possible because (1) the vocal folds are located within a fixed laryngeal framework; (2) muscles within the larynx (intrinsic laryngeal muscles) facilitate vocal fold abduction and adduction; (3) some of these intrinsic laryngeal muscles cause changes in the elastic properties of the vocal folds, thus affecting their rate of vibration; and (4) an outgoing airstream also affects vocal fold vibration. The myoelastic aerodynamic theory of phonation takes these factors into account and will be described later in this chapter. First, however, we turn our attention to providing an overview of laryngeal anatomy, including changes affecting voice across the lifespan.

The Laryngeal Framework

The larynx is a constricted tube with a smooth surface. It is located deep within the strap muscles of the neck and is situated vertically at the level of vertebrae C4–C6 in adults, but is higher in children, at the level of vertebrae C1–C3. The larynx is approximately 44 mm long (1.7 inches) in adult males and approximately 36 mm long (1.5 inches) in adult females. The circumference of the larynx in adults is approximately 120 mm (5 inches). A framework of cartilage, ligaments, membranes, and folds gives the larynx form. Connected to this framework are extrinsic and intrinsic laryngeal muscles that facilitate movement of either the laryngeal frame (in the case of the extrinsic muscles) or the vocal folds within (in the case of the intrinsic muscles).

Ligaments and membranes connect the larynx superiorly to the hyoid bone, inferiorly to the cricoid cartilage, and anteriorly to the epiglottis. These attachments of the larynx loosely position it at midline in the neck. Because the larynx is not rigidly fixed in the neck, it is capable of limited up-down and side-to-side movements (see Sidebar 2.10). The vertical and horizontal movements of the larynx are considered normal, and lack of such movements during a head and neck examination can be indicative of neurological damage, degenerative changes, blunt force trauma, the presence of a tumor or other mass, or possibly muscle tension dysphonia.

SIDEBAR 2.10

To illustrate, put the first three fingers of your right hand on your larynx and swallow. You should feel the larynx elevate and move forward slightly and then glide back to its resting position. If you apply a little firmer grip, you can move the larynx from side to side. Also, if you raise your tongue within the oral cavity, or protrude your tongue, you will feel the larynx elevate slightly; this is partially because the base of the tongue inserts into the hyoid bone. As the tongue contracts, it lifts the hyoid bone slightly.

The Extrinsic Laryngeal Muscles

The extrinsic laryngeal muscles have one attachment to the larynx and another attachment to some structure external to the larynx. Along with the hyoid bone, they are located in an area of the neck called the anterior triangle, which is bounded by the mandible, the sternocleidomastoid muscles, and the midline platysma muscle. The extrinsic laryngeal muscles have a role in supporting and stabilizing the larynx and in changing its position within the neck. Muscles within this group include the sternothyroid, thyrohyoid, and inferior constrictors.

The Supplementary Laryngeal Muscles

In addition to the extrinsic laryngeal muscles, two major groups of muscles attach to the hyoid bone and originate from either above or below the hyoid bone. The suprahyoid muscle group includes the digastric, stylohyoid, mylohyoid, geniohyoid, hyoglossus, and genioglossus. The infrahyoid muscle group includes the sternohyoid and omohyoid.

It is clinically useful to understand how each extrinsic and supplementary laryngeal muscle contributes to raising or lowering the larynx and moving it forward and backward, as listed below:

Raise	Lower	Forward	Backward
Digastrics	Omohyoid	Sternothyroid	Omohyoid
Geniohyoid	Sternohyoid	Digastric	Digastric
Mylohyoid	Sternothyroid	Mylohyoid	Stylohyoid
Stylohyoid		Geniohyoid	
Genioglossus		Genioglossus	
Hyoglossus			
Thyrohyoid			

The raising and lowering of the larynx is observable and noted mainly during the pharyngeal stage of swallowing. These movements serve primarily to help protect the airway from aspiration of food or liquid (see Sidebar 2.11). The extrinsic laryngeal muscles also come into play slightly during production of higher and lower pitches (especially in untrained singers) (see Sidebar 2.12). Conversely, if you lower your pitch dramatically, your larynx will lower. A good speaking voice does not apparently require much active muscle involvement of the extrinsic laryngeal muscles. Trained singers keep the height of the larynx nearly constant while singing a range of high and low notes (Sataloff, 1981).

An understanding of the laryngeal framework and muscles is critical when engaging in digital manipulation. In the first brief **video** segment, the clinician uses digital manipulation to assess the vertical position of the larynx in a case of functional aphonia. In the second segment, he gently pushes one aspect of the thyroid lamina to attempt to medialize the vocal folds in a case of suspected unilateral vocal fold paralysis. Grand Rounds: Cite three reasons why digital manipulation would be selected as a diagnostic probe.

CHECK YOUR KNOWLEDGE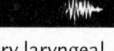

1. What is the difference between the extrinsic laryngeal muscles and the supplementary laryngeal muscles?
2. What role do the extrinsic and supplementary laryngeal muscles play in voice production?

Laryngeal Cartilages

Five major laryngeal cartilages are important for voice production and airway protection: the cricoid, the thyroid, the paired arytenoids, and the epiglottis. These are shown in Figures 2.7 through 2.9. Two other small paired cartilages, the corniculates (cone-shaped, elastic cartilages on the apex of the arytenoids extending into the aryepiglottic folds) and the cuneiforms (cone-shaped, elastic nodules located in the aryepiglottic folds), apparently play only a minimal role in the phonatory functions of the larynx. The larynx develops in utero from paired branchial arches, so slight asymmetries in structure are often observed, particularly as one ages (Lindestadt and colleagues, 2004). Such asymmetries typically do not affect voice, though.

The cricoid, thyroid, and arytenoid cartilages are intricately connected to one another by joints, ligaments, membranes, and muscles (we will describe these connecting structures in later sections of this chapter). The cricoid is the second largest of the three cartilages and is a signet-shaped ring connected to the first tracheal ring. The two pyramid-shaped arytenoid cartilages sit atop its high posterior wall. The base of each arytenoid cartilage has two concave and smooth surfaces, called processes, to which muscles attach. One of these surfaces, the muscular process, is laterally directed and is the attachment for those intrinsic laryngeal muscles that cause the arytenoid cartilage to rock, rotate, and slide on the cricoid cartilage. The other process, the vocal process, is anteriorly directed and is the posterior attachment for the vocal ligament and vocalis muscle. The remaining major cartilage, the thyroid cartilage, is the largest of the three listed. It has several parts: two laminae, a superior thyroid notch, two superior horns, two inferior horns, and two oblique lines. The two laminae fuse anteriorly in the midline and form the laryngeal prominence (commonly called the Adam's apple). In postpubertal males, the angle of the laryngeal prominence is approximately 90°, and in females, the angle is approximately 120°. If you feel your Adam's apple with your middle finger oriented horizontally and then place your index finger right next to it, you should feel a v-shaped notch between the laminae; this is the superior thyroid notch, present because the laminae are incompletely fused. The superior horns are posterior points of attachment for

FIGURE 2.7 Anterior View of the Laryngeal Cartilages, Hyoid Bone, and Epiglottis

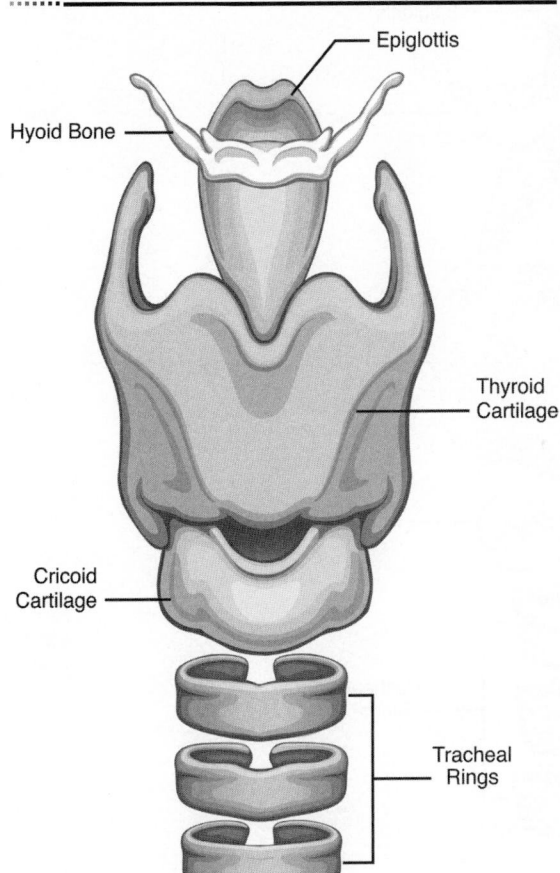

FIGURE 2.8 Posterior View of the Laryngeal Cartilages, Hyoid Bone, and Epigolottis

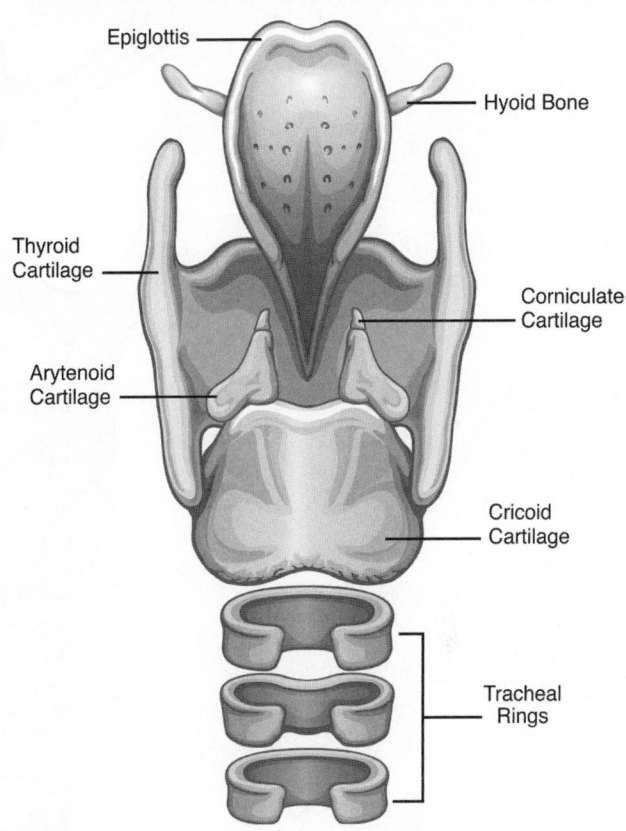

Four spectograms of the same speaker producing the /i/ vowel under four conditions: breathy, normal, harsh, and hoarse. The relative spacing of the formants stays the same as the signal source changes.

ligaments connecting the thyroid cartilage to the hyoid bone above. The inferior horns are also posterior points of attachment and connect the thyroid cartilage to the cricoid cartilage below via a joint. Each laminae also contains an oblique line, a ridge that descends diagonally from superior to inferior; this ridge is a line of attachment for some of the extrinsic laryngeal muscles and the inferior pharyngeal constrictor muscle. Similar to cartilage throughout the skeletal system, all the laryngeal cartilages are coated with a tough leathery covering (the perichondrium), which gives the larynx a waxy look. This perichondrium is thicker on the outside than the inside of the larynx.

CHECK YOUR KNOWLEDGE

1. List and describe the location of the five major laryngeal cartilages.
2. List the anterior, superior, and inferior borders of the larynx.

FIGURE 2.9 Lateral View of the Laryngeal Cartilages, Hyoid Bone, and Epiglottis

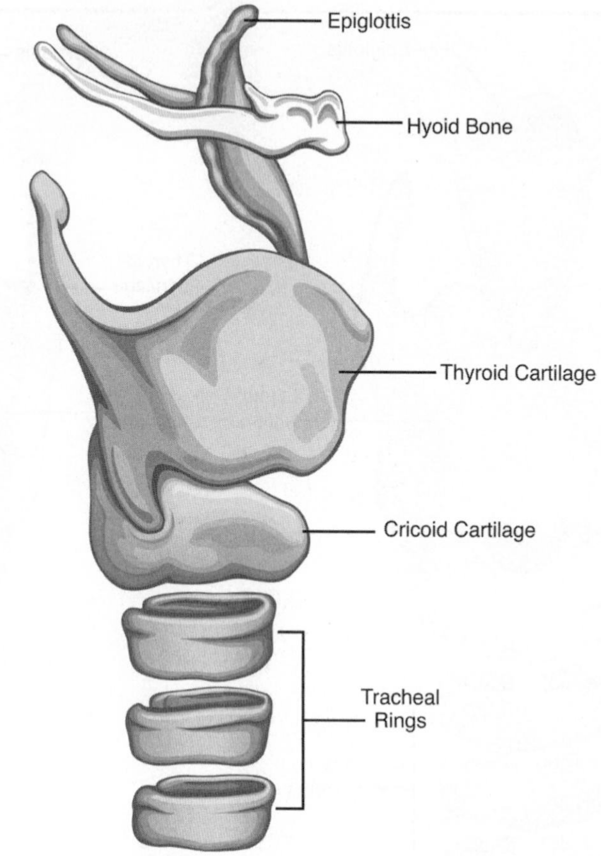

- Epiglottis
- Hyoid Bone
- Thyroid Cartilage
- Cricoid Cartilage
- Tracheal Rings

Extrinsic Laryngeal Ligaments and Membranes

Ligaments and membranes also connect parts of the larynx to adjacent support structures. Some of these ligaments and membranes connect laryngeal cartilages to the epiglottis, some connect laryngeal cartilages to the hyoid bone, some connect the epiglottis to the hyoid bone or tongue, and some connect laryngeal cartilages to the trachea. It is helpful in gaining an understanding of some of these ligaments and membranes if one refers again to Figures 2.7, 2.8, and 2.9 and notes that there are spaces between some of the major laryngeal cartilages and their adjacent external structures. For example, the medial and lateral thyrohyoid ligaments, along with the thyrohyoid membrane, connect the thyroid cartilage to the hyoid bone (see Figure 2.10). The cricotracheal ligament and cricotracheal membrane connect the cricoid cartilage to the uppermost tracheal ring. The cricothyroid membrane connects the cricoid and thyroid cartilages (see Figure 2.10). One can appreciate the thyrohyoid space, for example, with palpation (touch) (see Sidebar 2.13). Keep in mind too that we have previously described the

FIGURE 2.10 Extrinsic Laryngeal Membranes and Ligaments

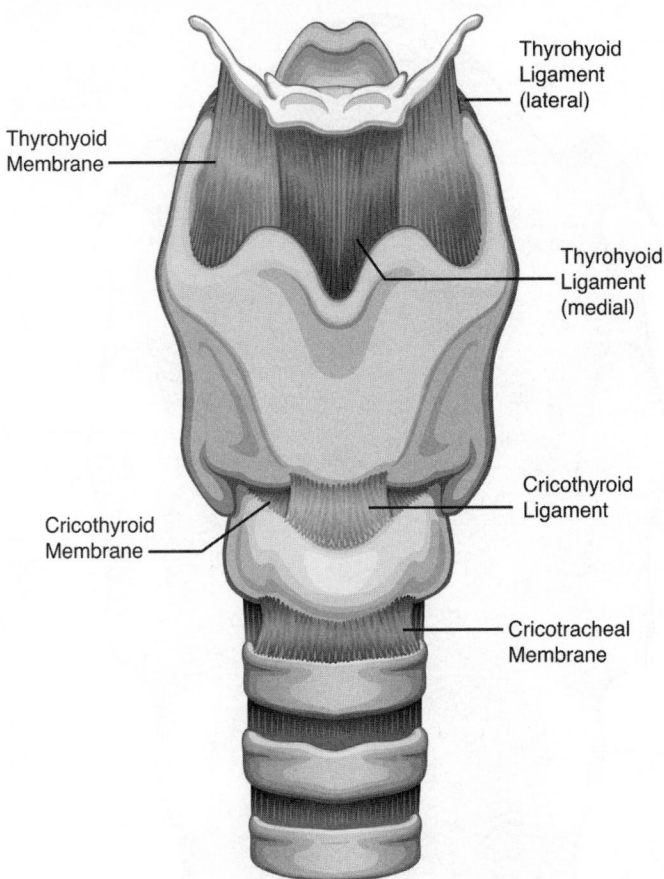

Thyrohyoid Ligament (lateral)

Thyrohyoid Membrane

Thyrohyoid Ligament (medial)

Cricothyroid Ligament

Cricothyroid Membrane

Cricotracheal Membrane

larynx as a closed tube. Therefore, there must be membranes spanning the space between cartilages. The interested reader is referred to Zemlin (1998) for a complete listing and description of all the extrinsic laryngeal ligaments and membranes.

The Laryngeal Cavity

The laryngeal inlet (aditus laryngis) is the entrance into the larynx (see Figure 2.11). It is a triangular opening, wider in front than in back, that slopes obliquely down and back. Its boundaries are the epiglottis in the front, the aryepiglottic folds on each side, and the arytenoid cartilages behind. Its shape is variable, depending on the position of the arytenoid cartilages and the epiglottis. The laryngeal vestibule is immediately beneath the inlet and contains two protruding sets of mucosal folds—the ventricular folds (more commonly referred to as the false vocal folds) and the true vocal folds (more commonly referred to simply as the vocal folds). (We will describe these folds later in this chapter.) The area between the false vocal folds and the true vocal folds is the ventricular space; within this pocketlike space are sacs that secrete mucus to coat the surface of the vocal folds below. The area between the vocal folds is the rima glottidis; the glottis refers to the vocal folds and the space in between them. The laryngeal cavity can thus be divided into the supraglottic (above glottis) space and subglottic (below glottis) space. The subglottis is narrower than

FIGURE 2.11 Cross Section of the Laryngeal Cavity

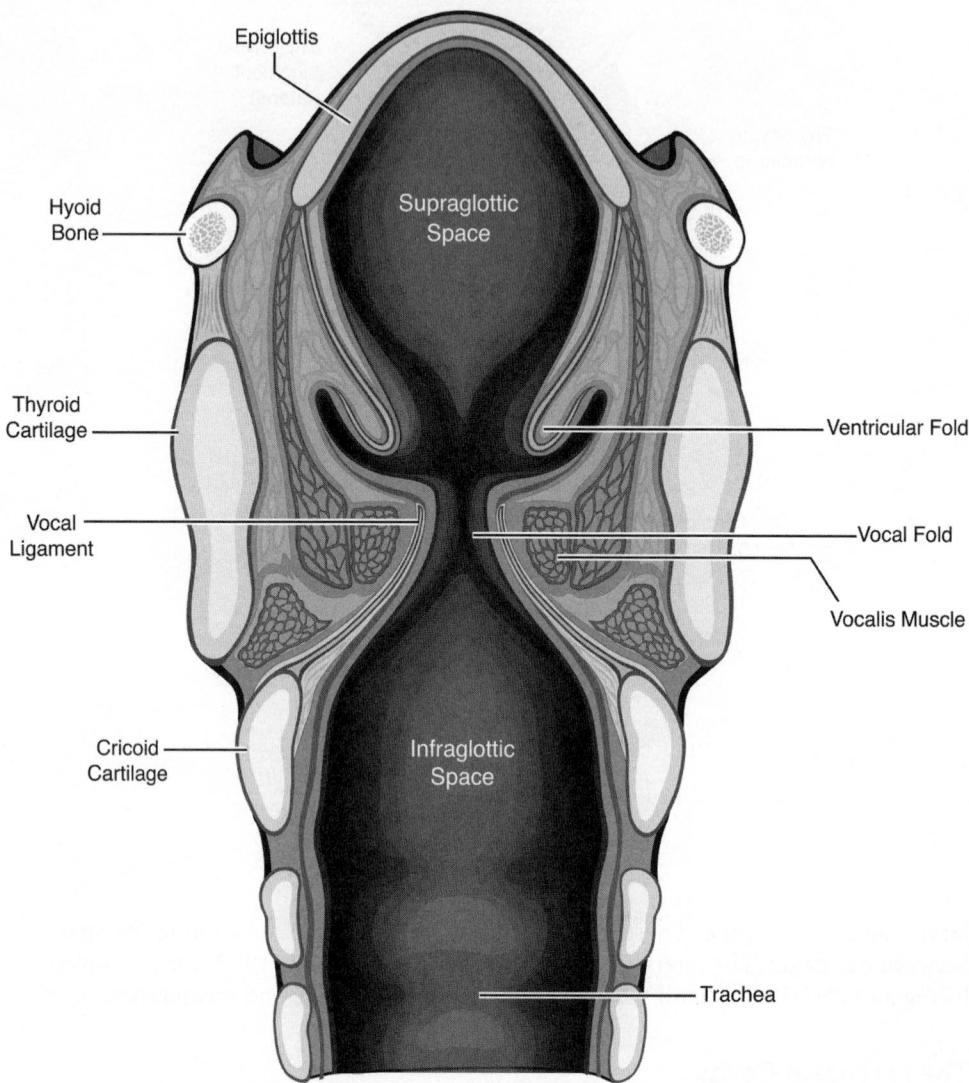

the supraglottis but eventually widens as it joins the tubular trachea. The laryngeal cavity is lined with a wet mucosa that is continuous with the mucosa of the tongue, pharynx, and trachea. This mucosa covers the laryngeal cartilages, membranes, ligaments, and muscles and is rich with sensory receptors and mucus-secreting glands. Irritation or drying of this lining can often contribute to a hoarse voice quality. In a more serious condition, the epithelial cells constituting this lining can become malignant, necessitating possible removal of all or part of the larynx.

Laryngeal Joints

The two laryngeal joints are the cricothyroid joint and the cricoarytenoid joint (see Figure 2.12). Both are synovial joints (filled with a lubricating fluid) that achieve movement at the point of contact of the articulating cartilages. Without these two

FIGURE 2.12 The Laryngeal Joints

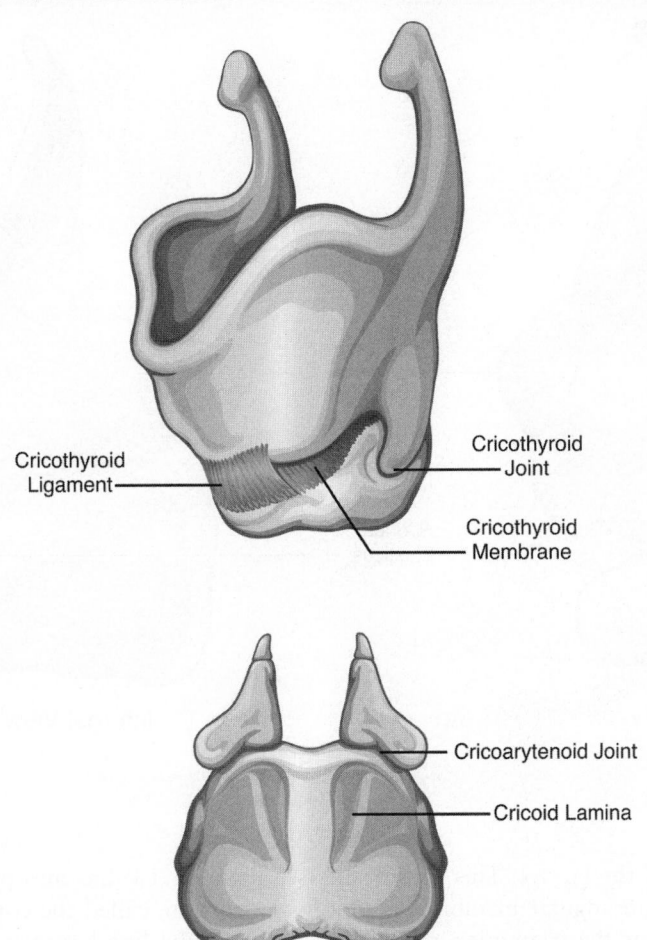

Cricothyroid Ligament

Cricothyroid Joint

Cricothyroid Membrane

Cricoarytenoid Joint

Cricoid Lamina

joints, the vocal folds would not be able to approximate (make contact) nor change their length. The cricothyroid joint is formed between the inferior horns of the thyroid cartilage and the posterior cricoid arch. Rotation at this joint results in the thyroid cartilage tilting downward and also gliding forward and back relative to the cricoid. This provides the major adjustment for change in pitch. The cricoarytenoid joints are formed between the superior borders of the cricoid cartilage and the arytenoid cartilages. The movement at the joint is described primarily as a rocking-gliding motion. The rocking motion at this joint primarily results in the vocal processes of the arytenoid cartilages swinging downward and inward (for adduction), or upward and outward (for abduction). The gliding motion primarily results in changes in vocal fold length. Arthritis or trauma can result in limited or absent motion of the arytenoid cartilages, resulting in vocal fold immobility (Speyer and colleagues, 2008).

Intrinsic Laryngeal Ligaments and Membranes

Ligaments and membranes connect the laryngeal cartilages to each other. Beneath the mucous membrane on each side of the larynx is a broad sheet of fibrous tissue containing many elastic fibers—it is sometimes referred to as the fibroelastic

FIGURE 2.13 Conus Elasticus and Quadrangular Membrane

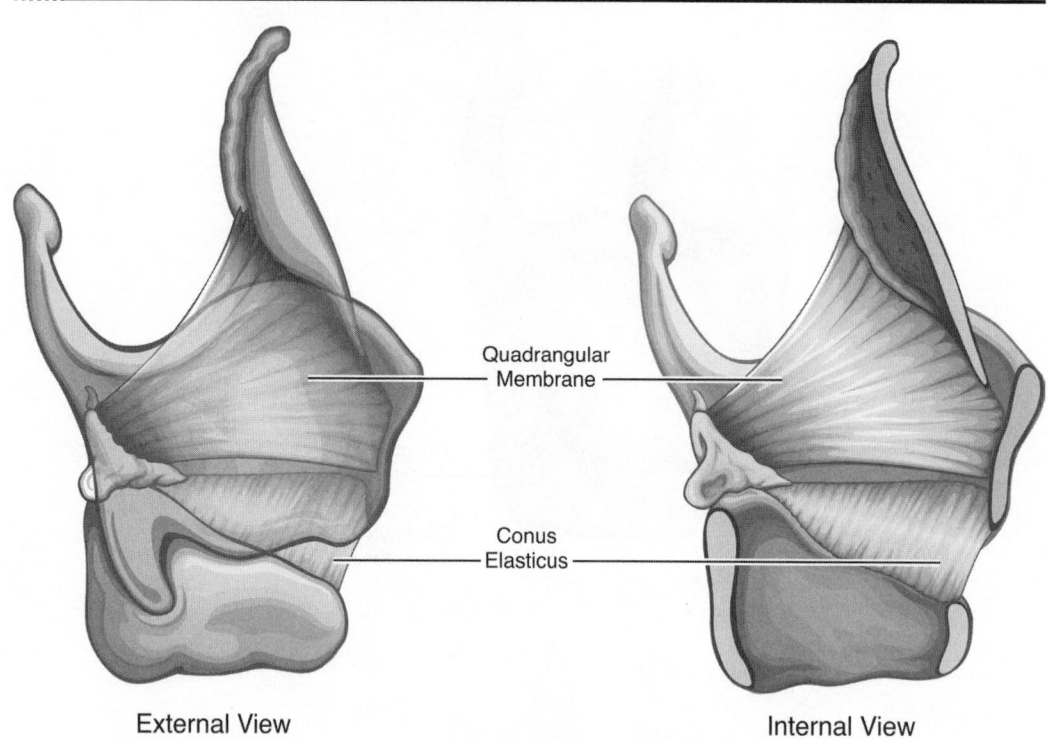

Quadrangular
Membrane

Conus
Elasticus

External View   Internal View

membrane of the larynx. This membrane (see Figure 2.13) has an upper portion, called the quadrangular membrane and a lower portion, called the conus elasticus (also known as the triangular membrane). The dividing line between these upper and lower membranes is the ventricular space. The paired quadrangular membrane originates in the lateral margins of the epiglottis and adjacent thyroid cartilage (at a midpoint between its upper and lower borders) and attaches to the corniculate cartilage and the lateral surface of the arytenoid. The free superior margins of the quadrangular membranes form the aryepiglottic folds, which drape an underlying aryepiglottic muscle. The free inferior borders of the quadrangular membranes form the ventricular ligaments, also known as the false vocal folds. The conus elasticus connects the cricoid cartilage with the thyroid and arytenoid cartilages via the medial and lateral cricothyroid ligaments. The free superior borders of the conus elasticus form the vocal ligaments.

The Intrinsic Laryngeal Muscles

The intrinsic laryngeal muscles connect the laryngeal cartilages to each other. Collectively, the contraction or relaxation of these muscles results in either the adduction, abduction, tensing, or relaxing of the vocal folds. These muscles are innervated by various branches of the Vagus nerve (CN X). The following brief descriptions identify each muscle in Figure 2.14; these muscles are named according to their attachments.

FIGURE 2.14 Superior View of the Intrinsic Laryngeal Muscles

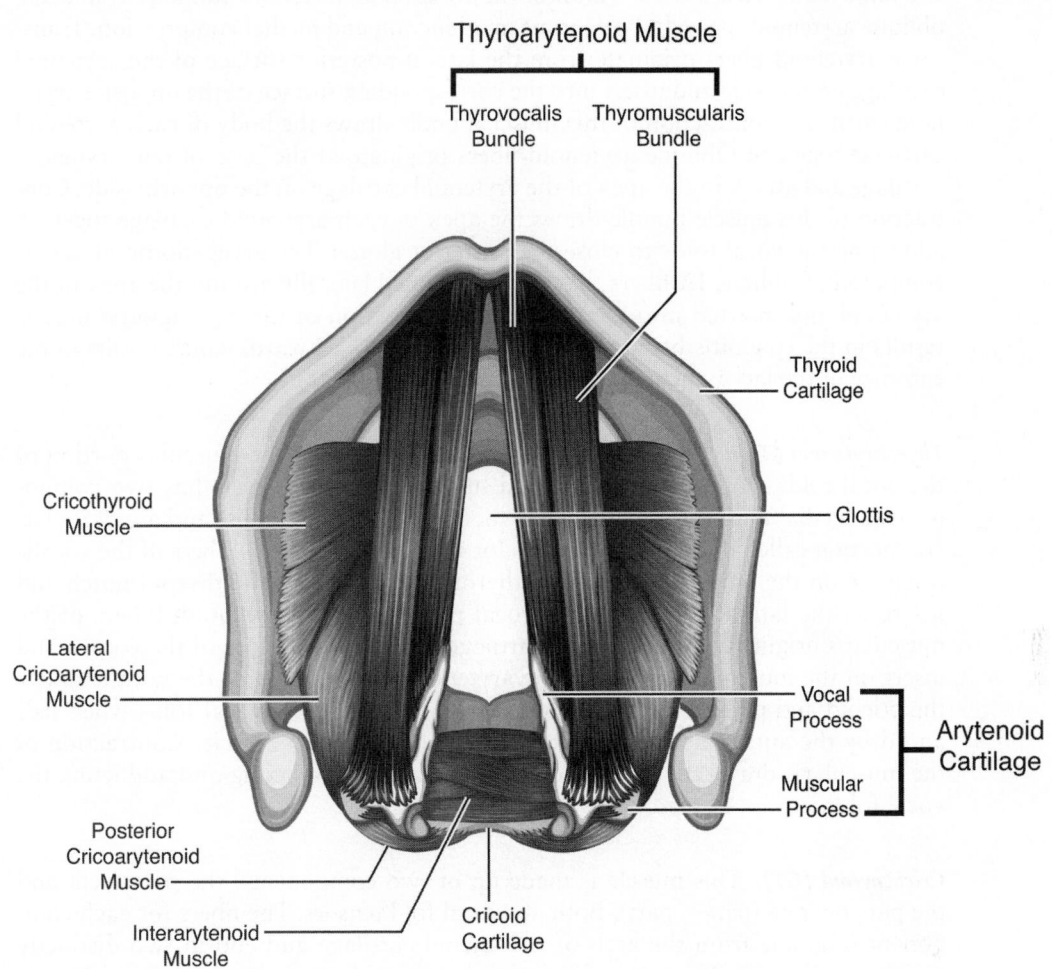

Posterior Cricoarytenoid (PCA). This paired muscle is the lone abductor muscle. Its fibers originate from the quadrate lamina of the cricoid and insert into the postero-medial surface of the muscular process of the arytenoid on that side (right-sided fibers go to the right muscular process, and so on). Contraction of this muscle draws the muscular process posteriorly, which pivots the arytenoid cartilage laterally. This results in abduction of the vocal folds and opening of the glottis. This muscle is particularly active during more active abduction, such as when needed for a quick or deep inhalation.

Lateral Cricoarytenoid (LCA). This paired muscle functions as a direct antagonist to the posterior cricoarytenoid muscle as it plays its adductor role. Its fibers originate from the arch of the cricoid and insert into the anterolateral surface of the muscular process of the arytenoid on that side. Contraction of this muscle draws the muscular process anteriorly, which pivots the arytenoid cartilage medially. This results in adduction of the vocal folds and closing of the membranous glottis. It also results in stiffening of all layers of the vocal folds (Sataloff, 2005).

Interarytenoid (IA). The only unpaired instrinsic laryngeal muscle, the interarytenoid is composed of two muscle bundles, the transverse arytenoid (unpaired) and the oblique arytenoid (paired). Both assist in adduction and medial compression. Transverse arytenoid fibers originate from the lateral posterior surface of the arytenoid cartilage on one side and insert into the corresponding surface of the opposite arytenoid cartilage. Contraction of this muscle bundle draws the body of each arytenoid cartilage together. Oblique arytenoid fibers originate at the base of one arytenoid cartilage and attach to the apex of the arytenoid cartilage on the opposite side. Contraction of this muscle bundle draws the apex of each arytenoid cartilage together, adducting the vocal folds to close the posterior glottis. The aryepiglottic muscle is composed of oblique IA fibers that have continued laterally around the apex of the arytenoid and inserted into the epiglottis. Contraction of the aryepiglottic muscle results in the epiglottis being pulled downward and backward, which results in the entrance of the larynx being covered.

Thyroarytenoid (TA). This paired muscle forms the bulk of the muscular portion of the vocal folds. Both anatomically and functionally, this muscle has two components: a medial muscle called the thyrovocalis (or simply, vocalis) and a bulkier lateral portion called the thyromuscularis (or simply, muscularis). Fibers of the vocalis originate on the inner surface of the thyroid cartilage near the thyroid notch and insert on the lateral surface of the vocal process of the arytenoid. Fibers of the muscularis originate on the thyroid cartilage just lateral to those of the vocalis and insert on the muscular process of the arytenoid. Contraction of the vocalis draws the cricoid and thyroid cartilages further apart, tensing the vocal folds when balanced by the antagonistic contraction of the cricothyroid muscle. Contraction of the muscularis draws the arytenoid cartilages forward, relaxing and adducting the vocal folds.

Cricothyroid (CT). This muscle is made up of two components: the pars recta and the pars oblique (pars = part). Both are vocal fold tensors. The fibers for each component originate from the arch of the cricoid cartilage and end in two distinctly different insertions. The lower fibers (pars oblique) insert near the thyroid lamina and the inferior horn of the thyroid cartilage. The upper fibers (pars recta) insert into the lower surface of the thyroid lamina. When the pars recta contracts, the thyroid cartilage is tilted downward, and when the pars oblique contracts, the thyroid cartilage is drawn forward. As a result, the distance between the anterior thyroid cartilage and the arytenoid cartilages is increased—because the vocal folds are passively strung between the thyroid and arytenoid cartilages, their length increases, their tension increases, and their mass per unit of length decreases. This results in faster vibration, which is perceived by the listener as an increase in pitch. The CT is the only intrinsic laryngeal muscle to receive innervation from the superior laryngeal nerve (SLN), thus the partial or total inability to change pitch when the SLN is compromised.

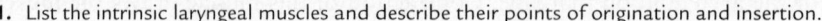

CHECK YOUR KNOWLEDGE

1. List the intrinsic laryngeal muscles and describe their points of origination and insertion.
2. For each intrinsic laryngeal muscle, describe whether it is an abductor, adductor, tensor, or relaxer.

The Ventricular (False) Vocal Folds

The ventricular folds (also known as false vocal folds) are two thick, membranous folds, each enclosing a narrow band of fibrous tissue, the ventricular ligament (see Figure 2.11). The ventricular folds contain numerous mucous glands that help to moisten and lubricate the true vocal folds beneath them, which is important for laryngeal health and normal voice (Sataloff, 2005). The ventricular ligament is attached to the thyroid cartilage (immediately below the attachment of the epiglottis) and to the arytenoid cartilage (a short distance above the vocal process). The lower border of the ventricular folds is the upper boundary of the laryngeal ventricle. The space between the ventricular folds is called the rima vestibuli. The ventricular folds should not adduct during normal phonation; in rare and clinically significant cases, they adduct during phonation, resulting in what is called ventricular phonation.

The True Vocal Folds

The vocal folds (also known as true vocal folds) are also two membranous folds, each enclosing a narrow band of elastic tissue, the vocal ligament. The vocal ligament (see Figures 2.11, 2.14, and 2.15) is attached anteriorly to the thyroid cartilage (midway between its upper and lower borders) at the anterior commissure, and posteriorly to the vocal process of the arytenoid cartilage. The upper border of the true vocal folds is the lower boundary of the laryngeal ventricle. The space between the vocal folds is called the rima glottides (or glottis). Laterally, the vocalis muscle lies parallel with it. The vocalis is covered by a mucous membrane, which is extremely thin and closely adherent to its surface. In adult males, the vocal folds are 17 to 20 mm

FIGURE 2.15 The Vocal Ligaments and Thyroarytenoid Muscles

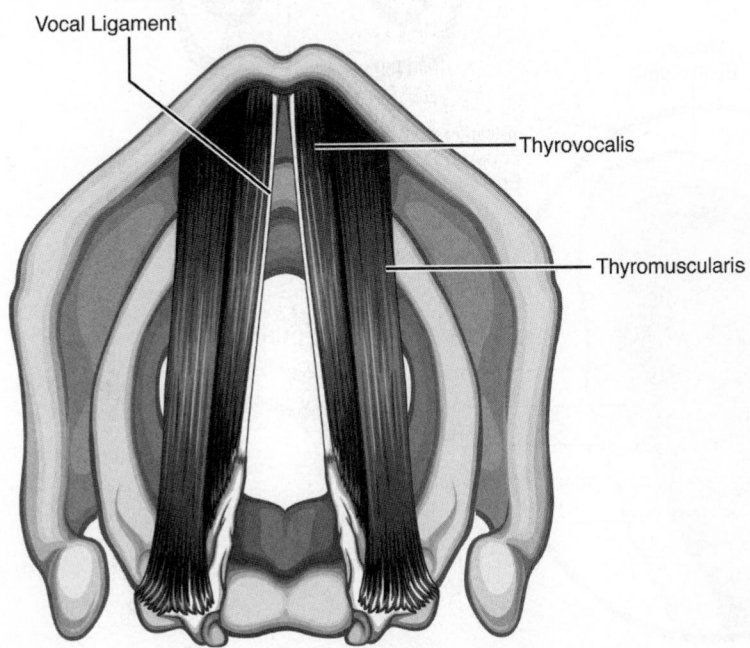

Vocal Ligament

Thyrovocalis

Thyromuscularis

long; in adult females, they are 11 to 15 mm long; and in infants, they are around 3 mm long. The anterior three-fifths of the vocal fold is generally described as being more membranous, while the posterior two-fifths is described as being more cartilaginous, although the ratio of the membranous to cartilaginous portions differs by age and gender. The midpoint of the membranous part vibrates with the greatest amplitude during phonation; the cartilaginous part is where the vocal fold attaches to the vocal process of the arytenoid cartilage, and this part does not participate much in phonation (except at very low pitches). During quiet breathing, the glottis is somewhat open, with the vocal folds in a paramedian position (that is, halfway between abduction and adduction). During deep inhalation (forced abduction), the width may double. During phonation of voiced sounds, the glottis is closed, with the vocal folds in a median position (adducted). During whispering, the glottis is closed along most of its length, but with a small posterior opening (chink).

The true vocal fold is comprised of mucosa and muscle; interwoven throughout are blood vessels. From top to bottom, the vocal fold has five layers (see Figure 2.16), each with a different cellular makeup and biomechanical properties. The layers are the (1) epithelium; (2) superficial lamina propria (also known as Reinke's space);

FIGURE 2.16 The Vocal Fold in Cross Section

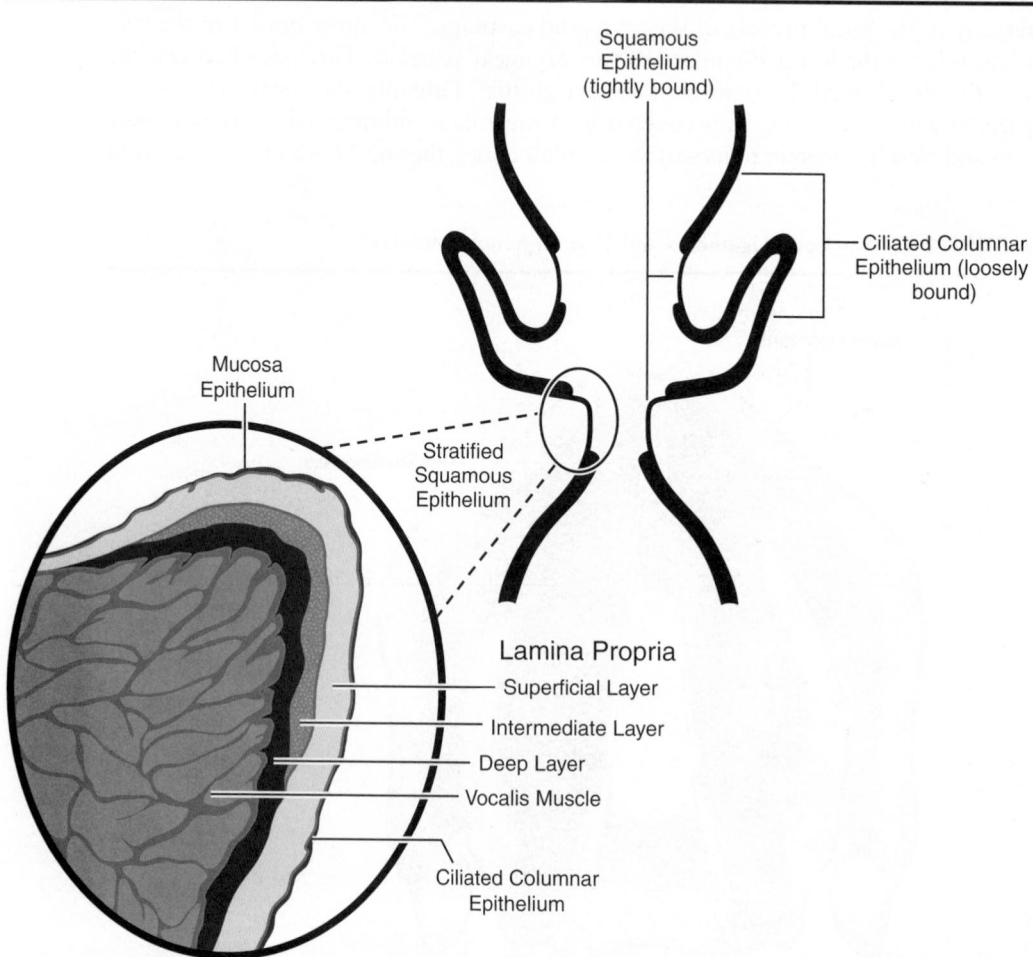

(3) intermediate lamina propria; (4) deep lamina propria; and (5) vocalis muscle, which is the medial portion of the thyroarytenoid muscle. The epithelium and superior and intermediate lamina propria are composed of elastin fibers, which allow for stretching and recoil, thus permitting movement during vocal fold vibration. The deep layer of the lamina propria is composed of collagen fibers, which prohibits stretching. The vocalis fibers make up the bulk of the vocal fold. Alternative descriptions, such as the cover-body model (Hirano and colleagues, 1983) places these five layers under three headings based on their biomechanical properties: (1) the compliant cover (epithelium and superficial lamina propria), (2) a stiffer transitional zone (intermediate and deep layers of the lamina propria), and (3) the least compliant body (vocalis muscle). Regardless of which description one uses, it is clear that the vocal fold is not comprised of the same tissue from top to bottom; that is, there is a loosely adherent cover, an underlying vocal ligament providing some stiffness and support, and a further underlying bulky muscle. The cover gives the vocal fold a glistening, white appearance and vibrates most markedly during phonation. During a laryngostroboscopic examination, the cover can be seen moving during vocal fold vibration, a phenomenon known as the mucosal wave (Hirano and Bless, 1993). Even when the vocalis muscle is weak or paralyzed, the cover may still vibrate passively (and to a more limited degree) because of exhaled air flowing over it. However, if the vocal fold is stiff and edematous (swollen), there may be an absent or markedly decreased mucosal wave.

CHECK YOUR KNOWLEDGE

1. From top to bottom, list the five layers of the vocal fold cover and body.
2. What effect does an abnormal vocal fold cover have on the voice?

Laryngeal Blood Supply and Lymphatic Drainage

There is a dual blood supply to and from each side of the larynx (see Figure 2.17). The two major arteries supplying the larynx are the inferior and superior laryngeal arteries, branches of the thyroid artery. The two veins draining the larynx are the inferior and superior laryngeal veins. The inferior arteries and veins serve the upper larynx, that is, the arytenoid cartilages, the false vocal folds and the laryngeal ventricle. The superior arteries and veins serve the lower larynx, that is, the piriform sinus and the quadrangular membrane. The laryngeal lymphatic vessels drain into the cervical lymph nodes. Abnormalities in laryngeal blood flow can be observed clinically, most dramatically in the case of a vocal fold hemorrhage, resulting in immediate and severe dysphonia.

Nervous System Control of the Larynx

Speech production is one of the most complex and rapid motor behaviors, and it involves a precise coordination of more than 100 laryngeal, velar, orofacial, and respiratory muscles. The paired vagus nerve (CN X), also known as the wanderer, is a complex and extensive nerve that plays a crucial role in speech and swallow production. This nerve serves both sensory and motor functions, sending motor signals to the soft palate, pharynx, and larynx, and picking up sensation from the entire vocal tract viscera. The sensory branches of the vagus are responsible for informing the speaker with muscle tension dysphonia that she has the sensation of fullness at the level of the larynx (globus) after speaking at the bottom of her pitch range. The vagus sends motor impulses to innervate the muscles of the velum, pharyngeal

FIGURE 2.17 Laryngeal Arterial Circulation

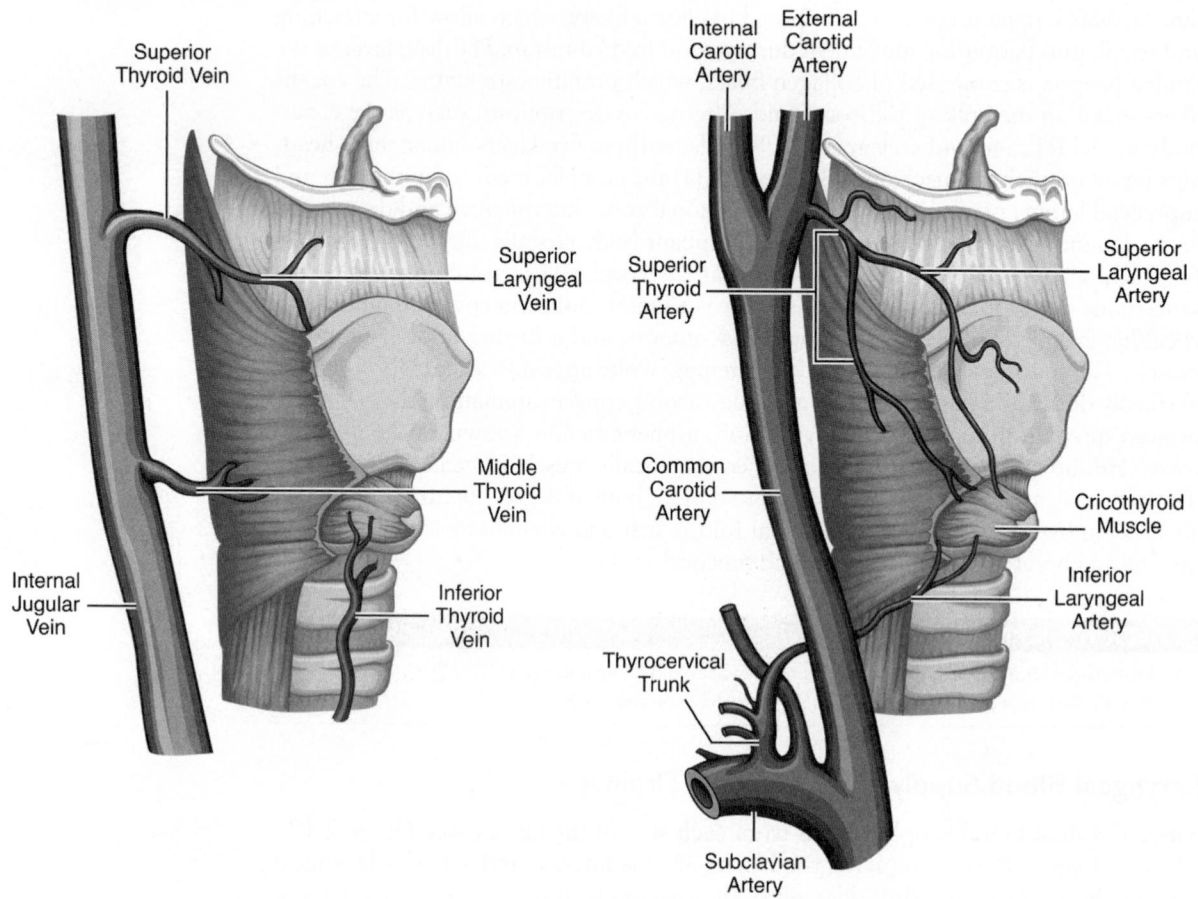

constrictors, and the larynx that are so finely tuned that the average speaker is able to produce 14 sounds per second.

Central control of voice production is conducted by two parallel pathways: (1) the limbic vocal control pathway, which is responsible for the control of innate nonverbal and emotional vocalizations, and (2) the laryngeal motor cortical pathway, which regulates the fine motor control of voluntary voice production, such as speech and song, as well as voluntary production of innate vocalizations (Simonyan & Horowitz, 2011). The ability to control various laryngeal behaviors voluntarily is most prominent in humans, whereas other species, including nonhuman primates, have limited ability to produce their vocalizations voluntarily. The laryngeal motor cortex, located within the motor homunculus in the primary motor cortex, executes voluntary laryngeal control through the multiple pathways both directly and indirectly descending to the brain stem laryngeal motor neurons in the medulla.

The vagus nerve originates in the nucleus ambiguous of the medulla (see Figure 2.18). As it descends, it splits into the pharyngeal branch, which innervates the soft palate and upper pharyngeal constrictors. It then courses inferiorly and splits off into the superior laryngeal and recurrent laryngeal branches, the latter of which is so named because it doubles back on itself before ascending to innervate

FIGURE 2.18 The Vagus Nerve

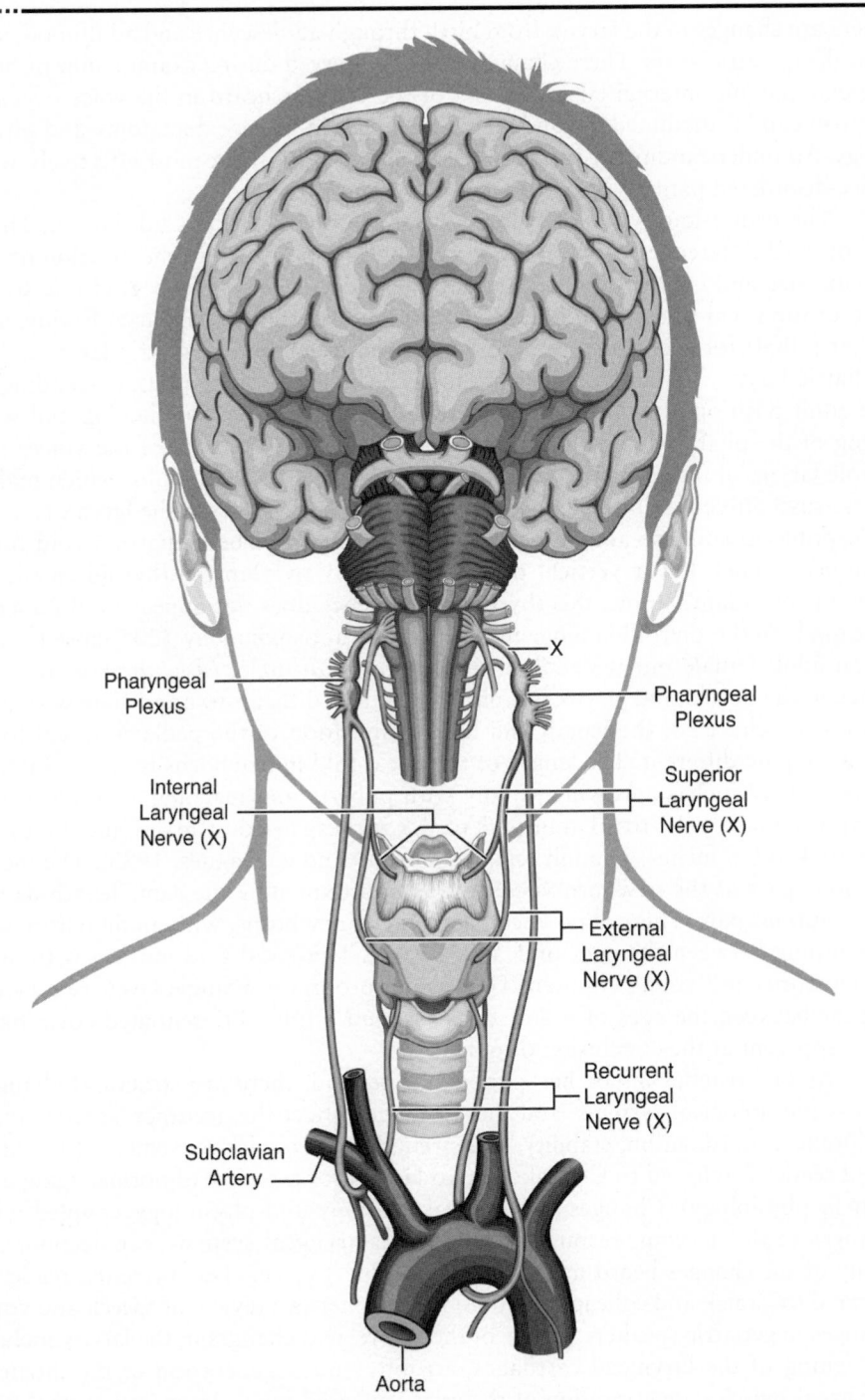

Pharyngeal Plexus

X

Pharyngeal Plexus

Internal Laryngeal Nerve (X)

Superior Laryngeal Nerve (X)

External Laryngeal Nerve (X)

Recurrent Laryngeal Nerve (X)

Subclavian Artery

Aorta

the larynx. Both the right and left recurrent laryngeal nerves innervate all of the intrinsic muscles of the larynx except for the cricothyroid. This is innervated by the superior laryngeal nerve (SLN). The extrinsic muscles are primarily innervated from the ansa cervicalis. Innervation of the soft palate, pharynx, and larynx will be explored further in Chapter 5.

Lifespan Changes in the Larynx

There are changes in the larynx from birth through adolescence and adulthood, and into the geriatric years. These changes can be observed during examination of both the external and internal larynx. Many of the changes heard in the voice over the lifespan can be attributed to fundamental changes in laryngeal anatomy and physiology. An understanding of such changes helps the SLP work most effectively with voice-disordered patients of all ages.

The pediatric larynx is not just a smaller version of the adult larynx. There are marked differences between the two, primarily in regard to the position of the larynx, size and configuration of the laryngeal cartilages, and size and fine structure of the vocal folds. (The interested reader is referred to Sapienza, Ruddy, and Baker [2004] for a complete description of the developing pediatric larynx.) The pediatric larynx is situated higher in the neck than that of an adult, descending to the adult position after puberty. With this descent comes a lengthening and widening of the pharynx, contributing to changes in the resonance of the voice. The whole laryngeal framework in children is much softer than in adults, which makes it less susceptible to blunt trauma; by the same token, however, the larynx is more susceptible to collapse and compromise of the airway. The pediatric hyoid bone assumes a much lower vertical position and may overlap the thyroid cartilage. There is no Adam's apple; this thyroid prominence does not appear until puberty. The angle of the thyroid laminae in newborns is approximately 120°, close to that of an adult female but wider than that of an adult male. Also, the cricothyroid space in the developing larynx is a narrow slit and difficult to appreciate with palpation (touch). Last, the length and fine composition of the pediatric vocal folds are also quite different. The length of the vocal fold in newborns is 2.5 to 3.0 mm (0.10 to 0.12 inches), growing rapidly with puberty and reaching an adult length of approximately 17 to 21 mm (0.7 to 0.8 inches) in adult males and 11 to 15 mm (0.4 to 0.6 inches) in adult females (Hirano and colleagues, 1983). The membranous part of the newborn vocal fold is approximately the same length as the cartilaginous part. There is no vocal ligament in newborns, with an immature one developing between the ages of 1 and 4 years. The vocal fold mucosa is thinner in newborns and young children. The lamina propria is a single layer; two layers appear between the ages of 6 and 12 years, and a fully differentiated covering is only apparent at the conclusion of puberty.

As one reaches his or her sixties and beyond, there are structural changes across physiological systems, and these changes affect the accuracy, speed, range, endurance, coordination, stability, and strength of muscular movements (the interested reader is referred to Chodzko-Zajko [1997] for a review of normal aging and human physiology). Changes in laryngeal anatomy and physiology, coupled with changes in the nervous, respiratory, and supralaryngeal systems, can account for many of the changes heard in the senescent (older) voice. (The interested reader is referred to Zraick and colleagues [2006] for an extensive review of speech and voice changes in geriatric speakers.) Some of the age-related changes in the larynx include hardening of the laryngeal cartilages, atrophy and degeneration of the intrinsic laryngeal muscles, deterioration of the cricoarytenoid joint, degeneration of glands in the laryngeal mucosa, degenerative changes in the lamina propria, degenerative changes in the conus elasticus, and decreased laryngeal blood flow (Kendall, 2007; Linville, 2001; Orlikoff, 1990; Thomas and colleagues, 2007). These changes can lead to what is commonly referred to as presbyphonia—an age-related voice disorder characterized by recognizable perceptual changes in the pitch, pitch range, loudness, and quality of the older speaker's voice (Roy and colleagues, 2007). Presbyphonia is described in Chapter 8.

CHECK YOUR KNOWLEDGE

1. List and describe five differences among the pediatric, adult, and geriatric larynx.
2. How can changes in the larynx brought about with advanced age potentially affect the voice?

PRINCIPLES OF PHONATION

In this section, we go into further detail about laryngeal functioning for voice production. We first summarize the myoelastic-aerodynamic theory of phonation (van den Berg, 1958). This is followed by brief descriptions of the major laryngeal adjustments needed to accomplish phonation. An overview of voice registers is then presented. We conclude with discussions of the mechanisms for changing vocal pitch, loudness, and quality. It is our hope that the reader will use the material presented in this chapter thus far (and that which follows) as a basis for understanding both normal and abnormal voice production.

The Myoelastic-Aerodynamic Theory of Phonation

According to van den Berg (1958), the myoelastic-aerodynamic theory of phonation "... deals with the control of the larynx by the higher centers of phonation" (p. 227). This theory is generally regarded as the most accurate model to explain the mechanics of vocal fold vibration. The major elements of this theory are embedded in its title: *Myo* refers to involvement of muscles, *elastic* refers to the ability of those muscles to return to their original state, *aero* refers to airflow and pressure, and *dynamic* refers to movement and change. The major principles of this theory can be summarized as follows: (1) the vocal folds adduct (come to midline) by contraction of certain intrinsic laryngeal muscles; (2) when fully approximated, there is an increase in subglottal air pressure relative to supraglottal air pressure; (3) the increased subglottal air pressure causes the vocal folds to separate first on their inferior border and then their superior border, eventually abducting completely (but not necessarily widely); (4) when abducted, the velocity of airflow between the vocal folds increases and the pressure between the vocal folds decreases (the Bernoulli principle); (5) the decreased air pressure, coupled with the elastic recoil of the vocal folds, causes them to move back toward midline; and (6) the vocal folds approximate first on their inferior border and then their superior border, eventually adducting (but not necessarily tightly or forcefully). Thus, the vocal folds have completed one cycle of vibration (closed-open-closed) due to *both* myoelastic and aerodynamic forces, not simply repetitive muscle contraction. This cycle of vibration will repeat as long as sufficient subglottal air pressure (on the order of 3 to 5 cm H2O at minimum) can build up to blow the vocal folds apart again (see Sidebar 2.14). This cycle is repeated approximately 125 times per second (Hz) in the habitual phonation of an adult male, approximately 225 Hz in an adult female, and approximately 265 Hz for a prepubertal child.

SIDEBAR 2.14

To appreciate the role of air pressure, do the following: Hum an /i/ and while holding the tone, occlude the nose with your thumb and forefinger. Note that the sound stops. Why? Because the cross glottal pressure drop is eliminated. You cannot have phonation without the airflow, which is created by the transglottal pressure drop.

CHECK YOUR KNOWLEDGE

1. Describe the five major elements of the myoelastic-aerodynamic theory of voice production.
2. What is the minimum subglottic air pressure needed to set the vocal folds into vibration?

SIDEBAR 2.15

To illustrate each of these, look again at the two phrases and do this: Place your right index finger on your Adam's apple and your left index finger just in front of (but not touching) your lips. Now, say the first word of each phrase (*he* versus *I*), paying close attention to the sensations on each finger during each utterance. When saying *he,* you should feel exhaled air on your left finger prior to feeling vibration of the vocal folds on your right finger. This is an example of breathy vocal attack; that is, air begins to flow before the vocal folds adduct. When saying *I* you should feel the opposite sensation; that is, exhaled air on your left finger is felt after vibration of the vocal folds is felt on your right finger. This is an example of glottal attack; that is, air begins to flow after the vocal folds are firmly adducted (much like in a cough). A third type of attack, called simultaneous vocal attack, can be appreciated by examining the word *zoos* in the first sentence. During production of the /z/ phoneme in the initial word position, you should feel exhaled airflow and vocal fold vibration at the same time.

Laryngeal Adjustments for Speech

The larynx is capable of making remarkably fast and accurate phonatory adjustments during speech. To illustrate, examine the following two written phrases: "He went to seven zoos" and "I wore seven shoes." When saying these phrases aloud, one can appreciate that each phrase consists of a combination of voiced and voiceless phonemes (sounds), in different sequences. For these phrases to "sound right" when spoken aloud, the larynx must adjust to the phonetic demands placed upon it. That is, the laryngeal musculature must adjust so that the voice turns on when it should, stays on when it should, and turns off when it should. On top of that, the voice that is produced must be acceptable in terms of pitch, loudness, and quality.

Moore and von Leden (1958) have described three types of vocal onset (or attack) (see Sidebar 2.15): breathy (also known as aspirate), glottal, and simultaneous (also known as easy, gentle). These three types of attack are all normal. Problems arise, however, when a particular type of attack (typically, glottal or breathy) is misused. For example, hard glottal attack is a misuse of normal glottal attack. This abnormal laryngeal adjustment is often associated with the "drill sergeant" voice—a voice where the onset of each word is greatly punctuated in terms of attack and loudness. In another example, breathy phonation is often associated with the "Marilyn Monroe" voice—a voice that is light and airy throughout an utterance, regardless of linguistic content. Simultaneous attack is considered the most optimal means of initiating phonation because it places less stress and strain on the vocal folds. In Chapter 7, we present Voice Facilitating Approaches to reduce hard glottal attack.

Looking again at the word *zoos* in the first sentence, one can also appreciate two additional laryngeal adjustments: sustained phonation and termination of phonation. Once simultaneous attack begins, the vocal folds must be actively held in a position within the airstream that allows their continued vibration. Placing your two index fingers in position again, you should feel ongoing airflow and vocal fold vibration throughout the utterance. Compare this to production of the word *vice,* where vocal fold vibration ceases just prior to production of the final /s/ phoneme.

Voice Registers

Consider for a moment whether your voice quality changes as you speak or sing at various pitch levels within your overall pitch range. Chances are it does. The voice quality near the bottom of your pitch range is likely very different from that near your habitual speaking pitch, and both are likely very different from the voice quality near the top of your pitch range. You probably also perceived a consistent voice quality within each of these three broad areas of your range, but not across them. That is, there may have been an abrupt change in voice quality as you moved through your range (particularly if you are an untrained singer). The concept of vocal register addresses the vocal phenomena we just considered. A vocal register is defined as a series of consecutive pitch values of approximately equivalent vocal quality (Hollien,

1974). There is a rich history of considerable debate about how to label, define, and differentiate among registers. (See Laver [1980]; Titze [1994]; Cleveland [1994] for recent discussions, and Luchsinger and Arnold [1965] for historical reference.) There is a general consensus that at least three recognizable registers exist: falsetto, modal, and glottal fry (or pulse). Each of these registers is characterized physiologically by different modes (or patterns) of vocal fold vibration (Laver, 1980). Thus, any change to the pattern of vocal fold vibration may result in a perceived change in voice quality.

The patterns of vocal fold vibration largely result from the degree of longitudinal tension on the vocal folds, the degree of medial compression of the vocal folds, and the degree of adductive force. Active longitudinal tension is achieved through the contraction of the vocalis muscle, whereas passive longitudinal tension is achieved through contraction of the cricothyroid muscle. Medial compression is obtained by contraction of the lateral thyroarytenoid muscles. The adductive force is caused by contraction of the interarytenoid muscles and the lateral cricoarytenoid muscles. Each register differs in terms of these physiological parameters (Laver, 1994).

Modal phonation is the register we use for most of conversational speech. The span of frequencies in this register for adult women is approximately 150 to 500 Hz; for adult men, it is approximately 80 to 450 Hz, with habitual speaking pitch falling in the low-to-mid part of the range. There is moderate longitudinal tension, moderate medial compression, and moderate adductive force. Vocal fold vibration is periodic, with very little audible frication (breathiness). The minimum subglottal pressure needed to maintain this pattern of vibration is approximately 3 to 5 cm H_2O. Average airflow rate is between 100 and 350 cc/s. According to Cleveland (1994), singers may divide the modal register into a lower and heavier chest voice and a higher and lighter head voice.

The glottal fry (or pulse) voice usually occupies the frequencies below the modal register, although there may be some overlap between the two registers in adult males. The span of frequencies in this register for both women and men is approximately 35 to 90 Hz (Sorenson, 1984). There is minimal longitudinal tension on the vocal folds, which are short and thicker, with a lax cover. There is moderate medial compression of the vocal folds, and mild adductive force. Vocal fold vibration is characterized by a double (or sometimes triple) closure pattern for each cycle (Chen and colleagues, 2002). The vocal folds close, bounce open, and then rapidly close again before finally opening to complete the cycle (Behrman, 2007). This generates a syncopated, secondary beat that is perceived as a crackling sound, much like bacon frying in a pan of oil or the sound of a stick being dragged along a picket fence. The minimum subglottal pressure needed to maintain this pattern of vibration is approximately 2 cm H_2O, a value often seen at the end of long phrases. Average airflow rate is between 12 and 20 cc/s. Excessive use of pulse phonation can be harmful to the vocal fold mucosa. The Voice Facilitating Approaches of respiration training, and pitch change, discussed in Chapter 7, are often effective in helping patients eliminate chronic use of glottal fry phonation. We also describe the use of glottal fry as a Voice Facilitating Approach to eliminate muscle tension dysphonia.

The falsetto voice usually occupies the frequencies above the modal register, though there may be some overlap. Falsetto is most easily recognized in the adult male voice at a speaking pitch of 300 to 600 Hz. There is moderately high longitudinal tension on the vocal folds; they are long and stiff, thin along the edges, and often bow-shaped. There is moderately high medial compression of the vocal folds, and high adductive force. The posterior cartilaginous portion of the glottis is so tightly adducted that little or no posterior vibration occurs while the anterior portion vibrates rapidly. The vocal folds make contact only briefly as compared to modal phonation, which gives falsetto its characteristic "breathy" quality. At times there may also be a posterior chink during the production of falsetto that contributes to the breathy quality. The amplitude of vocal fold excursion (lateral movement) is reduced. As a result of the limited lateral movement, the mucosal wave is confined to the medial edge of the vocal folds. The minimum subglottal pressure needed to maintain this pattern of vibration is less than that for modal phonation. This voice is perceived as not only being high-pitched, but thin and airy, with very little attack.

Teachers of voice strive to blend the various registers so that the difference in quality of the voice becomes almost imperceptible as the singer transitions from one register to the next. Some singers seem to have only one register; no matter how they change their pitch, their voice always seems to have the same quality, with no discernible break toward the upper part of the pitch range. This is no small accomplishment and requires considerable voice training. It is a highly regarded attribute in the professional singing voice.

How We Change Vocal Pitch

In this **video**, we observe a patient who presents with strained, strangled vocal quality and monopitch and monoloudness associated with spastic dysarthria due to a series of small ischemic strokes. Note how the Voice Facilitating Approach of pitch inflection increases the inflection of target words. Grand Rounds: What is happening at the laryngeal level to produce words that are longer, louder and elevated in pitch?

Vocal pitch is a perceptual attribute that is correlated with the frequency (rate) of vocal fold vibration. As fundamental frequency changes, the listener perceives a change in pitch. The primary biomechanical determinants of the rate of vocal fold vibration are: (1) the length of the vocal folds, (2) the tension of the vocal folds, and (3) the mass of the vocal folds per unit of length. Changes in subglottal pressure also occur as one changes frequency. All these factors interact with one another to achieve a target frequency of vibration.

As the vocal folds lengthen, their tension increases and their mass per unit of length is decreased (think of a rubber band that becomes thinner as it is stretched). As a result, the vocal folds vibrate faster. Which muscles contribute to this change, and how? The primary intrinsic laryngeal muscle involved in pitch change is the cricothyroid muscle. When this muscle contracts, there is an increase in the distance between the anterior thyroid cartilage and the arytenoid cartilage. The thyrovocalis also contributes to pitch change. When it contracts, the cricoid and thyroid cartilages are drawn further apart, tensing the vocal folds (when balanced by the antagonistic contraction of the cricothyroid muscle). As the vocal folds become shorter, less tense, and thicker, they vibrate slower. This change in frequency of vibration is perceived as a lowering of pitch. The thyromuscularis is the primary muscle responsible for this change. When it contracts, the arytenoid cartilages are drawn forward, relaxing and adducting the vocal folds.

Near the upper end of the natural pitch range, increased elasticity of the vocal folds results in increased glottal resistance, requiring increased subglottal air pressure to produce higher frequency phonations. Increased tension of the vocal folds requires greater air pressure to set the folds into vibration. According to van den Berg (1958), the average person must slightly increase subglottal air pressure in order to increase voice pitch; however, because increasing subglottal pressure has an abducting effect on the vocal folds, the folds must continue to increase in tension (longitudinal tension) to maintain their approximated position. Although the primary determinants of vocal frequency are the length, mass, and tension adjustments of the vocal folds, increases in frequency are usually characterized by increasing subglottal pressures, increased medial compression of the vocal folds, and increased glottal airflow rates.

CHECK YOUR KNOWLEDGE

1. Describe mass, length, and tension of the vocal folds during low- versus high-pitched phonation.
2. Which intrinsic laryngeal muscles are primarily responsible for changing the frequency of vocal fold vibration?

How We Change Vocal Loudness

Vocal loudness is a perceptual attribute that is correlated with the intensity of the sound wave generated during phonation. As intensity changes, the listener perceives a change in loudness. The primary biomechanical determinants of intensity are (1) subglottal pressure; (2) medial compression of the vocal folds; and (3) the duration, speed, and degree of vocal fold closure. Supraglottal adjustments also contribute to changes in vocal loudness.

SIDEBAR 2.16

Place your fingertips on your rib cage and feel what happens as you count aloud from 1 to 10 at a normal and constant loudness level. Repeat this exercise, steadily increasing loudness as you say the numbers 6 to 10. What you likely felt was an expansion of your rib cage.

SIDEBAR 2.17

Think of the sound of a hairdryer and how much louder the air is coming out of the nozzle when the dryer is set to a higher fan speed compared to a lower fan speed.

Hixon and Abbs (1980) have written: "Sound pressure level, the primary factor contributing to our perception of the loudness of the voice, is governed mainly by the pressure supplied to the larynx by the respiratory pump" (p. 68) (see Sidebar 2.16). More air in the lungs results in a greater buildup of subglottal air pressure when the vocal folds adduct, particularly the longer they remain adducted. As vocal intensity increases, the vocal folds tend to remain closed for longer periods of time during each vibratory cycle. When the vocal folds are eventually blown open, they abduct more widely. This allows more and more air molecules to escape—air that is explosively turbulent and that generates more acoustic power (see Sidebar 2.17).

CHECK YOUR KNOWLEDGE

1. Describe the subglottal pressure, medial compression, and degree of vocal fold closure during soft versus loud phonation.
2. Which intrinsic laryngeal muscles are primarily responsible for changes in vocal loudness?

How We Change Vocal Quality

Voice quality is a perceptual attribute related to the sound of the voice beyond its pitch and loudness (Behrman, 2007). The "quality" of one's voice is what distinguishes it from other voices of similar pitch and loudness. Changes in voice quality appear to result from changes at two levels of the speech production system: (1) the glottal source, and (2) the resonant characteristics of the vocal tract (Pershall and Boone, 1987). The principles of voice quality change are not as well understood as those of pitch change and loudness change. Further complicating matters is the subjective nature of voice quality judgments: What sounds acceptable to one listener may not be acceptable to another. On a related note, even when two listeners agree about the quality of a particular voice, they each may use a different term to describe that voice. Last, there is considerable debate about which objective measures of voice quality correlate with subjective measures.

Abnormal voice quality may be a hallmark feature of dysphonia, regardless of etiology. In our clinical practice, we see patients who present with a voice that is breathy, rough, strained, harsh (strained + rough), or hoarse (strained + rough + breathy). Each of these vocal qualities can result from either functional, organic, or neurological causes, or some combination of causes. Most of the Voice Facilitating Approaches described in Chapter 7 can be used to improve voice quality, particularly the abnormal voice qualities that result from vocal hyperfunction.

Breathy voice quality is often associated with incomplete glottal closure. When the vocal folds are loosely or incompletely approximated, turbulent airflow contributes noise to the vocal signal. Intensity is diminished. Rough voice quality is often associated with aperiodic vocal fold vibration. The irregular mucosal wave movement adds spectral noise. Intensity may be increased. Strained voice quality is often associated with considerable medial compression of the true (and perhaps false) vocal folds. Strained voice quality is also often associated with aperiodic vocal fold vibration, which adds spectral noise. Intensity may be increased. The four spectrograms in Figure 2.19 contrast the breathy voice, the harsh voice, the hoarse voice,

FIGURE 2.19 Spectrograms

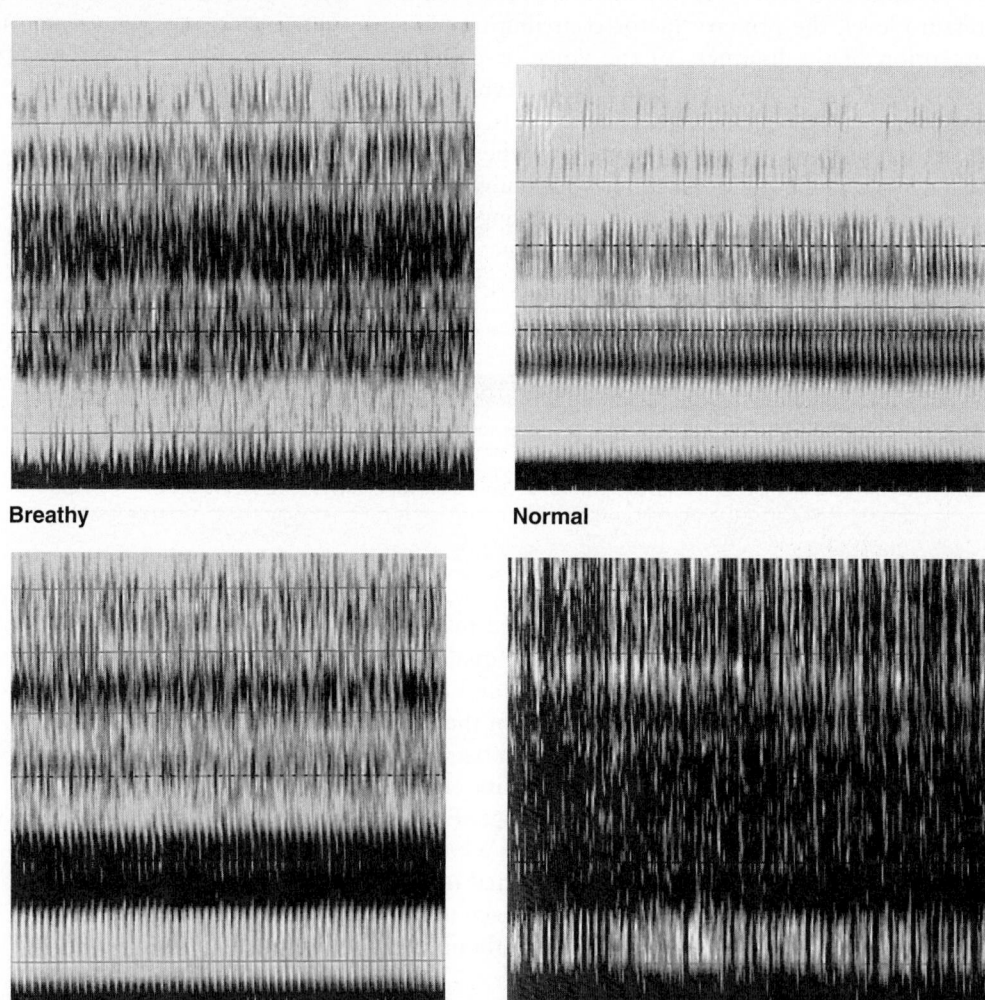

Breathy

Normal

Harsh

Hoarse

and the normal voice. Each of the spectrograms was produced by the same normal speaker prolonging an /i/.

Perkins (1983) has added constriction and vertical as well as horizontal focus to the concept of voice quality production. He describes the Voice-Facilitating Approach of yawn-sigh, discussed in Chapter 7, which demonstrates the clinical value of these physiological configurations of the supraglottal vocal tract. Imagery or feeling is used to determine the vertical focus of the voice, "the perception associated with the placement of the focal point of the tone in the head" (Perkins, 1983, p. 113). At the low end of the vertical focus, speakers or singers feel their voice is being squeezed out of the throat, whereas at the high end, the focus seems to be high in the head. The sensation is described as if the tone were "floating in the head." Vocal efficiency seems to occur best at the higher end of the vertical placement. The Voice-Facilitating Approach of focus discussed in Chapter 7, makes use of these observations. It has been our experience that subjects given these instructions relative to the imagery of constriction and verticality produce voices with greater aperiodicity (hoarseness) at the low end of the vertical scale and greater vocal clarity at the high end. In time, Perkins's construct of constriction and horizontal as well as vertical focus may well have greater measurement potential and utilization.

RESONANCE

The acoustic signal produced by the vocal folds would be a weak-sounding reedy voice without the additional component of resonance. Years ago, one of the authors of this text observed a patient who had been cut from ear to ear with a massive wound that opened immediately superior to his thyroid cartilage. Before the wound was sutured, we heard the patient's feeble attempts at phonation. Much of his airflow and sound waves escaped through the wound. The result was a voice that was truly unique. Someone even likened it to the thin bleat of a baby lamb. Apparently, what is perceived as the quality, timbre, richness, fullness, and loudness of the voice is largely produced by the supraglottal resonators. Even though the structures of the chest and trachea may play some role in resonance, this role is not as clearly defined as that of the supraglottal resonators of the pharynx, oral cavity, and nasal cavity. Figure 2.20 shows a line drawing and cadaver head that demonstrate the F-shaped vocal tract.

STRUCTURES OF RESONANCE

The vocal tract begins, for all practical purposes, at the level of the glottis. The airflow and sound waves probably have some beginning passage in the ventricular space (in Figure 2.20B) between the true folds (A) and the ventricular folds (C). In Figure 2.20 the cavities of the vocal tract have been shaded darker. The epiglottis (D), by its concavity, probably serves as a deflector or sounding-board resonator as sound waves travel between the aryepiglottic folds (E) into the hypopharynx (F). The hypopharynx is the cavity directly above the esophagus (G). Its anterior border comprises the structures and opening of the larynx; its sides and back wall are composed of the inferior pharyngeal constrictors. Superior to the inferior pharyngeal constrictors are the middle pharyngeal constrictors (H). The oropharynx (J) begins at the tip of the epiglottis and extends to the level of the velum and hard palate. The small angular

FIGURE 2.20A The F-Shaped Vocal Tract

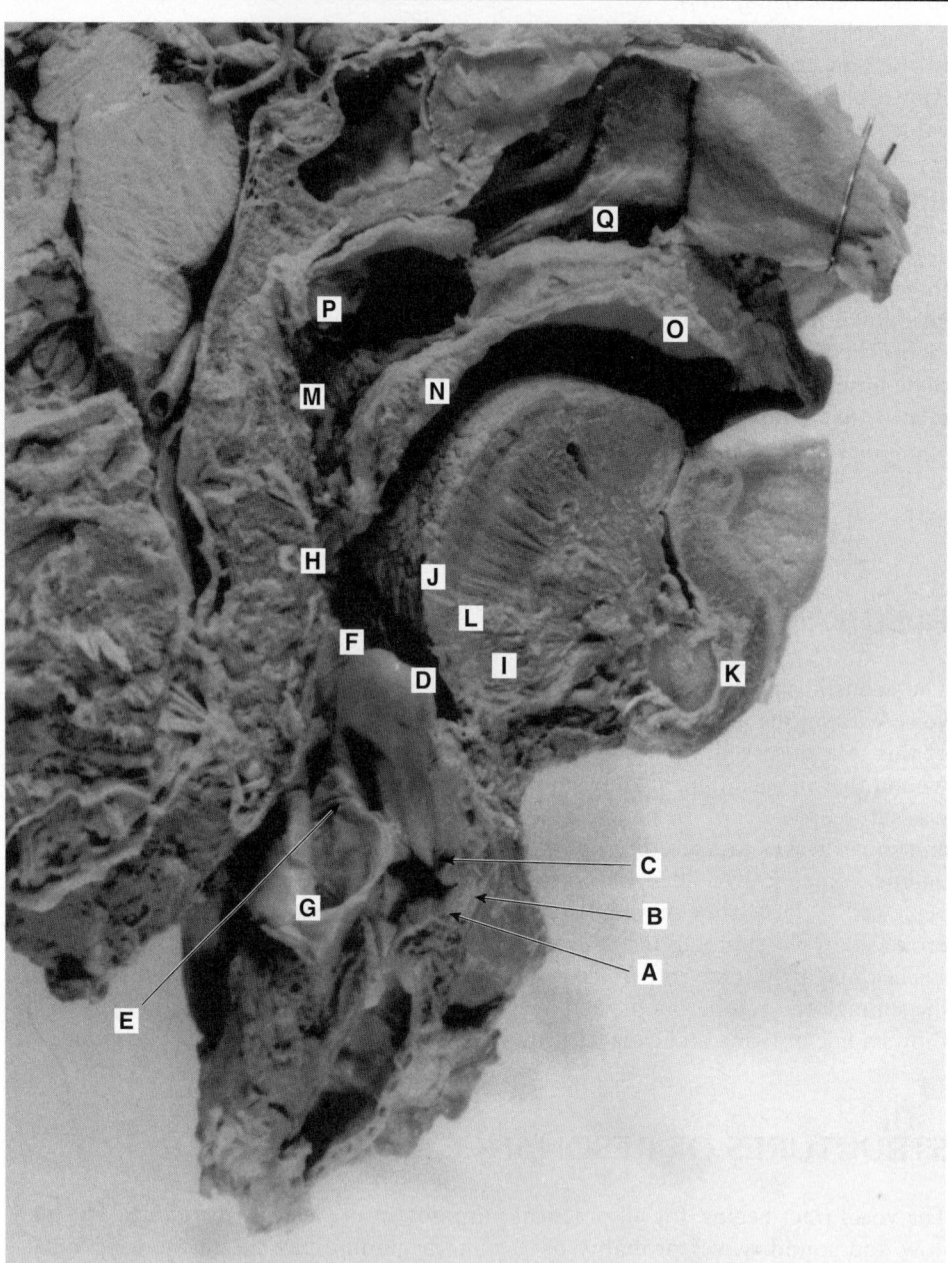

The F-shaped vocal tract is shown in both the photograph of a cadaver head in part A of this figure and the line drawing in part B. Letters A through Q identify various structures of the vocal tract: (A) True folds; (B) ventricular space; (C) ventricular folds; (D) epiglottis; (E) aryepiglottic folds; (F) hypopharynx; (G) inferior pharyngeal constrictors and upper esophageal sphincter; (H) middle pharyngeal constrictors; (I) valleculae; (J) oropharynx; (K) mandible; (L) tongue; (M) Passavant's pad; (N) soft palate (velum); (O) hard palate; (P) nasopharynx; (Q) nasal cavity.

FIGURE 2.20B

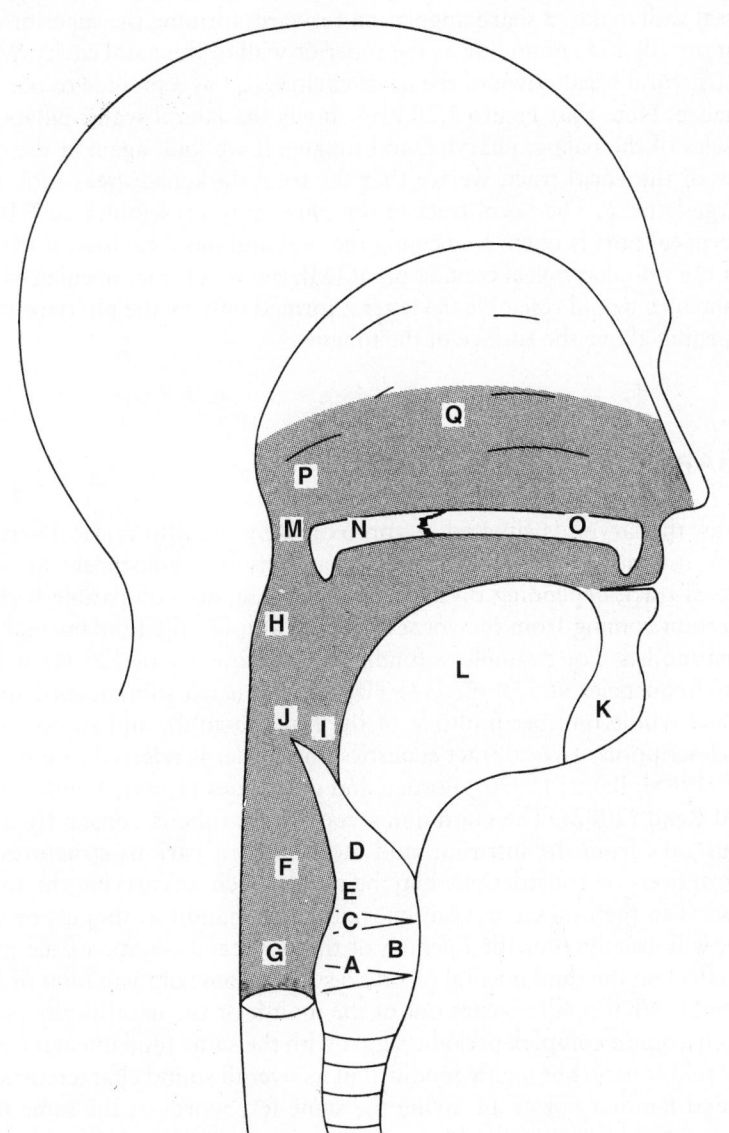

spaces between the front of the epiglottis and the back of the tongue (L) are called the valleculae (I). Cutting away the mandible (K) in a lateral view is the great body of the tongue, which occupies most of the oral cavity and forms the constantly changing floor of that cavity. The hard palate is designated (O), with the soft palate or velum (N) forming the roof of the oral cavity. The lips, teeth, and cheeks play obvious front and lateral roles in shaping the oral cavity. The middle and superior pharyngeal constrictors form the lateral and posterior muscular wall of the oropharynx (J). The site of the velopharyngeal closure, necessary for the separation of the oral and nasal cavities required for oral resonance, is the Passavant's pad (M) area of the superior pharyngeal constrictor; most people do not have much Passavant area enlargement. As shown in Figure 2.20, superior to the velopharyngeal contact point, the posterior pharyngeal wall makes a sharp angulation forward, forming the superior wall of the nasopharynx (P) and continuing as the superior wall of the nasal cavity. We make no further structural breakdown of the nasal cavities (Q) as a prelude to our discussion of resonance. Note that Figure 2.20 also shows the lateral walls, pillars of fauces, and muscles of the palate, pharynx, and tongue. If we look again at the overall lateral view of the vocal tract, we see that the total darkened areas look something like a large letter *F*. The vocal tract in the photograph resembles an *F* because the velopharyngeal port is open, connecting the oral and nasal cavities. If the port were closed at the velopharyngeal contact point (M), the vocal tract opening available for voice resonance would resemble the letter *r*, formed only by the pharynx and the oral cavity opening above the surface of the tongue.

MECHANISM OF RESONANCE

In humans, the larynx is situated at approximately the fifth cervical vertebra, thus creating a resonating chamber to filter and amplify the acoustic signal. Some areas of the vocal tract, depending on their configuration, are compatible with the periodic vibration coming from the vocal folds and amplify the fundamental frequency and its harmonics. For example, a fundamental frequency of 125 Hz will resonate harmonic frequencies at 250 Hz, 375 Hz, 500 Hz (each subsequent harmonic frequency is a whole number multiple of the fundamental), and so on. For a more detailed description of vocal tract acoustics, the reader is referred to sources such as Daniloff (1985), Baken (1996), Borden and colleagues (1994), Minifie (1994), and Kent and Read (2002). The continuous vocal tract tube is constantly interrupted at various sites from the intrusion and movement of various structures. Some of the interruptions or constrictions may be severe, such as carrying the tongue high and forward in the oral cavity. Any movement of mandible, tongue, or velum, for example, will greatly alter the opening of the oral cavity. Some of the movements have no effect on the fundamental or sound source; some of them filter or inhibit the fundamental. What finally comes out of the mouth or the nasal cavity perceived as voice has become a complex periodic signal with the same fundamental frequency as the vocal fold source, but highly modified in its overall sound characteristics. We can hear several familiar voices all saying the same few words at the same fundamental frequency, and we are still able to differentiate each voice and assign it to each familiar person. Even if we do not know the speaker, we can fairly accurately tell the approximate age and the gender of the speaker. Perhaps even more important, by filtering the glottal tone, we can tell if the person has a cold or is upset or angry, tired, or frightened. Or the meaning could even be changed by the change in quality or emphasis while saying the same words. The vocal characteristics related to the individualization of each person's vocal tract has given each voice its own unique characteristics (vocal quality) as the result of the amplification and filtering unique to each vocal tract.

The *F* configuration of the supraglottal vocal tract is constantly changing. What happens in any one portion of the tract influences both the total flow of air and sound waves through the total tract and the sound that eventually issues out from the mouth (or nose). By action of the pharyngeal constrictors and other supraglottal muscles, the overall dimensions of the pharynx are always changing. The membranes of the pharynx and the degree of relaxation or tautness of the pharyngeal constrictors have noticeable acoustic filtering effects. Higher frequency vocalizations seem to receive their best resonating effects under a fairly high degree of pharyngeal wall tension. Lower frequencies appear to be better amplified by a pharynx that is somewhat larger and more relaxed. This appears to be related to the short wavelength of high-frequency sounds and the long wavelength of the low-frequency components.

The oral cavity, or mouth, is as essential for resonance as the pharynx. Of all our resonators, the mouth is capable of the most variation in size and shape. It is the constant size–shape adjustment of the mouth that permits us to speak or, more accurately, allows us to be understood. Our vowels and diphthongs, for example, are originated by a laryngeal vibration, but shaped and restricted by the size and shape adjustment of the oral cavity. The mouth has fixed structures (teeth, alveolar processes, dental arch, and hard palate) and moving structures (tongue, velum, cheeks, mandible, and lips). We are most concerned with the moving structures, primarily the tongue, velum, and mandible, in our study of voice resonance. The mouth and other supraglottal resonators give us the perception of a regional dialect to help identify the speaker and, more important, allow for the formation of distinguishable vowels.

The tongue is the most mobile articulator, and it possesses both extrinsic and intrinsic muscles to move it. Each of the extrinsic muscles can, on contraction, elevate or lower the tongue at its anterior, middle, or posterior points and extend it forward or backward. The intrinsic muscles control the shape of the tongue by narrowing, flattening, lengthening, or shortening the overall tongue body and elevating or lowering the tongue tip. The various combinations of intrinsic and extrinsic muscle contractions can produce an unlimited number of tongue positions with resulting size–shape variations of the oral cavity. In addition to the tongue movements, the lowering and closing of the mandible contributes to the formation of specific vowels. The relationships of these cavities to vowel formants have been well described in several references, such as Peterson and Barney (1952) and Kent and Read (2002).

The structural adequacy and normal functioning of the velum are also important for the development of normal voice resonance. The elevation and tensing of the velum, as well as some pharyngeal wall movement, are vital for achieving velopharyngeal closure. A lack of adequate palatal movement, despite adequacy of velar length, can cause serious problems of excessive nasality. Although the velum probably serves as a sounding-board structure in resonance, it plays an obviously important role in separating the oral cavity from the nasal cavity (Abdel-Aziz, 2008). The movement and positioning of the velum changes the size and shape of three important resonating cavities: the pharynx, the oral cavity, and the nasal cavity. Therefore, any alteration of the velum (such as a soft-palate cleft or velar weakness) may have a profound influence on resonance. Velar movement is only one component contributing to velopharyngeal closure (Dworkin and colleagues, 2004). Closure patterns that separate the oral and nasal cavities from one another may include velar action coupled with posterior pharyngeal wall movement, or velar action coupled with active lateral and posterior pharyngeal wall movement. Watterson and McFarlane (1990) describe five classes of velopharyngeal closure and their various effects on speech and voice. Regardless of the type of closure pattern (velar-posterior-lateral pharyngeal wall), the site of closure is generally in the Passavant's area (designated as M in Figure 2.20). More will be said of nasal resonance and of the treatment of hypernasality and hyponasality in Chapters 7 and 10.

CHECK YOUR KNOWLEDGE

1. What structures are responsible for coupling and decoupling the oral and nasal cavities?
2. What would you hear with abnormal coupling of the oral and nasal cavities?

SUMMARY

In this chapter, we have reviewed the respiratory, phonatory, and resonance aspects of voice, and we also discussed the five aspects of voice (loudness, hygiene, pleasantness, flexibility, and representation). We found that the outgoing airstream is the primary driving force of voice. A description of the physiology of respiration reviewed the structures and mechanisms of normal breathing for speech. The efficient user of voice develops good expiratory control. The value and magnitude of respiratory volumes were discussed. A description of the physiology of phonation reviewed the structures and mechanisms of normal phonation, including frequency, intensity, and quality-shaping mechanisms. Supraglottal structures and functions specific to quality and resonance were also reviewed. The entire vocal tract contributes to the amplification and filtering of the fundamental frequency into the final unique voice of any speaker. The understanding of these processes provides the underpinning for effective voice therapy for patients with dysphonia.

CLINICAL CONCEPTS

The following clinical concepts correspond with many of the objectives at the beginning of this chapter:

1. Many voice-disordered patients will come to you because one or more of the five aspects of voice are abnormal. Some examples include: a speaker with Parkinson's disease (PD) who has a soft voice (see Chapter 5); a speaker who is a Marine drill sergeant and has a voice that gives out before lunch each day (see Chapter 3); a speaker with a 20-year history of smoking who has Reinke's edema, resulting in a rough/harsh voice quality (see Chapter 4); a speaker with a traumatic brain injury whose affect is (emotions are) perceived as flat because he or she cannot use the voice to express emotion effectively (see Chapter 5) ; and a transgender client who is mistaken for the wrong gender in person and over the telephone (see Chapter 8).
2. Some voice-disordered patients will come to you because they have inadequate respiratory function for speech/voice. Some examples include: a speaker with a high spinal cord injury who cannot time inhalation/exhalation with voice onset, resulting in unusual breath group phrasing (see Chapter 5); a speaker with lung disease, such as chronic obstructive pulmonary disease, who cannot produce a loud enough voice (see Chapter 4); a geriatric speaker with weak respiratory muscles who has to take more frequent breaths during talking (see Chapter 8); and a speaker with spastic dysarthria who cannot control the flow of air through the glottis, resulting in loudness bursts and harsh voice quality (see Chapter 5).

3. Some voice-disordered patients will come to you because they simply have forgotten how to "take a breath before and/or during speaking." These patients talk too long on a single breath, which results in strained voice quality and decreased loudness (see Chapter 3).

4. Some voice-disordered patients will come to you because they cannot control or change the pitch of their voice. Some examples include: speakers who have a paralyzed vocal folds (see Chapter 5); speakers who have nodules, a polyp, or other mass on their vocal folds (see Chapters 4 and 9); a patient who is using excessive laryngeal muscle tension (see Chapter 3); and a male speaker who has gone through puberty but still maintains his juvenile voice (see Chapter 8).

5. Some voice-disordered patients will come to you because they cannot control or change the loudness of their voice. Some examples include: speakers with Parkinson's disease (PD) (see Chapter 5); speakers with flaccid dysarthria (see Chapter 5); speakers who have a paralyzed vocal fold (see Chapter 5); speakers who have nodules, a polyp, or other mass on their vocal folds (see Chapters 3 and 9); speakers with a high spinal cord injury (see Chapter 5); speakers with hearing loss (see Chapter 8); and geriatric speakers (see Chapter 8).

6. Some voice-disordered patients will come to you because they have an imbalance of oral and nasal resonance. Some examples include: speakers with dysarthria (see Chapter 5), speakers with cleft palate (see Chapter 10), and speakers with muscle tension dysphonia (see Chapter 3).

GUIDED READING

Read the following articles:

Sapienza, C. M., Ruddy, B. H., & Baker, S. (2004). Laryngeal structure and function in the pediatric larynx. *Language, Speech, and Hearing Services in Schools, 35*, 299–307.

Zraick, R. I., Gregg, B. A., & Whitehouse, E. L. (2006). Speech and voice characteristics of geriatric speakers: A review of the literature and a call for research and training. *Journal of Medical Speech-Language Pathology, 14*, 133–142.

Describe four ways in which the information reported in the articles might influence your clinical practice.

PREPARING FOR THE PRAXIS™

Directions: Please read the case study and answer the five questions that follow. (Please see page 319 for the answer key.)

Harriet is a 75-year-old woman with a history of smoking one pack of cigarettes per day for more than 50 years. Her chief voice complaints are rough voice quality, low speaking pitch, weak voice, and running out of air when she speaks. She saw an otolaryngologist (ENT), who diagnosed her with emphysema and Reinke's edema.

1. The ENT's report of his stroboscopic laryngeal exam noted "Reinke's edema, bilaterally." Based on this information, which of the following laryngeal structures were affected?
   A. Superficial layer of the lamina propria
   B. Intermediate layer of the lamina propria
   C. Deep layer of the lamina propria
   D. The vocalis muscle
   E. The vocal fold epithelium

2. Which of the following laryngeal findings would also likely be noted by the ENT?
   A. Vocal fold paralysis
   B. Vocal fold nodules
   C. Vocal fold atrophy
   D. Subglottic stenosis
   E. All of these

3. Which of the patient's following pulmonary function test values are abnormal?
   A. Tidal volume of 300 ml
   B. Vital capacity of 2,500 ml
   C. Expiratory reserve volume of 600 ml
   D. Total lung capacity of 5,000 ml
   E. Both A and B

4. Which of the following mechanisms primarily accounts for the patient's low speaking pitch?
   A. Decreased mass of the vocal folds
   B. Increased mass of the vocal folds
   C. Incomplete glottic closure
   D. Decreased subglottic air pressure
   E. None of these

5. Which of the following mechanisms primarily accounts for the patient running out of air when she speaks?
   A. Poor respiratory support for speech
   B. Talking too fast
   C. Incomplete glottic closure
   D. Psychological stress
   E. Reinke's edema

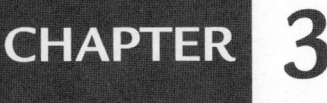

CHAPTER 3

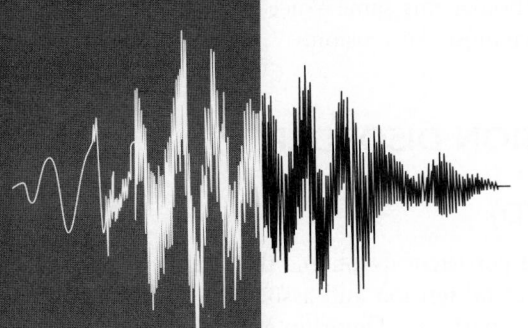

Functional Voice Disorders

■ ■ ■ ■ ─────────────── **LEARNING OBJECTIVES** ─────────────── ■ ■ ■ ■

After reading this chapter, one should be able to:

- Define the term *functional voice disorders*.
- Define the term *psychogenic voice disorders*.
- Describe the benign pathologies that may result from excessive laryngeal tension.

- Describe the voice symptoms of muscle tension dysphonia (MTD).
- Describe the treatment options for MTD.

This chapter describes functional voice disorders. Most voice problems seen by the speech-language pathologist (SLP) have no organic or neurological cause. Although the mechanisms of respiration, phonation, and resonance appear physically capable of normal voicing function, they lack the proper functional balance. This results in a voice disorder classified by many as a *functional voice disorder*. Sometimes an adult elects to habitually use a voice with hard glottal attack (such as the "drill sergeant" voice). Many times a child plays with his or her voice by making odd sounds (such as truck noises, animal noises, etc.). Or the actor may elect to speak with excessive loudness, or pitch that is excessively high or low, or speak with hoarseness or excessive nasality. When not playing a role, however, the actor's voice is immediately normal. In other instances, an adult "puts too much effort" into his or her voice as a result of physical or emotional stress, or as a compensation for laryngitis.

To promote the study of therapy outcome, we find two different causes under the "functional voice disorder" label: (1) excessive muscle tension or (2) psychogenic origin. In cases of excessive muscle tension, benign vocal fold masses such as nodules, polyps, and Reinke's edema may result. To evaluate the effectiveness of a particular Voice Facilitating Approach, a single technique could produce different outcomes, depending on which of these two causes exist. For example, the Voice Facilitating Approach of change of loudness (see Chapter 7) in the patient with psychogenic voice disorder might result in the rejection of the approach because the change might be in direct conflict with the patient's emotional needs. Conversely, for the patient with muscle tension dysphonia, this same Voice Facilitating Approach may be excellent for reducing excessive muscular tension.

EXCESSIVE MUSCLE TENSION DISORDERS

Muscle Tension Dysphonia (MTD)

Muscle tension dysphonia (MTD) is a persistent dysphonia that results from excessive laryngeal and related musculoskeletal tension and associated hyperfunctional true and/or false vocal fold vibratory patterns (Dworkin and colleagues, 2000). Morrison and colleagues (1983) first described MTD as the occurrence of vocal dysfunction in the absence of laryngeal structural abnormalities. In patients with MTD, the larynx is often noted to be elevated in the neck due to increased extrinsic laryngeal muscle tension (Van Houtte and colleagues, 2011), and pain is often reported in the neck, jaw, and shoulders (Stemple and colleagues, 2000).

Muscle tension dysphonia can be categorized as primary or secondary based on whether organic pathologic conditions contribute to trigger the muscle tension behavior (Rosen and Murray, 2000a). Primary MTD occurs *in the absence* of current organic pathology, without obvious psychogenic or neurologic etiology. Patients with primary MTD represent up to 40% of the dysphonias seen in voice clinics (Altman and colleagues, 2005; Dromey and colleagues, 2008). Secondary muscle tension dysphonia occurs *in the presence* of current or recent organic pathology, or psychogenic or neurologic etiology. Secondary MTD is believed to originate as a compensatory response to the primary etiology. Muscle tension dysphonia may be seen in both children and adults (Lee and Son, 2005).

Auditory-perceptual features of MTD can include strained or effortful voice quality, aberrant pitch, breathiness, and vocal fatigue (Roy and colleagues, 2008). Physiologic features considered core traits of MTD are generally based on subjective measures and include laryngeal elevation, decreased space between the hyoid bone and larynx, increased extrinsic laryngeal muscle tone, and the presence of one or more patterns of excessive laryngeal or supralaryngeal constriction (Lowell and colleagues, 2012). Constriction patterns include anterior-posterior compression, medial compression, and a sphincter-like combination of these two (Koufman and Blalock, 1991). Excessive vocal fold tension resulting in an underapproximation of the vocal folds may also be observed (Hillman and Verdolini, 1999). In some patients, medial compression may be a normal configuration, however, and must be interpreted in light of other laryngoscopic findings (Behrman and colleagues, 2003).

Numerous factors may contribute to the development of MTD, including deviant body posture and misuse of neck and shoulder muscles, high stress levels, excessive voice use, persistently loud voice use, and laryngopharyngeal reflux disease (Altman and colleagues, 2005; Van Houtte and colleagues, 2011). Patients frequently demonstrate significant emotional stress or conflict (Deary and Miller, 2011) suggesting an interaction between personality and psycho-emotional status and the voice (Seifert and Kollbrunner, 2005; Dietrich and colleagues, 2008; Mersbergen, 2011). Understandably, voice-related quality of life is diminished in persons with MTD (Kooijman and colleagues, 2005).

For the inexperienced and experienced voice clinician alike, MTD can sometimes be difficult to differentiate from other forms of dysphonia, such as adductor spasmodic dysphonia and vocal tremor. This is because some patients with adductor spasmodic dysphonia, vocal tremor, or MTD present with symptoms that overlap to such a degree that a correct diagnosis is not easy. Findings from a number of recent studies examining diagnostic elements such as patient interview, visualization of the larynx, acoustic and aerodynamic evaluation, and perceptual judgments may help the clinician arrive at the correct diagnosis in a timely manner (see Barkmeier and Case [2000], Dworkin and colleagues [2000], and Roy [2010] for reviews). For example, comparison of laryngeal behaviors during quiet breathing, counting from 1 to 10 in usual voice compared with falsetto and whispered speech, comparison of all-voiced versus all-voiceless utterances, variation of pitch and loudness during sustained phonation versus connected speech, and singing or crying may elicit differing patterns between adductor spasmodic dysphonia and MTD. The key difference between laryngeal behaviors in individuals with adductor spasmodic dysphonia versus MTD is the consistency of laryngeal postures across and within each of the examination tasks. Patients with MTD maintain hyperadduction of the involved laryngeal structures across all tasks, whereas those with adductor spasmodic dysphonia tend to demonstrate more intermittent hyperadduction (Leonard and Kendall, 1999). In patients with adductor spasmodic dysphonia, voice severity is perceived to be worse for connected speech than sustained vowels; this is not the case in patients with MTD, where no difference is usually heard (Roy and colleagues, 2005). In patients with MTD, voice severity is generally perceived to be the same on connected speech regardless of whether the sentences are all voiced or all voiceless; this is not the case for patients with adductor spasmodic dysphonia (Roy and colleagues, 2007). In Chapter 4, comparisons are made between MTD and problems such as essential tremor and adductor spasmodic dysphonia.

Treatment for MTD typically focuses on relaxation of the head and neck muscles. In Chapter 7, we present the Voice Facilitating Approaches of chant talk, chewing, digital manipulation, focus, laryngeal massage, relaxation, and yawn-sigh, all of which can be effective in minimizing or eliminating MTD. Studies investigating the effects of laryngeal massage have been appearing in the literature since the early 1990s, but the evidence base remains extremely small. A recent review by Mathieson (2011) indicates that there is evidence that laryngeal manual therapy, in various forms, can be a useful primary intervention in cases of MTD (see also Van Houtte and colleagues, 2011).

CHECK YOUR KNOWLEDGE

1. What is the difference between primary and secondary MTD?
2. What are the perceptual voice characteristics in MTD?

Ventricular Dysphonia

Ventricular dysphonia, sometimes known as *dysphonia plicae ventricularis*, refers to the pathological interference of the false vocal folds during phonation. Sataloff (2005) defines ventricular dysphonia as ". . . phonation using false vocal fold vibration rather than true vocal fold vibration, most commonly associated with severe muscular tension and occasionally may be an appropriate compensation for profound true vocal fold dysfunction."

Maryn and colleagues (2003) describe four types of ventricular phonation under two broad headings: compensatory and noncompensatory. The first type, compensatory, is a reaction to true vocal fold disease (paralysis, true vocal cord surgery etc.). In the three noncompensatory types, the vocal folds are capable of normal vibration. Of these, the first type, habitual, is caused by excessive vocal use; the second type, psycho-emotional, is provoked by physical and psychogenic tension and distress; and the third type has no known origin and is classified as idiopathic.

Although the first anatomic illustrations of the ventricular (also known as false) vocal folds (see Figure 2.11) were done in 1775 by Santorini, their role in phonation was not completely understood (Arnold and Pinto, 1960). In 1860, Czermak was the first to recognize that involvement of the false folds in phonation is a pathological phenomenon (Saunders, 1956). Although the ventricular folds physiologically move with the arytenoid cartilages and are brought together to assist in glottic airway closure, they do not approximate the median line (covering the true vocal folds) during normal voice production and they normally do not participate in vocal vibration (Nasri and colleagues, 1996). While ventricular dysphonia is most commonly produced by the vibration of the approximating ventricular folds, it is often heard when the true vocal folds vibrate in an abnormal fashion due to the false folds riding or loading them.

Sometimes the ventricular voice becomes the substitute voice of patients who have had resection due to severe disease of the true folds (such as cancer, severe recurrent respiratory papilloma, or large polyps). The ventricular voice is usually low-pitched because of the large mass of vibrating tissue of the ventricular bands (as compared to the smaller mass of vibrating tissue of the true folds) or from the combined mass of the true and false vocal folds. In addition, the voice has little pitch variability and is therefore monotonous. Finally, because the ventricular folds have difficulty in making a good, firm approximation for their entire length, the voice is usually quite hoarse and may also be breathy. This combination of low pitch, monopitch, and hoarseness makes most ventricular voices sound very unpleasant. If no persistent true cord pathology continues to force patients to use their ventricular voices, this disorder usually responds well to voice therapy. Sometimes, however, hypertrophy (enlargement) of the ventricular folds is present, which makes their normal full retraction somewhat difficult. Ventricular phonation is impossible to diagnose by the sound of the voice alone (Maryn and colleagues, 2003). Laryngoscopic examination during phonation shows the ventricular folds moving laterally toward one another, covering (partially or completely) from view the true folds that lie below (Nemetz and colleagues, 2005).

Some ventricular dysphonias display a special form of diplophonia (double voice), which results when the true and false vocal folds vibrate because the false vocal folds are sitting atop the true folds (loading the true folds with the ventricular folds). That is, the ventricular folds often do not vibrate as a sole source of sound, but load the true vocal folds and alter the sound they produce. Identification and confirmation of which vibrating structures the patient is using for phonation can be made by flexible or rigid laryngostroboscopy (McFarlane and colleagues, 1990). In ventricular phonation, the true vocal folds are slightly abducted, with the ventricular folds in relative approximation and very possibly resting on the true vocal folds. In normal phonation, the opposite relationship between the true and ventricular vocal folds occurs; that is, the true vocal folds are adducted and the ventricular folds are abducted. Once ventricular phonation is confirmed by laryngoscopy, any physical problem of the true vocal folds that might make normal phonation impossible should be eliminated. For example when one true fold is paralyzed or is too stiff (due to postsurgical scarring) to vibrate, the false fold is brought into the phonatory act. Figures 3.1 and 3.2 show ventricular fold vibration would be possible from a prolapsed right ventricle. Note how the Voice Facilitating Approach of inhalation phonation (see Chapter 7) decreases the impingement.

FIGURE 3.1 Ventricular Fold Phonation

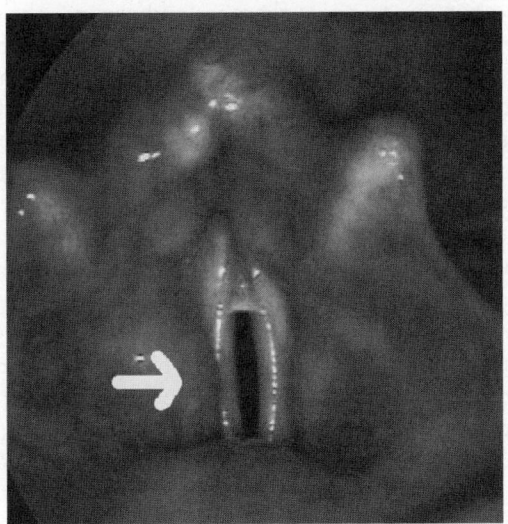

Prolapsed right ventricle in a 75- year-old trumpet player. Voice is low in pitch, hoarse, and breathy due to the ventricular (false) vocal fold impinging on the true vocal fold.

FIGURE 3.2 Intervention Using Inhalation Phonation

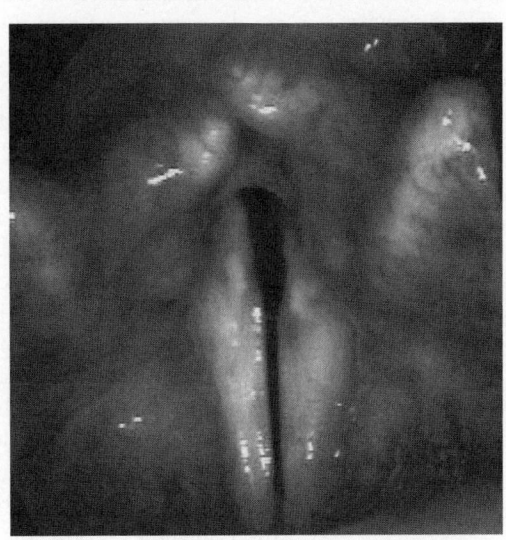

With the Voice Facilitating Approach of inhalation phonation, the ventricular (false) vocal fold impinges less on the true vocal fold.

We have known ventricular phonation to become habituated after a bout of flu when the true vocal folds were too swollen to vibrate. Ventricular fold phonation in such cases is a compensation used by the patient. It is usually not the best compensation for the problem and is generally responsive to voice therapy, such as inhalation phonation, pitch elevation, or breathy voice onset (see Chapter 7). In those rare cases where voice therapy alone is not effective in eliminating ventricular phonation, treatment options include pharmacological therapy (injection of anesthetics or botulinum toxin) (Kendall and Leonard, 1997; Theodoros and colleagues, 2007) and surgery (Friedrich and colleagues, 2010).

BENIGN PATHOLOGIES RESULTING FROM EXCESSIVE MUSCLE TENSION DISORDERS

Vocal Fold Nodules

Vocal fold nodules are the most common benign lesions of the vocal folds in both children and adults (Rosen and colleagues, 2012). They are caused by continuous abuse of the larynx and misuse of the voice. Nodules are generally bilateral, whitish protuberances on the glottal margin of each vocal fold, located at the anterior-middle third junction. However, McFarlane and Watterson (1990) demonstrate in their study of 44 cases of vocal nodules that there can be considerable variation in the size, number, and location of vocal nodules in both children and adults. Of the variations that can be observed and documented in vocal nodules, perhaps the

This **video** shows a comprehensive approach to vocal nodules in a young male patient. The clinician supplements intervention by using visual examples of different loudness levels; demonstrates good vocal production and then directs the patient to imitate; and finally, asks the patient to reflect on the level of vocal loudness that would be appropriate for various scenarios in his life. Again, appreciate how the patient becomes a full partner in his own voice intervention. Grand Rounds: How do vocal nodules develop?

most striking is that nodules can range from singular to two, three, and even four (quad nodules) in number. While these variations are interesting, two important facts remain. First, nodules are responsive to voice therapy, and second, the classic description of number and location (juncture of anterior and middle third) is generally accurate. Vocal nodules are typically characterized as bilateral, mid-membranous vocal fold lesions of the basement membrane zone and the superficial layer of the lamina propria (McFarlane and Von Berg, 1998; Rosen and Murry, 2000a; Martins and colleagues, 2010). In the early stages of development, the nodule is soft and pliable. With continuous phonotrauma, the nodule becomes more fibrotic and may be slightly larger, or it may become more focused, smaller, and harder.

As the bilateral nodules approximate one another on phonation, there is usually an open glottal chink anterior and posterior to the nodule contact point, which results in a glottal hourglass figure. This open glottal chink (produced by the nodules coming together in exact opposition to one another) results in a lack of complete vocal fold adduction. This faulty approximation leads to breathiness in the voice and air wastage, the perception of which increases as nodule size increases (Shah and colleagues, 2005, p. 93). Also, the increased mass of the vocal folds as a result of the nodules contributes to the perception of a lower habitual speaking pitch and hoarseness, which again is positively correlated with nodule size (Shah and colleagues, 2008, p. 723). This leads to a breathy, flat kind of voice that often seems to lack appropriate resonance. Patients complain that they need to clear their throat continually and often perceive that they have excessive mucus or something on the vocal folds (Bonilha and colleagues, 2012). Excessive throat clearing often becomes an identified vocal abuse, which may lead to further enlargement or further organization and consolidation of the nodules (Leydon and colleagues, 2009). Typical patients with vocal nodules complain that their voices seem to deteriorate with continuous voicing; they may start the day with fairly good voices that become increasingly dysphonic with continuous vocal usage. With prolonged speaking and singing, perhaps coupled with vocal abuse and misuse, phonation rapidly deteriorates.

Vocal nodules in children before puberty are more common in boys. In their review of 254 cases of children with vocal nodules, Shah and colleagues (2005) reported that nodules were most commonly observed in males between the ages of 3 and 10 years. Laryngopharyngeal reflux disease was present in one-fourth of the cases reviewed by Shah and colleagues, and in three-fourths of the cases there was evidence of vocal hyperfunction (p. 903). As boys get older, there is less evidence of nodules, with adolescent and adult females showing the highest prevalence of nodules (Herrington-Hall and colleagues, 1988; Nagata and colleagues, 1983). However, in discussing the fact that vocal fold lesions are more common in women than men, Koufman and Belafsky (2001) suggest that differences in incidence may be multifactorial and related to hormonal, anatomic, inflammatory, and aerodynamic factors. Shah and colleagues (2007) and Nuss and colleagues (2012) have developed reliable scales for grading the size of vocal nodules in children, which should facilitate objective analysis of outcomes when studying and following pediatric patients with vocal nodules.

Small nodules and recently acquired ones can be successfully treated with voice therapy (Ruotsalainen and colleagues, 2007; Leonard, 2009), which is usually the first choice of treatment by SLPs (Signorelli and colleagues, 2011). Holmberg and colleagues (2001), reporting on voice therapy success with 11 adult females with vocal nodules, found a significant decrease in severity of dysphonia following behavioral voice therapy. In addition, videolaryngostroboscopy at the end of therapy showed that the nodules had decreased in size and that edema was reduced for nearly all clients. McFarlane and Watterson (1990) reported success in 44 cases presenting both large and small nodules in children and adults, and in both singers and nonsingers. They also document with pictures the before-and-after therapy conditions of the larynx of a child and an adult singer. The nodules were completely resolved via voice therapy. Boone (1982) developed a four-point program for adults with vocal nodules that focuses on identifying abuse-misuse; reducing the occurrence of such abuse-misuse; searching with the patient for various Voice Facilitating Approaches that seem to produce an easy, optimal vocal production (see Chapter 7); and using the Voice Facilitating Approach that works best as a practice method. Although we strongly recommend voice therapy as the primary treatment for nodules, we also acknowledge that larger nodules and long-established ones may be treated by surgery, followed by a brief period of complete voice rest and then voice therapy (Pedersen and McGlashan, 2001). However, a trial period of voice therapy is an appropriate conservative course of treatment prior to surgery for nodules in nearly all cases (Pedersen and colleagues, 2004). Because voice therapy must follow if surgery is the treatment, then one might ask, "Why not begin with a period of voice therapy?" It is not unusual for new nodules to reappear after surgical removal of nodules or injection of steroids into the nodules (Lee and colleagues, 2011). Unless the underlying hyperfunctional vocal behavior is identified and reduced, vocal nodules have a stubborn way of reappearing (Ferrand, 2012).

It is generally accepted that nodules result from continuous and prolonged MTD and are therefore often observed in individuals who exhibit hyperfunctional vocal behaviors. Some could be referred to as vocal overachievers. Green (1989) found that children with vocal nodules demonstrated more aggressive behaviors, acting out, and disturbed relationships with peers compared to children with normal voices. This finding was not supported, though, in a study by Roy and colleagues (2007), who reported no evidence of amplified aggressiveness or immature behavior in children with vocal nodules compared to children with normal voices. Roy and colleagues did report, however, that children with nodules use their voice for socializing more so than those children with normal voices.

Although symptomatic voice therapy has been effective in reducing or eliminating vocal nodules, young patients with vocal nodules often require strong psychological support by the voice clinician (Andrews and Summers, 2002). Merati and colleagues (2008) studied voice-related quality of life of children with voice disorders and reported that it is significantly impaired in those with vocal nodules, particularly in the social-emotional and physical-functional domains. The effect of vocal nodules on children may depend on the age of the child. Connor and colleagues (2008) assessed the attitudes of children with dysphonia across four age groups (toddler: ages 2 to 4; preschool: ages 5 to 7; school age: ages 8 to 12; and adolescent: ages 13 to 18) and found that as the children got older, social and emotional handicap became greater as a result of having vocal nodules and other forms of dysphonia. Providing therapy to children with vocal nodules is important because children do not simply "outgrow" the problem. De Bodt and colleagues (2007) questioned 91 adolescents who were diagnosed with nodules in childhood and found that 21% had voice complaints persisting into postpubescence, with a statistically significant difference between boys and girls. Nodules were still present in 47% of the girls and 7% of the boys, with significant higher long-term risks for dysphonic girls with allergy.

Vocal Fold Polyps

A vocal fold polyp is a focal abnormality of the superficial lamina propria, usually at the same site where vocal fold nodules occur. This lesion, however, is thought to be slightly deeper within the superficial lamina propria. Vocal fold polyps are usually unilateral, but a reactive lesion is often found on the vocal fold immediately across from the polyp. Unlike vocal nodules, which result from continuous or chronic vocal fold irritation, polyps are often precipitated by a single vocal event. For example, a patient may have indulged in excessive vocalization, such as screaming for much of an evening, which produced some hemorrhaging on the membrane at the point of maximum glottal contact. Such hemorrhagic irritation eventually results in formation of either a translucent, fibrotic, hyaline, hemorrhagic, or mixed polyp that adds mass to the vocal fold. Once a small polyp begins, any continued phonotrauma will irritate the area, contributing to its continued growth (Petrovic and colleagues, 2009; Nakagawa and colleagues, 2012).

Kleinsasser (1982) reviewed 900 cases of polyps and developed an excellent description of vocal fold polyps, their formation, and their treatment. Three-fourths of patients were male and one-fourth female, with the mean age of both being around 40 years. In 90% of the cases, polyps were unilateral; in 5%, they were bilateral; and in 5%, they were both multiple and unilateral. Over 80% of patients smoked; other contributing factors included inhaled allergens and irritants. As described by Rubin and Yanigisawa (2003, p. 74), the gross appearance of vocal fold polyps varies: they may be reddish or white, large or small, and sessile (broad-based) or pedunculated (narrow-necked on a stem). Most are small and sessile, however. As polyps become more advanced, they become increasingly more pedunculated. Polyps are associated with other vocal fold pathologies in 15% of cases (Bouchayer and Cornut, 1991).

Kleinsasser (1982) further described vocal fold polyps as being responsive to surgery. Surgery can sometimes be performed in the office as opposed to the hospital (Woo, 2006). The goal of vocal fold surgery is to preserve as much superficial lamina propria as possible and to disrupt the glottal margin as little as possible. Thus, microflap surgery designed to raise a flap of mucosa, remove a benign lesion via suction, and then lay the flap back down on the vocal fold is common (Courey and colleagues, 1997; Hirano and colleagues, 2008). Another technique, epithelial cordotomy, involves microdissection between the polyp and the residual normal superior lamina propria while disturbing as little of the epithelium as possible (Benninger, 2000; Hochman and Zeitels, 2000). Cohen and Garrett (2007) examined the utility of voice therapy alone for patients with vocal fold polyps and cysts. In their study of 57 patients, almost half experienced an improved voice. Factors such as length of dysphonia, smoking status, allergy, and gastroesophageal reflux treatment were not associated with treatment outcome. They also found that the type of polyp was associated with voice improvement. Specifically, patients with translucent polyps were more likely to experience an improved voice than were those with fibrotic, hyaline, or hemorrhagic polyps. Klein and colleagues (2009) followed 13 patients with polyps of varying sizes who underwent voice therapy only while waiting for an optimal time for surgical polyp removal. They reported that slightly more than half the patients experienced spontaneous resolution of their polyps, in all cases within 4 to 7 months. Patients who were more likely to experience resolution of the polyp were women with small polyps. Nakagawa and colleagues (2012) compared the outcomes of voice therapy only versus surgery for polyp removal. Of the 13, 2 patients treated with voice therapy only, nearly half experienced complete polyp disappearance at a 5-month follow-up visit, and nearly one-fourth showed polyp shrinkage at a 4-month follow-up visit; all were satisfied with the outcome in terms of their voice. Patients who were more likely to experience resolution of the polyp were women with small polyps and a shorter duration of voice symptoms (3 weeks versus 14 weeks for those who did not experience polyp resolution or shrinkage). Taken together, the findings reported by Klein and colleagues and Nakagawa and colleagues suggest that conservative treatment (that is, voice therapy only) is warranted as a first course of treatment for those patients who are willing to "wait it out" in hopes of avoiding surgery. This opinion is additionally supported by research by Zeitels and colleagues (2002) and Lavorato and McFarlane (1983), who suggest that successful management of vocal fold lesions depends on prudent patient selection and counseling, ultraprecise surgical technique, and vigorous vocal rehabilitation using various Voice Facilitating Approaches (see Chapter 7).

CHECK YOUR KNOWLEDGE

1. What characteristics differentiate a polyp from a nodule?
2. Should one undergo immediate surgery to remove polyps?

Reinke's Edema

Chronic diffuse swelling of the superficial lamina propria of the vocal fold is known as Reinke's edema (Thibeault, 2005). This edema is also referred to as polypoid degeneration of the vocal fold (Martins and colleagues, 2009). Within the lamina propria (see Figure 2.16), the collagen architecture is disrupted, and a thick, gelatinous, fluid-like material develops in Reinke's space (Sakae and colleagues, 2008). There may also be an altered number and size of microvessels within the subepithelial space (Sugumaran and colleagues, 2011). Reinke's edema is usually bilateral but can be more pronounced on one side. It is associated strongly with smoking, frequently with chronic vocal hyperfunction, and occasionally with laryngopharyngeal reflux (Kamargiannis and colleagues, 2011; Marcotullio and colleagues, 2002). Branski and colleagues (2006) suggest that Reinke's edema may result from prolonged exposure to inflammatory stimuli, accompanied by abnormal healing.

Reinke's edema and related forms of vocal fold thickening are conditions often affecting the anterior two-thirds of the glottal margin (the vibrating portion of the vocal folds) or the membrane covering the muscular portion of the vocal fold. This is in contrast to vocal nodules and polyps, which usually affect a localized area of the vocal fold. The more extensive the condition, the more likely it is that the voice will be affected.

Dysphonia resulting from Reinke's edema and related conditions is often responsive to voice therapy. Success from voice therapy is highly dependent on eliminating the cause of the problem, such as smoking. A behavioral program that promotes easy and proper use of the vocal mechanism (vocal reeducation), along with reducing the source of the irritation (such as eliminating an allergy, eliminating smoking, reducing laryngopharyngeal reflux, or curbing vocal abuse) is probably the best management of the problem. Many of the voice therapy facilitating approaches presented in Chapter 7 have been effective in reducing Reinke's edema and related conditions. Surgical treatment of vocal fold thickening, without removing the cause of the problem, will not usually be a permanent solution to the dysphonia. Our strong preference is to have a serious course of voice therapy first. This will generally eliminate the need for phonosurgery (surgery to improve the voice).

If Reinke's edema is extensive and a first course of voice therapy (as described above) is not effective, then medical-surgical intervention may be warranted (supplemented still by voice therapy). In a study by Dursun and colleagues (2007), 15 patients with Reinke's edema who underwent microlaryngoscopic surgery were reported to experience significant positive changes in voice quality and laryngeal status. These researchers further reported no recurrence of Reinke's edema one year following surgery, speculating that the removal of redundant mucosa of the vocal fold reduced the risk of the recurrence of Reinke's edema and resulted in better voice quality (p. 1027). Voice rest after surgery is often prescribed to promote vocal fold healing. Voice therapy is also prescribed to promote positive vocal use behavior.

CHECK YOUR KNOWLEDGE

1. Reinke's edema is most likely to be seen where on the vocal fold?
2. What would you expect to hear in the voice of the person with Reinke's edema?

Laryngitis

In a retrospective U.S. database review of the charts of over a half-million patients with a diagnosis of dysphonia (Cohen and colleagues, 2012), it was discovered that the most frequent diagnosis overall was acute laryngitis, comprising nearly half of the cases. Chronic laryngitis occurred in about 10% of the cases. Primary care physicians were reportedly more likely to diagnose acute laryngitis than were otolaryngologists, the latter being more likely to diagnose chronic laryngitis. Common comorbid conditions included upper airway inflammatory conditions such as acute pharyngitis, acute bronchitis, pneumonia, and upper respiratory illness. There were no age or gender differences in regard to the diagnosis of laryngitis.

In traumatic laryngitis, patients experience swelling of the vocal folds as a result of excessive and strained vocalization. Phonotrauma, such as yelling, screaming, abrupt and strained voice usage, chronic coughing, habitual throat clearing, and forceful singing are common causes of traumatic laryngitis. Typical traumatic laryngitis is heard in the voices of excited spectators after a sporting event or rock music concert. In the excitement of the event, with their own voices masked by the noise of the crowd, fans scream at pitch levels and intensities they normally do not use. Under these speaking conditions, the surface tissues of the true (and possibly the false) vocal folds experience intense friction, thermal agitation, and molecular breakdown (Dworkin, 2008). Irritation (erythema) accompanies the fold edema.

The acute stage of laryngitis is at its peak during the actual yelling or traumatic vocal behavior, with the vocal folds much increased in size and mass. In general, the greater the irregularity, size, and consistency of the gap between the vocal fold free edges during the closed phases of vibration, the more severe the dysphonia. Variably hoarse, breathy, harsh, strained, and low-pitched voice abnormalities result from the underlying glottal incompetence. In the case of laryngitis secondary to yelling or a similar form of vocal abuse, eliminating the abuse usually permits the vocal mechanism to return to its natural state. The temporary laryngitis experienced toward the end of a sporting event or concert is usually relieved by a return to normal vocal activity, and most of the edema and irritation vanish after a good night's sleep or two.

Chronic laryngitis may produce serious vocal problems if the speaker attempts to speak above the laryngitis. The temporary edema of the vocal folds alters the quality and loudness of the phonation, forcing the speaker to increase vocal efforts. This increase in effort only increases the irritation of the folds, thereby compounding the problem. If such hyperfunctional behavior continues over time, what was once a temporary edema may become a more permanent polypoid thickening, which sometimes develops into vocal fold polyps, vocal fold nodules, hyperkeratosis, or a vocal fold scar. For this reason, functional laryngitis should be promptly treated by eliminating the causative abuse and, if possible, by enforcing a short period (less than one week) of complete voice rest. Voice rest in itself is not a cure for most voice disorders. This is not true, however, for acute laryngitis. Complete or absolute voice rest, which means no phonation or whispering for several days, is usually enough for irritated vocal fold margins to lose their swelling and return to their normal shape. It is important that voice rest designed to promote healing of irritated vocal fold surfaces *not* include whispering; whispering (as most people do it) still causes too much vocal fold vibration, and irritation from the rubbing together of the approximating surfaces of each vocal fold is still possible. Studies have shown that, during forced whisper, there are increases in expiratory muscle activity and airflow, and the ventricular folds often may be brought into function (Pearl and McCall, 1986). Again, one must identify and curb the events that cause acute laryngitis.

CHECK YOUR KNOWLEDGE

1. What kinds of phonotrauma may result in acute and/or traumatic laryngitis?
2. What should be the first course of treatment for acute laryngitis?

VOICE CHARACTERISTICS WITH EXCESSIVE MUSCLE TENSION DISORDERS

Diplophonia

The term *diplophonia* means "double voice." A diplophonic voice is produced with two distinct frequencies occurring simultaneously. Diplophonia is the consequence of irregular vocal fold vibration. It may be produced by some normal speakers voluntarily, but is more likely to be heard in patients with mass lesions, vocal fold paralysis, vocal fold scarring, laryngitis and other inflammatory conditions, muscle tension dysphonia, puberphonia, or paradoxical vocal fold movement (Ishi and colleagues, 2006; Vertigan and colleagues, 2007). As mentioned in our previous look at ventricular phonation, the ventricular voice is often a false fold/true vocal fold double-pitch vibration. The two pitch levels heard simultaneously are labeled *diplophonia*. Auditory-perceptual and acoustic analyses usually form the basis for a diagnosis of diplophonia. Laryngostroboscopy is of limited diagnostic value because the tracking of the frequency of vocal fold vibration depends on a single frequency (Kendall and colleagues, 2005).

 The clinician in this **video** segment encourages the patient to replace functional dysphonia behaviors with the redirection approaches of focus and nasal/glide stimulation. Note how the clinician extends (generalizes) these successful productions into functional phrases so the patient can appreciate that she has the techniques to re-find her voice. Grand Rounds: Which properties of nasals and glides are conducive to reducing muscle tension dysphonia?

The treatment of diplophonia is geared toward eliminating the source of the second voice. Sometimes, surgical removal of a mass lesion or surgical repositioning and tensing of a paralyzed vocal fold eliminates diplophonia (Tsukahara and colleagues, 2005). More often, though, diplophonia is corrected by voice therapy (which we discuss in Chapter 7). This is accomplished by reducing any laryngeal hypertension that may be contributing to production of a second sound source. Videoendoscopy is helpful in identifying the source of the undesired vibration and in guiding voice therapy in reestablishment of normal voice production.

Phonation Breaks

A phonation break is a temporary loss of voice that may occur for only part of a word, a whole word, a phrase, or a sentence. The individual is phonating with no apparent difficulty when suddenly a complete cessation of voice occurs. Such a fleeting voice loss is usually situational, and it usually happens after prolonged hyperfunction. Typical patients with this problem work too hard to talk, often speaking with great effort, and suddenly experience a complete voice break. Such patients usually struggle to find their voice by coughing, clearing their throat, or taking a drink of water. In most cases, phonation is restored and remains adequate until the next phonation break, which may occur in only a few moments or not for days. Other than continued vocal hyperfunction, no physical condition seems to cause these phonatory interruptions. They may result from a variety of physiological sources: reduced subglottal air pressure near the end of a phrase, loading of the true vocal fold or by the ventricular fold, or mucus on the true vocal fold. Most of the time, breaks result from excessive laryngeal muscle tension and inappropriate adjustments of the otherwise normal mechanism. Phonation breaks can be experienced by children as well as adults (Lee and Son, 2005).

Voice patients who experience phonation breaks rarely show them during voice evaluation sessions. In their histories, however, such patients report the occurrence of phonation breaks, often with much embarrassment when they occur. Occasionally patients have been told by their employers that they must learn to use their voices correctly (without voice breaks) or they will lose their jobs. Fortunately, the treatment of phonation breaks secondary to MTD is relatively simple: taking the work out of phonation and eliminating inappropriate vocal behaviors such as excessive coughing and violent throat clearing. The Voice Facilitating Approaches of chant talk, nasal/glide stimulation, and pitch inflections (see Chapter 7), designed to reduce vocal hyperfunction, are most effective in eliminating the phonation breaks. Phonation breaks due to abductor spasms, such as those seen in persons with spasmodic dysphonia, are discussed in Chapter 5.

Pitch Breaks

There are two kinds of pitch breaks. One is a developmental phenomenon seen primarily in boys experiencing marked pubertal growth of the larynx, and the other is caused by prolonged vocal hyperfunction, particularly while speaking at an inappropriate (usually too low) pitch level. The rapid changes in the size of the vocal folds and other laryngeal structures produce varying vocal effects during the pubertal years. Boys experience a lowering of their fundamental frequency of about one octave; girls, a lowering of only about two or three semitones (Ferrand, 2012). This change does not happen in a day or two. For several years, as this laryngeal growth is taking place, boys experience temporary hoarseness and occasional pitch breaks. Wise parents or seasoned voice clinicians witness these vocal changes with little comment or concern. These mass-size increases of puberty tend to thwart any serious attempts at singing or other vocal arts. Luchsinger and Arnold (1965) point out that much of the European literature on singing makes a valid plea that the formal study of singing be deferred until well after puberty. Until a male child experiences some stability of laryngeal growth, the demands of singing might be inappropriate for his rapidly changing mechanism. Laryngeal strain is a real concern when serious singing is attempted during this period. One of the authors was told by Beverly Sills, the most famous of recent sopranos, that she stopped singing altogether for three years during puberty. Interestingly, Beverly Sills, unlike any other opera singer we know, had only a single voice teacher for her entire child and adult career.

The age and rate of pubertal development varies markedly. From the pediatric literature we find that the main thrust of puberty for any one child seems to take place in a total time period of about four years, six months (Hacki and Heitmuller, 1999). The most rapid and dramatic changes occur toward the last six months of puberty, when pitch breaks, if they occur, may be observed in some boys (Pribusiene and colleagues, 2011). Most pubertal changes begin at age 12 in boys, a little earlier in girls, and are completed by age 16 (Meurer and colleagues, 2009).

Younger children and adults might experience a different kind of pitch break, one in which the voice breaks an octave (sometimes two octaves) up or an octave down when speaking at an inappropriate pitch level (Lee and Son, 2005). When individuals speak at an inappropriately low frequency, their voice tends to break one octave higher; if they speak too high in the frequency range, their voice may break one octave down.

Pitch breaks can also result from overall vocal fatigue. Heavy users of voice, such as actors after long rehearsals or during long-running performances, may begin to experience pitch breaks after hours of prolonged voicing. Such continued vocal hyperfunction, speaking with too much effort, sometimes results in either pitch or phonation breaks. Such pitch breaks are usually warnings that the vocal mechanisms are being overworked and being held at an inappropriate pitch level for a prolonged period of time. We refer to such pitch or phonation breaks as *vocal limping*, just as one limps when walking with an injured foot. With a little temporary voice rest (two or three days) and initiation of Voice Facilitating Approaches targeting easy phonation, such as glottal fry or yawn-sigh (see Chapter 7), fatigue-induced pitch and phonation breaks usually disappear.

 The yawn-sigh approach is one of the most powerful techniques for reducing muscle tension dysphonia and increasing ease of phonation. In the **video,** we see multiple approaches to the technique, but commonalities of yawn-sigh are the lowering of the larynx and dilation of the pharynx. Grand Rounds: How does dilation of the pharynx increase the potential for greater vocal resonance?

CHECK YOUR KNOWLEDGE

1. With which laryngeal conditions is one likely to hear diplophonia?
2. What vocal use behaviors likely result in pitch and phonation breaks?

PSYCHOGENIC VOICE DISORDERS

The emotional and psychological state of the individual can affect voice production. Each person's voice is highly individual and unique in terms of pitch, loudness, and quality. As introduced in Chapter 1, voice can reflect an individual's emotions, mood, and self-image, while listeners draw inferences about a person from the way he or she sounds. Laryngeal musculature works in balance to express emotion in the voice, providing a psychological impact that conveys meaning to the listener. Psychological upset can interfere with normal voice production. Voice disorders can result from emotional stresses, while voice disorder itself can produce its own emotional stresses with consequent psychological impact (Butcher, 1995). Individuals can feel their personality change when they are unable to access their voice, experiencing a "loss of self," which returns only when their own voice is restored (House and Andrews, 1987).

In the classic definition of psychogenic voice disorders, the voice problem is typically resistant to change from various symptomatic voice therapy approaches. The patient's psychological trauma or conflicts may be strong enough to cause and maintain the vocal symptoms (Seifert and Kollbrunner, 2006). Psychological counseling or therapy may have to play a primary role in the total voice rehabilitation process. However, psychological factors sometimes are reactive to the emergence of a voice problem and are not the cause of the disorder; for these cases, voice therapy can play a primary and successful role.

To simplify for the reader the role of the SLP in working with children or adults with psychogenic voice disorders, we have identified four different types of clinical voice problems: puberphonia, functional aphonia, functional dysphonia, and somatization dysphonia. The SLP trained in counseling or clinical psychology may well combine needed psychological support with voice therapy for most of these psychogenic patients. Or appropriate psychological or psychiatric referral may be indicated. The first three disorders listed may well have psychogenic causation but still have successful voice therapy outcomes. Somatization dysphonia is primarily a psychiatric conversion problem and requires psychiatric management.

Puberphonia

Puberphonia is inappropriate use of high-pitched voice beyond pubertal age in males. It is usually seen in the immediate postpubescent period when the male laryngeal mechanism has undergone significant changes in size and function caused by hormonal changes. Other names for puberphonia are falsetto, mutational falsetto, juvenile voice, and incomplete voice mutation. From a singing point of view, some men and women can extend the singing voice well beyond the chest register, producing the falsetto or loft register. Some classical singing includes the counter-tenor voice where the singing voice extends well above middle-C (260 Hz). The high lyric soprano sings several octaves higher. Our concern with the falsetto voice is not in singing but in the speaking voice. Falsetto may also occur in females; Verdolini and colleagues (2006) cite a form of puberphonia referred to as juvenile resonance disorder in postpubescent females.

Occasionally, young men with falsetto voices have found the transition from boy to manhood to be difficult. Increased adultlike feelings and responsibilities may be complicated by the rapid physical changes they have experienced. As an overall coping mechanism, these young men may continue to use their prepubescent voices. For this occasional puberphonic patient, some psychological counseling or therapy is a required part of overall voice management. Most young men with mutational falsetto (we use the interchange of the words *falsetto, puberphonia,* and *mutational falsetto* deliberately as synonyms) are very accepting of voice therapy that helps them find and establish an appropriate lower voice pitch. The vast majority of young men with puberphonia achieve normal pitch levels and vocal quality after only brief exposure to voice therapy (Desai and Mishra, 2012).

Voice therapy for puberphonia (Dagli and colleagues, 2008) first requires a thorough review of the medical chart and perhaps medical evaluation confirming that the client has reached postpuberty status. When asked to cough, the cough usually sounds like that of an adult; both male and female patients will present a much lower pitch level than that of children when asked to cough. The SLP generally begins therapy for the puberphonic patient by demonstrating a cough and then extending phonation beyond the cough to a hum for a few seconds. Following the SLP cough demonstration, the patient is asked to do the same thing: cough and then extend the phonation after the cough on the same outgoing breath. In most cases, it is best to record the patient's cough response and then provide the patient with an auditory feedback model. The SLP then explains that the vocal folds are able to produce the lower phonation, and a brief, all-voiced word list can then be presented, with each word said on the extended phonation following the cough.

If the cough is not successful in uncovering the patient's natural pitch, light digital pressure against the thyroid cartilage often "uncovers" the lower pitch. The patient is asked to say and prolong an "ah" for more than five or six seconds. During this extended phonation, the SLP applies light finger pressure on the patient's anterior thyroid cartilage, usually producing an immediate lowering of voice pitch. After several finger pressure productions, the patient is then asked to see if he or she can match the lower voice pitch. The therapy session should be recorded for immediate playback and discussion. The Voice Facilitating Approaches of masking and glottal fry (see Chapter 7) are useful in eliminating the falsetto speaking voice.

Counseling should supplement the positive commentary about the appropriateness of using the newly found lower pitch (Aronson, 1990). The majority of patients with puberphonia have an excellent therapy outcome in one or two clinical sessions and seemingly rejoice in finding a voice that sounds like that of their peers. Only a few anecdotal reports exist about an occasional patient with puberphonia who requires counseling or psychotherapy before releasing the need for continuing with the falsetto voice. Following the successful elimination of the high-pitched voice, the SLP should schedule all patients with puberphonia for a three- or four-week follow-up to determine how they are doing, both from a voice and emotional perspective. In the exceedingly rare instances where voice and other therapies are not successful, surgery to shorten and relax the true vocal fold (Isshiki and colleagues, 1983) or injection of Botox into the cricothyroid muscle may be considered; both are successful (Remacle and colleagues, 2010; Woodson and Murry, 1994).

Functional Aphonia

The unique aspect of functional aphonia is that the patient speaks in a whisper but continues speaking with the same rhythm and prosody of normal speech. Only voice is lacking. To rule out some form of organic involvement of the vocal folds, such as vocal fold paralysis (described in Chapter 5), these patients need a laryngoendoscopic examination to visualize vocal fold movement. When the aphonic patient says "ah," the normal vocal folds remain too far apart to permit phonation and often develop the open position used for a whisper production (Case, 2002). The visual examination usually confirms normal function for both the cough and the throat clearing. When swallowing, the aphonic patient exhibits both normal laryngeal elevation and vocal fold closure, both required to prevent aspiration into the airway below the larynx. When these patients are asked to speak, the larynx often appears to elevate excessively near the hyoid bone and is difficult to move manually in any direction.

Aronson, in his classic text, *Clinical Voice Disorders* (Aronson, 1990), describes a persistent functional aphonia as a possible "conversion aphonia." Aronson goes on to write that a conversion disorder is the "somatization" of an emotional disorder and can be "created by anxiety, stress, depression, or interpersonal conflict" (Aronson, 1990, p. 142). In somatization, it is believed that an unresolved psychological conflict results in a dysfunction of some bodily system. We will consider the somatization of laryngeal function in greater detail later in this chapter. It appears clinically, however, that the majority of patients with aphonia do not seem to have a conversion causation; they respond favorably to symptomatic voice therapy in one or very few therapy sessions. While normal phonation is usually restored with minimal voice therapy with the SLP, emotional conflicts may require psychological or psychiatric therapy over a longer period of time (Gerritsma, 1991).

The onset of functional aphonia varies. Many aphonic patients say that their "loss of voice" came on gradually or occurs only sporadically. Under tight emotional situations, they might "lose" their voices in that particular situation but recover normal voice after subsequent stress reduction. Sometimes aphonia occurs after patients have experienced some kind of laryngeal pathology or severe systemic disease; perhaps laryngeal edema during an acute infection may render voice impossible. Days or weeks later, after the initial infection that caused the voice loss is gone, the aphonia continues. Two aphonic patients who developed aphonia originally from an acute infectious disease seemed subsequently to incorporate the lack of voice into their lives (Boone, 1966b). Months after the onset of their aphonia, both patients participated in voice therapy and had complete voice recoveries. For some patients, communication without voicing seems to help them meet their emotional needs temporarily.

A young boy age 7 years, found to have bilateral vocal nodules by his ENT physician, was told by this doctor to stop using his voice for a few weeks. The parents enforced voice rest for four weeks, and the boy was never heard to use his voice during that time. When the parents brought him back for another checkup, the nodules were gone but his voice was totally absent. Despite the physician's urgings and parental requests, the aphonia persisted for an additional month. Presented at a voice team conference, the child was presented as the "boy who had forgotten how to talk." He was subsequently scheduled for voice therapy and happily "found" his voice during the first therapy session. Over a four-year follow-up period, he continued to have a normal prepubescent voice in all situations.

Patients with functional aphonia communicate well by gesture and whisper or by a high-pitched, shrill-sounding weak voice. Typical aphonic patients whisper with clarity and sharpness. Aphonic patients rarely avoid communication situations; conversely, they communicate effectively by using facial expressions, hands, and highly intelligible whispered speech. What they lack in communication is voice. Embarrassed and frustrated by lack of voice, aphonic patients generally self-refer to a physician or SLP. Despite Greene's (1980) warning that many patients with functional aphonia may require psychological counseling, most aphonic patients, in our experience, completely recover their normal voice, with voice therapy alone (often in the first session of therapy). Aphonic patients as a group, in fact, have an excellent prognosis (Kollbrunner and colleagues, 2010). It is almost as if, for whatever reason, the patient has lost the set for phonation. The voice clinician's task is to help the patient find his or her voice primarily by helping the patient use nonspeech phonations, such as coughing and throat clearing, humming, or inhalation phonation or sometimes using masking noise (Chapter 7).

In Chapters 7 and 8, we consider in more detail some of the Voice Facilitating Approaches that are commonly used by the SLP in reestablishing voice in the functional aphonic patient. Therapy approaches include extending the cough and throat clearing, redirecting phonation achieved while singing or humming on a kazoo, and reading aloud with auditory masking. The patient's various responses to selected voicing tasks should be audio-recorded, affording immediate playback of any phonations the patient is able to produce.

The voice therapy provided for a nine-year-old girl who had lost her voice following severe influenza provides a good example of successful therapy for functional aphonia. For six weeks following a severe flulike infection, she communicated entirely by whisper with good facial animation and normal interactive communication with her listeners. In the therapy session, we had her read aloud. Using the old Lombard effect (Newby, 1972), which is used to detect a hearing loss of the malingering type, the patient is asked to read aloud in a whisper and continue reading aloud as about 75 dB of speech-range masking is introduced. The whispered reading changes immediately to voicing when the patient hears the masking noise. When masking was introduced as this girl read aloud in her whisper, she started reading in a light voice. This voice was recorded and played back as the SLP commented, "Now your vocal folds seem to be coming together well." The girl was overjoyed with the discovery of her lost voice. Once voice is established, the SLP moves slowly to increase loudness as a drill activity and then works "gently" to produce voice interactively. After voice is reestablished, psychological support should be offered to the aphonic patient, with strong SLP assurance that the voice is "back for good." It usually is.

Functional Dysphonia

Some of the most abnormal or strangest voices we may hear have no organic or structural causes. The voice patient may be using one's normal respiration system in an incorrect balance between initiating the airstream with the beginning of phonation, such as beginning voice after much expiratory air has been expelled. The patient may take in too small a breath or too large a breath for producing a normal voice. Or the patient with functional dysphonia may bring the vocal folds together in a lax manner, producing breathiness, or in a tight manner, producing symptoms of harshness or tightness. Or patients may be speaking at inappropriate pitch levels, voices too low or too high, for their age and sex. Excesses of mouth opening, head position, or jaw positioning may alter the quality of the voice. Or the sound of the voice can be easily altered by tongue positioning within the mouth, with the tongue positioned too far back or too far forward. Excessive nasality can be added to one's voice production by a slight alteration in velopharyngeal closure. In our use of the label "functional dysphonia," we are suggesting that these components for producing voice are in a physiologic imbalance that may be produced in part by the psychological needs of the patient.

The diagnosis of functional dysphonia implies that the patient has no physical or organic cause of the voice problem. In our evaluation and testing, this means that normal structure and capability for normal function should be demonstrated. The SLP should search with the patient to see if he or she can produce normal voice in some situations. One way to do this is to include a number of diagnostic probes (see Chapters 6 and 7) to determine if the patient can imitate the SLP's modeling of pitch, loudness, or quality change, demonstrating capability for producing some normal voice behaviors. If the patient can demonstrate a normal voicing function by performing some particular therapy approach, this is often a good place for the SLP to begin voice therapy intervention.

The patient often reports other somatic problems associated with functional dysphonia, such as weight loss, difficulty swallowing, throat and neck pain, excessive coughing, or other somatic abnormalities (Verdolini and colleagues, 2006). The SLP may uncover psychological complaints of worry, avoiding responsibility, shyness, excessive fears, and so on. Aronson (1990) states:

> A psychogenic voice disorder is broadly synonymous with a functional one but has the advantage of stating positively, based on exploration of its causes, that the voice disorder is a manifestation of one or more types of psychologic disequilibrium—such as anxiety, depression, conversion, or personality disorder—which interferes with normal volitional control over phonation (p. 131).

Even though the patient may be capable of producing a normal voice when requested to do so in the voice evaluation, the SLP must consider the relative weight of emotional factors possibly preventing the use of a normal voice in everyday living.

In functional dysphonia, there is often a mixture of emotional problems and faulty voice usage. The patient may demonstrate a weak soft voice, or symptoms of vocal hyperfunction, such as a loud, harsh voice. While the patient may demonstrate some emotional issues deserving of some counseling or therapy, he or she may also have the capability of using a normal voice after some voice therapy intervention. In Chapter 7, we will consider a few Voice Facilitating Approaches—such as counseling, hierarchy analysis, relaxation, respiration training, and vocal hygiene—that are particularly effective with this functional dysphonia group of patients. Stemple's *Vocal Function Exercises* were designed to strengthen and "balance the laryngeal musculature" and have been found to have a positive "holistic" effect for general voice improvement (Stemple, 2005). Faulty voice physiology may not necessarily have a strong emotional origin.

Emotionality may play a minimal role in some children and adults with faulty voices who live with their voicing difference (mild hoarseness, inappropriate voice pitch, etc.). They do not think of this difference as being a voice disorder. Listeners perceive their voices as different and perhaps unique but not as disordered (Zraick and colleagues, 2007).

In their classic look at efficacy of voice therapy, Ramig and Verdolini (1998) describe most voice disorders as caused by ". . . habits of vocal misuse and hyperfunction," medical/physical conditions, and/or psychological factors. We include voice misuse and vocal hyperfunction or MTD in the next major section of this chapter as representing most of what the SLP sees in patients with functional voice problems. The myriad of published studies that have considered the outcome of voice therapy for voice disorders have targeted the misuse-hyperfunctional type of disorders. The range of voice therapy methods for vocal hyperfunction include the accent method (Kotby and colleagues, 1991), resonant therapy (Verdolini, 2000), symptomatic therapy (Boone and colleagues, 2009), manual circumlaryngeal therapy (Roy and colleagues, 2001), and physiologic therapy (Colton and colleagues, 2011; Stemple, 2005). Vocal hyperfunctional behaviors often lead to tissue changes over time (Lee and Son, 2005) within the larynx, creating glottal margin disorders such as vocal fold thickening, nodules, and polyps (as we will see in our discussion of muscle tension dysphonia).

When functional dysphonia is classified as a psychogenic voice disorder, priority is given both to the emotional support of the patient and the concomitant voice differences. Sometimes the voice client does not have a voice disorder but only a voice difference, such as poor breathing, influencing a soft voice, or using a pitch level that is not appropriate. While vocal differences can be treated by the SLP using Voice Facilitating Approaches, there are other discipline-specific approaches (National Association of Teachers of Singing, 2010; Voice and Speech Trainers Association, 2012) that can be helpful in learning to optimize vocal function. The client with a "different" voice might be better served on occasion by a National Association of Teachers of Singing (NATS) or Voice and Speech Trainers Association (VASTA) member, rather than by an SLP. The singing teacher and members of NATS have long recognized the connection between emotions and the optimal usage of both speech and singing. Similarly, voice-speech teachers and members of VASTA have developed voice improvement methods that help the actor and speaker minimize speech differences that might negate performance. In the treatment of psychogenic dysphonia, there needs to be greater future interaction among the psychologist or psychiatrist, the SLP, and the teachers/coaches of the singing and speaking voice.

Somatization Dysphonia

In reviewing the clinical files of hospital and university voice clinics, we find rare clinical occurrences of voice patients who may be classified as having somatization dysphonia or who show symptoms of Briquet's dysphonia. In somatization dysphonia, the voice patient shows beyond dysphonia an array of possible conversion symptoms, such as laryngeal pain, neck and shoulder pain with stiffness, shortness of breath, depression, and extreme vocal fatigue (Verdolini and colleagues, 2006). Historically, these patients might have carried the diagnosis of Briquet's syndrome, but in recent years would be classified in the ICD-10 as a "Dissociative Motor Disorder" (F44.4), and in the DSM-IV under "Somatoform Disorders" as a "Conversion Disorder" (300.11) (Kollbrunner and colleagues, 2010). The SLP may be overwhelmed by the severity of patient symptoms, soon realizing that the presenting dysphonia is but a small part of the patient's overall problem. Such a patient should be referred for an extensive medical workup and psychiatric evaluation/treatment.

The voice evaluation of such patients may typically reveal an elevated voice pitch, or increased hoarseness with a reduced signal-to-noise ratio. Vegetative laryngeal functions (coughing, prevention of aspiration, etc.) may remain normal. The voice symptoms often begin in late adolescence extending into young adulthood, and from the beginning are surrounded by many other symptoms. The severity of these associated symptoms may present greater problems to the patient than the presenting dysphonia. The prevalence of somatization dysphonia is much greater in women than in men by a ratio estimated to be as high as 10 to 1 (Verdolini and colleagues, 2006). Critical to the diagnosis is the absence of any physical evidence that can support the cause of the dysphonia and the other related symptoms (Deary and Miller, 2011). Somatization dysphonia is a true conversion disorder, and management appears possible only with successful identification and reduction of emotional and psychological factors.

CHECK YOUR KNOWLEDGE

1. What are the major categories of psychogenic voice disorders?
2. What is the first course of treatment for puberphonia?

SUMMARY

This chapter reviewed functional voice disorders—those that have no organic or neurological cause. We described voice disorders due to excessive muscle tension, and the benign laryngeal pathology that may develop as a result. We also described voice disorders with a psycho-emotional basis or overlay. We presented some evidence-based practice (EBF) studies supporting the value of Voice Facilitating Approaches in treating most functional and psychogenic voice disorders.

CLINICAL CONCEPTS

The following clinical concepts correspond with many of the objectives at the beginning of this chapter:

1. The majority of voice-disordered patients you see will be those with a functional basis to their disorder. Most of these patients will exhibit excessive laryngeal muscle tension, resulting in a voice that does not meet their daily communication needs. Examples include a child who demonstrates repeated phonotrauma and develops vocal fold nodules (see Chapter 8), a speaker who is an auctioneer and has a voice that gives out before lunch each day, a speaker who has a weak or paralyzed vocal fold and compensates by "pushing the voice out" (see Chapter 5), and a speaker with glottic cancer who uses the false vocal folds to phonate (see Chapter 9).

2. Some voice-disordered patients will come to you because they have a strong psycho-emotional basis for their voice disorder, or a strong psycho-emotional reaction to their voice disorder. Examples include a postpubescent male who sounds like a little boy or little girl (see Chapter 8), a patient who was put on short voice rest after laryngeal surgery and whose voice did not "turn back on" easily after the period of voice rest (see Chapter 4), an adult female in a verbally abusive marriage who "loses her voice" in order to avoid angering her spouse and bringing on additional verbal abuse (see Chapter 8), a patient who perceives himself as being stuck in a high-stress job and who sees having a voice disorder as a way out of his job, and a patient who is deprived of emotional attention and who experiences emotional gain by having a voice disorder.

GUIDED READING

Read the following article:

Van Houtte, E., Van Lierde, K., & Claeys, S. (2011). Pathophysiology and treatment of muscle tension dysphonia: A review of the current knowledge. *Journal of Voice*, 25, 202–207.

Describe two ways in which the information reported in the article might influence your clinical practice.

Read the following article:

> Deary, V., & Miller, T. (2011). Reconsidering the role of psychosocial factors in functional dysphonia. *Current Opinion in Otolaryngology and Head and Neck Surgery, 19*, 150–154.

Using the information reported in the article, identify the factors one should consider before making a diagnosis of psychogenic voice disorder.

PREPARING FOR THE PRAXIS™

Directions: Please read the case study and answer the five questions that follow. (Please see page 319 for the answer key.)

> *Miranda is a 34-year-old woman with a 3-month history of dysphonia, which began after an upper respiratory infection. Her chief voice complaints are harsh and strained voice quality, high speaking pitch, and vocal fatigue by the end of the day. She saw an otolaryngologist (ENT), who diagnosed her with muscle tension dysphonia and laryngopharyngeal reflux disease (LPRD). Miranda also complains of being depressed because of the changes in her social life due to her dysphonia.*

1. The ENT's report of his stroboscopic laryngeal exam noted "moderate laryngeal constriction." Based on this information, which of the following constriction patterns were likely observed?
   A. Anterior-posterior compression of the true vocal folds
   B. Medial compression of the true vocal folds
   C. Both anterior-posterior and medial compression of the true vocal folds
   D. Medial compression of the ventricular folds
   E. All of these

2. Which of the following laryngeal findings would also likely be noted by the ENT?
   A. Swelling and redness of the vocal folds and arytenoid mucosa
   B. Vocal fold atrophy
   C. Vocal fold nodules
   D. Paresis

3. Which of the following acoustic voice parameters would likely be abnormal?
   A. Speaking intensity
   B. Speaking fundamental frequency
   C. Harmonic-to-noise ratio
   D. Maximum phonational frequency range
   E. All of these

4. Which of the following treatment options would serve this patient well?
   A. Use of medication to control her acid reflux disease
   B. Vocal hygiene education
   C. Voice rest
   D. Both A and B
   E. All of these

5. Which of the following observations would be made about this patient's performance on a standardized voice protocol?
   A. Her voice changed considerably across the speaking tasks.
   B. Her voice remained consistent across speaking tasks.
   C. Her voice was normal for certain speaking tasks.
   D. She presented with complete aphonia.

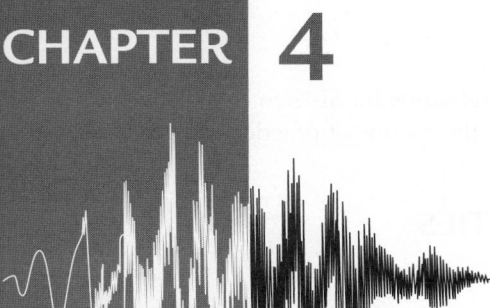

CHAPTER 4

Organic Voice Disorders

■ ■ ■ ■ ■ ————————————— **LEARNING OBJECTIVES** ————————————— ■ ■ ■ ■

After reading this chapter, one should be able to:

- Identify the major organic causes of voice disorders.
- Explain the underlying pathologies that cause and maintain these disorders.
- Explain the medical and pharmacologic approaches to these organic disorders.

- Describe how behavioral voice therapy intervention and lifestyle change counseling can reduce the recurrence of these disorders.
- List behavioral voice intervention techniques that may reduce some of the dysphonic characteristics that accompany these disorders.

■ ■ ■ ■

This chapter describes organic voice disorders. Tolerance by the public or an indifference to voice problems makes the early identification of voice pathologies difficult. Hoarseness that persists longer than several days is often identified by the otolaryngologist (ENT physician) as a possible symptom of serious laryngeal disease, and it may be. Hoarseness is certainly the acoustic correlate of improper vocal fold functioning, with or without true laryngeal disease. The distinction between organic disease of the larynx and functional misuse has been a prominent dichotomy in the classification of voice disorders (as described in Chapter 1). It is important for ENT physicians, in their need to rule out or identify true organic disease, to view the laryngeal mechanism by laryngoscopy in order to make a judgment about functional versus organic versus neurological involvement. In the absence of observable structural deviation or neurological involvement, the ENT physician generally describes the voice disorder as functional. In addition to the examination by the ENT physician, it is important for the speech-language pathologist (SLP) to view the larynx as part of the voice evaluation and in designing the voice therapy. Indeed, the American Speech-Language-Hearing Association (ASHA) (American Speech-Language-Hearing Association, 2004b) affirms the practice of visualization of the larynx by both ENT physicians and SLPs. It is an important milestone for SLPs to be able to count laryngeal visualization and imaging as within their scope of practice.

CONGENITAL ABNORMALITIES

Laryngomalacia

Laryngomalacia is the term most commonly used to describe ". . . inward collapse of the supraglottic structures of the larynx during inspiration" (Holinger, 1997). Laryngomalacia accounts for 75% of all congenital anomalies of the larynx and is the most prevalent cause of stridor in the neonate (Elluru, 2006). In most children with the condition, symptoms are evident at birth or within the first few hours or days of life (Andrews and Summers, 2002). Laryngomalacia is diagnosed and managed by an ENT physician, who normally confirms the condition using direct laryngoscopy under general anesthesia (without muscle relaxant) (Peggy, 2005) or via flexible nasopharyngolaryngoscopy (under topical anesthesia) (Whymark and colleagues, 2006). Children with laryngomalacia rarely present with acute airway compromise, and Tunkel and colleagues (2008) report that it is common for children to outgrow laryngomalacia by 18 to 24 months. However, for those 5% of patients who require surgical intervention for severe laryngomalacia, this occurs within one to two weeks of presentation (Elluru, 2006). Severe laryngomalacia is associated with the primary symptoms of inspiratory stridor, suprasternal retraction, substernal retraction, feeding difficulty, choking, postfeeding vomit, failure to thrive, and cyanosis (Lee and colleagues, 2007). The presence of concomitant gastroesophageal reflux disease (GERD) or laryngopharyngeal reflux disease (LPRD) contributes to the feeding- and swallowing-related symptoms (Thomson, 2010). Supraglottoplasty is currently the preferred surgical intervention, replacing tracheostomy (Fattaha and colleagues, 2011). Supraglottoplasty eliminates inspiratory obstruction by widening the supraglottis. It is a successful approach to correcting all anatomic abnormalities associated with laryngomalacia (Bedwell and Zalza, 2011).

Subglottic Stenosis

Subglottic stenosis is the narrowing of the space below the glottis and above the first tracheal ring. Although rare, it is one of the most common causes of chronic upper airway obstruction in infants and children. It can be congenital or acquired. Congenital subglottic stenosis is the second most common cause of stridor in neonates, infants, and children. Acquired subglottic stenosis is the most common acquired anomaly of the larynx in the pediatric age group, and is the most common abnormality necessitating tracheotomy in children below one year of age. This is because of the advent of endotracheal intubation in neonatal medicine and the need for long-term ventilation in premature babies (Choo and colleagues, 2010). The prognosis of acquired subglottic stenosis in infants and children is significantly poorer than that of the congenital type (Wei and Bond, 2011). Walner and Cotton (1999) introduced levels of stenosis grading that help determine levels of intervention by the ENT physician and SLP. For children with Grades I or II subglottal stenosis—that is, stenosis corresponding to 0 to 50% and 51% to 70%, respectively—careful observation rather than intervention may be appropriate. Stenosis of Grades III or IV, on the other hand—which correspond to 71% to 99%, and 100%, respectively—often present with either tracheal dependency or stridor and exercise intolerance. Children in these latter categories may require endoscopic or surgical intervention, usually with voice intervention to follow (Kelchner and colleagues, 2012).

Esophageal Atresia and Tracheoesophageal Fistula

Congenital esophageal atresia (EA) represents a failure of the esophagus to develop as a continuous passage. Instead, it ends as a blind pouch. Tracheoesophageal fistula (TEF) represents an abnormal opening between the trachea and esophagus. EA and TEF can occur separately or together. EA and TEF are diagnosed in the intensive care unit (ICU) at birth and are treated immediately. The standard intervention is surgery. However, surgery is not without risks, such as severe respiratory distress, recurrent aspiration pneumonia, failure to thrive, and dysphagia. Any attempt at feeding could cause aspiration pneumonia because the milk or other liquid collects in the blind pouch and overflows into the trachea and lungs. A fistula between the lower esophagus and trachea may allow stomach acid to flow into the lungs and cause damage. Because of these dangers, patients should be treated as soon as possible after birth. Treatment by the SLP focuses primarily on feeding (Khan and colleagues, 2009), and secondarily on voice (Oestreicher-Kedem and colleagues, 2008). The clinician may suspect dysphagia and dysphonia because unilateral vocal fold paralysis has been associated in a small percentage of patients treated surgically for EA or TEF (Morini and colleagues, 2011).

ACID REFLUX DISEASE

Over the past 25 years, there has been a growing acknowledgment that gastroesophageal reflux disease (GERD) and laryngopharyngeal reflux disease (LPRD) are etiologic factors in a high percentage of patients with laryngeal complaints (Altman and colleagues, 2011; Gupta and Sataloff, 2009). In adults, an estimated 4% to 10% of chronic nonspecific laryngeal disease seen in ENT and voice clinics is associated with GERD or LPRD (Gilger, 2003). This may be just the tip of the iceberg. In a review of clinical practice guidelines for reflux, Altman and colleagues (2011) found that gastroenterologists (GI physicians) and ENT physicians see only about one in five patients who might potentially experience GERD. Physicians in internal medicine and family practice see the remaining symptomatic patients.

GERD is the passage of gastric juices from the stomach into the esophagus (see Figure 4.1). Among other pathologies, GERD can lead to esophagitis; ulceration; dysphagia; and Barrett's metaplasia, which is a precancerous condition. If these contents move superiorly and through the upper esophageal sphincter, the disorder is identified as LPRD, as the contents spill into the pharynx. LPRD is synonymous with extraesophageal reflux disease (EERD), another accepted but older term for reflux upstream from the stomach (Sasaki and Toolhill, 2000). LPRD has been implicated in the occurrence of vocal fold erythema and edema, contact ulcers and granulomas, laryngitis, chronic rhinitis, sinusitis, globus pharyngeus, respiratory compromise, otitis media, laryngomalacia, and subglottic stenosis, to name a few (Arvedson, 2002; Belafsky and colleagues, 2002; Molyneux, 2011). Additional studies have suggested an association of LPRD and paradoxical vocal fold movement (Murry and colleagues, 2010).

Rather than simply describe the general symptoms of reflux, the clinician in this **video** uses time effectively by asking the patient to reflect on her own signs and symptoms of laryngopharyngeal reflux. See Voice Facilitating Approaches 13 and 19 for hierarchy analysis and pitch inflections. Not mentioned in the interview is that the patient has begun a regimen of proton pump inhibitors. Grand Rounds: Identify two additional behavioral precautions that this patient might initiate to reduce reflux and abusive voice behaviors.

FIGURE 4.1 Acid Reflux Disease

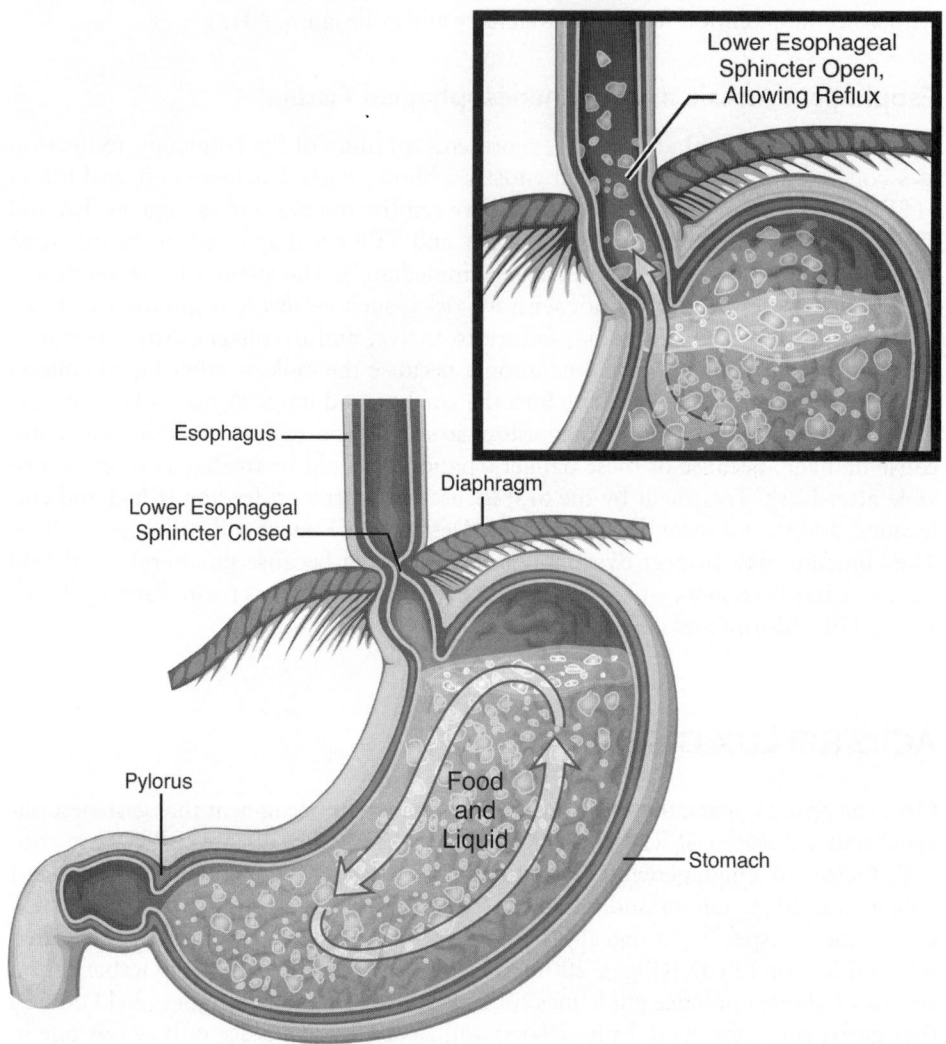

The symptoms of acid reflux vary considerably among voice patients, ranging from no symptoms to mild heartburn, to extreme burning or choking in the larynx, sometimes awakening the patient from a deep sleep. Typical symptoms of LPRD may include morning hoarseness, sour taste in mouth with bad breath, frequent throat clearing and coughing, and severe symptoms occurring when the head is lower than the abdominal area (such as in shoe tying, bungee jumping, or occupational tasks requiring bending over). Among the physical findings on laryngeal examination are posterior glottal redness, contact ulcers, pharyngeal irritation, and arytenoid hyperplasia with possible granuloma. The patient, on questioning, may be unaware of any symptoms related to LPRD; we have found that this is especially true among children. Altman and colleagues (2011) have also developed a clinical protocol for the identification and management of reflux disease.

With respect to children, GERD and LPRD are believed to be strongly associated with pediatric voice disorders (Theis, 2011) and, in some cases, middle ear infections (Tasker and colleagues, 2002). Several upper airway conditions have been attributed to GERD and LPRD, including stridor (Heatley and Swift, 1996), paradoxical vocal fold movement (PVFM) (Wilson and colleagues, 2009), chronic nasal irritation, and chronic cough and dysphonia. With respect to older adults, Gregory and colleagues (2012) reported that about 90% of the dysphonic patients they examined over age 65 years had evidence of LPRD.

Diagnostic reflux batteries include barium esophagram, bronchoalveolar lavage, radionuclide reflux scans, scintigraphy, multichannel intraluminal impedance monitoring, color Doppler sonography, and laryngeal biopsy (Stavroulaki, 2006). At present, 24-hour dual-probe esophageal pH monitoring is the most definitive study of LPRD, even for children (Chiou and colleagues, 2011). Esophageal pH monitoring involves passing a thin catheter transnasally into the esophagus. A special sensor records each reflux incidence over a 24-hour period. After the catheter is removed, the recorder is attached to a computer so that data it has gathered can be interpreted. Koufman (1991) reported on 225 patients with suspected reflux. Eighty-eight percent of the patients underwent 24-hour pH probe testing, with 62% of those demonstrating abnormal studies. Of these, 30% demonstrated LPRD. A more recent advance in pH monitoring involves the placement of an acid-sensing capsule introduced into the esophagus via a removable catheter (Javors and Buckman, 2011). The capsule transmits reflux events for two days to a recorder, and then detaches from the esophagus and passes in the stool.

Based on the knowledge that a negative pH probe test does not rule out reflux, some authorities advocate esophageal biopsy to rule in the disease. This can be performed on infants as young as two weeks of age (Coletti and colleagues, 1995; Stroh and colleagues, 1998). Upper gastrointestinal endoscopy is another diagnostic procedure. In addition to these instrumental assessments, questionnaires for determining the presence of reflux and the type of reflux present have been developed and refined for routine use in ENT practice (Habermann and colleagues, 2012). The Reflux Symptom Index (RSI) (Belafsky and colleagues, 2002b) raises the clinical suspicion of LPRD in patients presenting with ENT symptoms. The Reflux Finding Score (RFS) (Belafsky and colleagues, 2001b) characterizes morphologic lesions presumably associated with LPRD.

Reflux treatment can be divided into three categories: behavioral, pharmacological, and surgical, or a combination of these treatments. Behavioral therapy involves following a vocal hygiene program that includes elevating the head of the bed; remaining upright for at least 60 minutes after meals; avoiding spicy foods; not exercising after eating; and cutting down on caffeine, carbonated drinks, and alcohol, especially in the afternoons and evenings. We even recommend that patients avoid drinking excessive quantities of water right before bed because this can raise the level of acid in the stomach. Other treatment recommendations for controlling reflux are avoiding activities that compress the abdomen, weight loss, wearing looser clothing around the waist, and eliminating smoking. Following these management suggestions for reflux can often produce a dramatic lessening of symptoms, both in voice and pharyngeal–laryngeal mucosal irritation.

For those patients who do not readily respond to behavioral therapy, a combination of anti-reflux therapy with a proton-pump inhibitor (PPI) and a prokinetic agent has been shown to result in rapid symptomatic and endoscopic improvements in the majority of patients (Vaezi and colleagues, 2003; Arvedson, 2002; Hamdan and colleagues, 2001). A study by Park and colleagues (2005) found that PPIs taken twice a day (bid) appear to be more effective than once a day (qd) in achieving clinical symptom response. Greater acid suppression was achieved at four months compared with two months. In addition to LPRD, PPIs have been used in the treatment of postnasal drip (PND). Pawar and colleagues (2007) studied the effects of PPI on patients having postnasal drainage with no objective evidence to support a sinonasal or infectious etiology. Findings supported the potential benefits of PPI therapy to reduced PND frequency, hoarseness, and chronic cough.

Surgical laparoscopic fundoplication is effective in treatment of LPRD for patients who show poor response to PPI (up to 120 mg/day). Five years after laparoscopic surgery, a corpus of 445 patients with previous poorly controlled GERD revealed reduced acid reflux, lower esophageal sphincter pressure, and symptom control. The authors report that the patients also revealed a significant improvement in both the physical and mental health component of a quality of life assessment (Anvari and Allen, 2003).

The SLP usually encounters the dysphonic patient with LPRD initially at the time of the voice evaluation. If the signs of laryngeal irritation are present, the patient is referred to the ENT physician. The SLP, ENT physician, and patient work as a team to plan a successful reflux management regimen and a voice therapy program that can produce optimal vocal function. It is helpful to have access to a number of voice-related quality of life and reflux-related scales to document pre- and post-treatment scores (see Chapter 6). In a prospective study by Park and colleagues (2012), 100 patients diagnosed with LPRD with voice symptoms were divided into two groups: a control group of 50 patients were treated with medication alone, and an experimental group of 50 were treated with medication plus voice therapy. The following data were recorded before treatment and at one, two, and three months post-treatment: RSI, RFS, Voice Handicap Index (VHI), auditory-perceptual analysis, and acoustic analysis. Park and colleagues reported that "significantly more patients in the experimental group showed a clinically significant change in RSI, VHI, and perceptual scores at the 1-, 2-, and 3-month follow-up evaluations. Further, no clinically significant change in RFS was achieved in either group at 1 or 2 months, but a significantly greater change was achieved in the experimental group at 3 months" (p. 93). This study suggests that voice therapy may help to restore reversible mucosal change secondary to acidic reflux, inducing rapid resolution of symptoms and shortening of the treatment period.

Helping the patient reduce throat clearing and nonproductive coughing (more often habit than an effort to clear mucus), developing easy glottal attack, changing throat focus to facial mask focus, and sometimes elevating voice pitch one or two half notes are among the Voice Facilitating Approaches that help the reflux patient maintain a functional voice.

CHECK YOUR KNOWLEDGE

1. Why is it so important to investigate GERD and LPRD, even if patients deny symptoms on clinical interview?
2. What are the perceptual voice characteristics in LPRD?

CONTACT ULCERS (GRANULOMAS)

As we explained in Chapter 2, the total length of the glottis can be divided into thirds: The anterior two-thirds is muscular (vocalis portion of the thyroarytenoids) and covered by a membrane, and the posterior third is cartilaginous (arytenoids) and covered by a membrane. Contact ulcers are small ulcerations that develop on the medial aspect of the vocal processes of the arytenoid cartilages due to irritation. When granulated tissue forms over these ulcers as a protective mechanism, they are called contact ulcer granulomas.

The typical symptoms of contact ulcers are deterioration of voice after prolonged vocalization (vocal fatigue), accompanied by pain in the laryngeal area or sometimes pain that lateralizes out to one ear. Watterson and colleagues (1990) also found hoarseness or roughness reported 75% of the time and throat clearing in 65% of the 57 cases of contact ulcers they studied. Laryngoscopy usually reveals bilateral ulcerations with heavy buildup of granulation tissue along the approximating margins of the posterior glottis. Greene (1980) labeled the toughened membranous tissue changes on the posterior glottis as pachydermia, citing the work of Kleinsasser (1979), and wrote that "contact ulcers are not actually ulcers or granulomas but consist of 'craters' with highly thickened squamous epithelium over connective tissue with some inflammation (edema)" (p. 147).

Contact ulcers are multifactorial in nature and are a chronic inflammatory disease of the larynx. They seem to result from one of three causes or a combination of these: hard glottal attack along with throat clearing and coughing, LPRD, and endotracheal intubation. The first cause is excessive slamming together of the arytenoid cartilages during production of low-pitched phonation coupled with excessively hard glottal attack and perhaps increased loudness with frequent throat clearing and coughing. The speaker is usually a hard-driving person who speaks in a loud, controlling low pitch, often with words punctuated by sudden onset. However, Watterson and colleagues (1990) found that hard glottal attack was reported only 26% of the time by diagnosing clinicians, while pain was reported in 56% of the cases. Indeed, we now feel that those patients who develop contact ulcers and granuloma due to faulty vocal functioning alone are in the minority. These individuals may experience co-occurring organic factors such as LPRD.

Maier and colleagues (1994) and Emami and colleagues (1999) found that the majority of their patients with contact ulcers who received an anti-reflux regimen and voice therapy experienced a complete remission of the contact ulcers. In another group of patients, when the ulcers and granulomas were removed surgically, more than 90% of these patients experienced recurrence unless voice therapy was performed. This was also found by Hirano and colleagues (2002), who reported that for 23 surgeries performed to remove contact granulomas, 10 of the 23 recurred. After surgical removal of the offending lesion, Hirano suggests that voice therapy is needed to help the patient regain a normal voice.

Endotracheal intubation is a third cause of contact ulcers in a small number of cases, especially where large, protective granulomas are the presenting picture following the removal of the endotracheal tube. Any patient who is intubated during surgery or for airway preservation risks having a traumatized laryngeal membrane with the subsequent development of granuloma. The risk is particularly greater in children and women, who have smaller airways and are thus more often traumatized by large tubes. The physician places a tube down the pharynx into the airway, between the open (it is hoped) vocal folds, and into the trachea. If the tube is larger than the glottal opening, the patient runs the risk of trauma. Ellis and Bennett (1977) have recommended that, in order to prevent intubation granuloma or hemangioma, patients should be intubated with tubes one size smaller than what would be needed for a snug fit.

Any change in postsurgical voice should be investigated for intubation trauma with resulting irritation and granuloma. These complications from intubation may not appear immediately but rather develop over time (McFerran and colleagues, 1994). No voice therapy should be initiated until a laryngeal examination is completed. If postsurgical granulomas are identified along the posterior glottis, medical–surgical treatment will promote healing and preserve the airway.

The focus of voice therapy for patients with contact ulcers and/or granuloma is to take the effort out of phonation. The patients must learn to use a voice that can be produced with relatively little strain (which usually means a slight elevation in pitch), to speak with greater mouth and jaw relaxation, to speak at lower levels of volume, and to eliminate all traces of excessively hard glottal attack. Contact ulcers are rare today; according to Watterson and colleagues (1990), these cases comprise about 1% of total voice cases. Those patients who do have contact ulcers, however, seem to respond fairly well to voice therapy. Leonard and Kendall (2005) reported the effects of a unique behavioral voice therapy program in patients who had failed other treatments for vocal process granulomas related to LPRD. The researchers introduced a "phonoscopic" approach, whereby the patient observed his or her larynx endoscopically while voicing, and altered vocal fold vibration so that a small gap remained between the vocal processes. Of the 10 patients who received intervention, eight experienced full or a marked reduction in the granuloma.

CHECK YOUR KNOWLEDGE

1. Identify the three most common causes of contact granuloma.
2. Identify the various intervention approaches to contact granuloma.

CYSTS

Cysts in the larynx are usually unilateral, occurring on the vocal folds (inner margin, superior or inferior surface) or anywhere on the ventricular folds. They are often caused by an abnormal blockage of the ductal system of laryngeal mucous glands (Case, 2002), but there are other causes. Cysts may be congenital or acquired. The cyst often appears soft and pliable, in contrast to the hard, fibrotic structure of a vocal nodule. The SLP who identifies any kind of laryngeal lesion should refer the patient to an ENT physician. This is especially true for cysts because their management requires surgical excision rather than voice therapy per se. Courey and colleagues (1996) studied 41 benign laryngeal lesions (nodules, polyps, cysts, and corditis) and identified seven squamous cysts and seven mucous cysts. All 14 cyst lesions were found on histological examination to be benign. Depending on the site of the lesion, the patient may or may not experience dysphonia. Young and Smith (2012), in a retrospective review, reported that all of a large cohort of patients with saccular cysts reported dysphonia. Because cysts rarely resolve spontaneously, they should be removed surgically using a small superficial incision along the superior edge of the vocal fold, without disrupting the glottal margin. Voice therapy postsurgically is usually confined to helping the patient eliminate any voice compensations (such as increased glottal attack) that may have been used to minimize the negative voice consequences of the cyst.

ENDOCRINE CHANGES

Occasionally patients' voice problems are related to some kind of endocrine dysfunction. Endocrine disorders often have a major impact on developing larynges and cause excesses in fundamental frequency, so that an individual's voice is either too low or too high in pitch. For example, in hypofunction of the pituitary gland, laryngeal growth is retarded. A pubescent child with such a problem experiences a continued high voice pitch. Such a pituitary problem can prevent normal development of progesterone by the ovaries (in girls) and testosterone by the testes (in adolescent males). The resulting lack of secondary sexual characteristics (including a change in voice) is treated by endocrine therapy designed to stimulate normal pituitary function. The opposite problem, caused by some tumors of the pituitary gland, results in a "precocious puberty as well as acromegaly" (Strome, 1982, p. 18). Hypofunctioning of the adrenal glands (Addison's disease) can also contribute to lack of secondary sex characteristics, including a prepubescent voice in males. Sometimes tumors in the adrenal system cause adrenal hormone excesses, causing virilization and a deepening of the voice.

Hypothyroidism (insufficient secretion of thyroxin by the thyroid gland) can produce many physical changes over time, including increased mass of the vocal folds, which in turn lowers pitch. Aronson (1990) describes the dysphonia of hypothyroidism as "characteristically hoarse, sometimes described as coarse or gravelly and of excessively low pitch" (p. 60). Such symptoms can usually be well controlled by thyroid hormone therapy. In hyperthyroidism (excessive thyroid function), vocal symptoms are less severe, and the patients experience jumpiness and irritability, which result in a breathy voice that may lack sufficient loudness.

Premenstrual vocal syndrome, as described by Greene (1980) and Abitbol and colleagues (1999), is characterized by vocal fatigue, reduced pitch range, hypophonia, and loss of certain harmonics. The syndrome usually begins four to five days before menstruation in 33% of women. Videostroboscopic examination reveals congestion, microvarices, vocal fold thickening, and reduced vibratory amplitude. Some female opera singers avoid heavy singing obligations several days before and after menstruation. Two studies (Amir and colleagues, 2006; La and colleagues, 2007) suggest that oral contraceptive pills may reduce the irregularity of vocal fold vibration in professional and nonprofessional singers during menstruation. Another study by Hamdan and colleagues (2011) suggests that women undergoing in vitro fertilization (IVF) demonstrate increased throat clearing. Pregnancy has also been reported to be associated with vocal changes as a response to sex steroid hormonal variations (La and Sundberg, 2012).

The climacteric (menopause) is a time when some women may experience vocal changes, particularly a lowering of fundamental frequency. Because of the secretion of excessive androgenic hormones after menopause, the glottal membrane becomes thicker, increasing the size-mass of the folds, which in turn produces a lowering of voice pitch (Raj and colleagues, 2010) and sometimes vocal roughness. It would appear that, in any case in which the larynx is under- or overdeveloped for the age and sex of the patient, some endocrine imbalance might be suspected. If some kind of hormonal imbalance is discovered, the primary treatment, if possible, would be hormonal therapy. Voice therapy can be of help to the patient in developing the best vocal performance possible with the changing (because of hormone therapy) mechanism. Most of the Voice Facilitating Approaches presented in Chapter 7 are appropriate when applied to these patients.

HEMANGIOMA

Laryngeal hemangiomas are similar to contact ulcers and granulomas, differing only in type of lesion. Whereas a granuloma is usually a firm granulated sac, a hemangioma is a soft, pliable, blood-filled sac. Laryngeal hemangiomas are relatively rare and occur in two main forms: infantile and adult. While infantile hemangiomas are usually found in the subglottis, adult hemangiomas occur usually in the supraglottis (Prasad and colleagues, 2008). Like granulomas, hemangiomas often occur on the posterior glottis. They are frequently associated with vocal hyperfunction, LPRD, or intubation trauma. This blood-filled lesion, when identified, should be removed surgically (Yan and colleagues, 2010). As soon as glottal healing permits, a vocal hygiene program and voice therapy should be initiated (Erkan and colleagues, 2007).

HYPERKERATOSIS

Patients often come to their dentist or ENT physician because they are concerned about some oral or pharyngeal lesions they have observed. Once professionally identified, these lesions are often biopsied and found to be either malignant (cancerous) or nonmalignant (benign). Laryngeal examination may also locate and subsequently identify, by biopsy, additive lesions in the pharynx or larynx. Hyperkeratosis, a pinkish, rough lesion, is often the identified lesion, a nonmalignant growth that may be the precursor of malignant tissue change (Isenberg and colleagues, 2008). Hyperkeratotic growths are reactive lesions to continued tissue irritation. Therefore, hyperkeratotic lesions must be watched closely over time for any change in appearance. Favorite sites of hyperkeratosis include under the tongue, on the vocal folds at the anterior commissure, and posteriorly on the arytenoid prominences. Their effect on voice may be negligible or severe, depending on the site and the extent of the lesion. We once had an eight-year-old female voice patient with hyperkeratosis of the vocal folds who had experienced the secondhand smoke of both parents for those eight years.

It is generally believed that chronic irritants to the oral and laryngeal membranes over time are the primary etiologies of hyperkeratosis. Consequently, the most effective treatments are eliminating the sources of tissue irritation, that is, ceasing smoking and, in cases of LPRD, prescribing a PPI and encouraging lifestyle modifications. Sataloff and colleagues (1996) report on a case of severe hyperkeratosis mimicking cancer. The 50-year-old patient had smoked for 30 years and presented with complaints of persistent cough, throat clearings, and other symptoms of LPRD. Surprising to the authors, pathology revealed hyperkeratosis, inflammation, and viral changes suggestive of papilloma, but there was no carcinoma. The patient's voice improved after surgery, vocal hygiene, anti-reflux therapy, and smoking cessation. Garcia and colleagues (2006) described a case of tenacious hyperkeratosis that persisted in spite of aggressive anti-reflux therapy. After two months on a regimen, the patient still presented with surface irregularities and keratosis of both vocal folds. Biopsy was negative for malignancy, but the pathologist reported several areas of mild to moderate dysplasia (tissue changes). The dose of pantoprazole was increased to 40 mg twice a day, and ranitidine and GERD behavior modifications continued. Four months later, strobovideolaryngoscopy revealed an absence of keratosis and vocal fold inflammation.

INFECTIOUS LARYNGITIS

Some of the same people who experience traumatic laryngitis after only minor abuse and/or misuse of the voice also experience infectious laryngitis when they have an upper respiratory infection (URI). The case histories of such people often contain multiple entries of loss of voice, dysphonia, or laryngitis. In other individuals, infectious laryngitis is a very rare event that occurs as one of the symptoms of a severe head and chest cold. Infectious laryngitis often develops in a patient who has had a fever, headache, runny nose (rhinorrhea), sore throat, and coughing. Infectious laryngitis can also include complaints of odynophagia (sore swallowing), hyperemia (increased blood flow to area), and dysphonia (Dworkin, 2008). Although most problems of infectious laryngitis are viral in origin, the more severe problems (often accompanied by high fever and a very sore throat) may be caused by bacterial infections. Bacteria-caused laryngitis can often be dramatically treated, with relatively quick resolution, through antibiotic therapy. Unfortunately, most laryngitis experienced during a URI that is viral in origin does not respond to antibiotics. Amantadine appears to be useful against influenza (Wingfield and colleagues, 1969); however, it may not be effective against all types of viruses, and side effects include xerostomia and xerophonia, among others (Sataloff, 1997). Increased resistance among Americans to amantadine and other influenza-specific antiviral drugs underscores the need for novel prevention and treatment strategies (Rothberg and colleagues, 2008). Strome (1982) recommends voice rest, humidification, increased fluid intake (hydration), reduced physical activity, and analgesics.

From a voice conservation point of view, absolute voice rest—no attempts at spoken communication, including voice or whisper—should be initiated by the patient with such a laryngeal infection. Whispering should be discouraged because most people produce a glottal whisper by placing the vocal folds in close approximation to one another, which in effect produces a light voice. The irritated, swollen tissues continue to touch and to vibrate. What infectious laryngitis patients need is total voice rest for a period of two or three days, with the vocal folds in the open, inverted-V position, and increased fluids (hydration).

CHECK YOUR KNOWLEDGE

1. Why is whispering discouraged in cases of infectious laryngitis and other organic changes to the larynx?
2. Describe why infectious laryngitis might be accompanied by odynophagia.

LEUKOPLAKIA

Leukoplakias are whitish-colored patches that are additive lesions to the surface membrane of mucosal tissue and that often extend beneath the surface into the subepithelial space. Although the lesions are classified as benign tumors, similar to hyperkeratosis, they are considered precancerous lesions and must be followed closely. Within the vocal tract, common sites for leukoplakia are under the tongue and on the vocal folds. It is important to note that it is difficult or impossible to distinguish between leukoplakia and cancer of the larynx by visual inspection alone. The primary etiology of these white patches is continuous irritation of membranes. The most common cause is heavy smoking; a heroic effort must be initiated to prevent continued irritation, such as absolute insistence that the patient quit smoking and emotional support for the patient. More recently, LPRD has been a suggested cause (Beaver and colleagues, 2003), as has human papilloma virus (HPV) (Makowska and colleagues, 2001). Continued irritation and subsequent growth of leukoplakia often lead to squamous cell carcinoma.

Although leukoplakias on or under the tongue have only minimal effects on voice, leukoplakia on the vocal folds may dramatically alter voice. The added lesion mass to the vocal folds lowers voice pitch and frequently causes hoarseness and sometimes hypophonia. Because leukoplakias are also random in size and location, they often cause the vocal folds to be asymmetrical. The vocal fold asymmetry may result in diplophonia when each fold vibrates at a different frequency because of its different size or mass. Leukoplakias that occupy space on the glottal margin may prevent optimal approximation of the folds, contributing to breathiness, reduced loudness, and overall dysphonia. The treatment of leukoplakia is medical–surgical (Sieron and colleagues, 2001), and voice therapy only contributes to developing the best voice possible. In spite of lesion effects, a functional aspect of the dysphonia can often be lessened with therapy. These functional aspects may be the only vocal symptoms; thus, voice therapy is important to restore normal voice.

RECURRENT RESPIRATORY PAPILLOMATOSIS

Juvenile onset recurrent respiratory papillomatosis (JORRP) is the most common benign laryngeal neoplasm in children and the most common cause of pediatric hoarseness (Derkay, 2001). It is estimated to have an incidence of 1.7 to 2.6 children per 100,000 in the United States (Andrus and Shapshay, 2006). Papillomas are wartlike growths, viral in origin, that occur in the dark, moist caverns of the airway, frequently in the larynges of young children. The vast majority of JORRP lesions are due to human papilloma virus (HPV) types 6 and 11 (Goon and colleagues, 2008). Other extralaryngeal sites are the oral cavity, trachea, and the bronchi. JORRP can represent a serious threat to the airway, limiting the needed flow of air through the glottal opening. The majority of papillomas occur in children under the age of six; for this reason, hoarseness and shortness of breath in preschool children should be evaluated promptly. Harris and colleagues (2012) write that in their clinical experience, patients with JORRP are usually asymptomatic for the first six months of life. As the RRP develops, symptoms begin to develop. These range from hoarseness to inspiratory stridor.

Excessive loudness of voice is most often not the primary reason driving a voice problem, rather a secondary symptom. Although the child in this **video** does not present with a history of RRP, he is still a candidate for change of loudness intervention because of a history of screaming and yelling. Grand Rounds: Describe the changes that might occur to a child's larynx with surgical intervention to remove papilloma. How might the changes lead to the child's perceived need to speak more loudly?

Although the majority of papillomas stop recurring about the time of puberty, approximately 20% persist beyond puberty (Andrus and Shapshay, 2006). We have seen adults who developed RRP in adulthood without ever having it in childhood. When RRP occurs in the larynx, the additive mass often contributes to dysphonia. For this reason, the voice clinician should be particularly alert to any child who demonstrates dysphonia. Any child with continued hoarseness for more than 10 days, independent of a cold or allergy, should have the benefit of a laryngeal examination to identify the cause of the hoarseness.

Treatment of RRP is usually surgical, with the addition of adjuvant therapy following surgical removal. Treatment is considered *palliative*, not curative, because of the resiliency of the HPV genome in the tissue. Treatment focuses on eliminating the space-occupying lesions, ensuring a safe airway, and subsequently introducing key Voice Facilitating Approaches that offer the best voice possible. Surgical removal techniques include excision by a microdebrider, laser surgery, and conventional excision surgery (Burns and colleagues, 2007; Goon and colleagues, 2008; Roy and Vivero, 2008). Adjuvant therapies include interferon therapy, indole-3-carbinole, cidofovir, ribavarin, mumps vaccine, and photodynamic therapy (El Hakim and colleagues, 2002; Rosen and colleagues, 1998). A task force on RRP (Derkay, 1995) reported that 33% of children needed more than 20 operations, with 7% requiring more than 100 operations in their lifetime. A recent study of 30 cases of JORRP by Gandhi and Jacobs (2012) revealed that half the patients experienced remission, which was more likely in those whose RRP onset was earlier in childhood rather than later.

The SLP is sometimes asked to see a toddler or young child with obstructive RRP who has had to have a tracheostomy to permit adequate respiration. Developing functional communication with such a child and fostering normal language growth are the primary concerns of the clinician. Teaching the child to occlude the trach tube with a finger, or fitting the child with a one-way valve that covers the valve (to permit vocalization without finger occlusion), usually permits some voicing. In older children or adults who are being treated surgically for RRP, helping them to develop the best voice possible with the compromised laryngeal mechanisms is a realistic goal in voice therapy. Some work on respiration control (such as voicing with larger lung volumes of air); some work on loudness and pitch, which may improve vocal function.

CHECK YOUR KNOWLEDGE

1. What is the voice therapist's role in voice rehabilitation for patients after RRP removal?
2. List the various interventions for RRP.

PUBERTAL CHANGES

At about age nine, before the onset of puberty, the larynges of boys and girls are anatomically about the same size, and they produce about the same voice pitch (265 Hz). Pubertal growth changes in girls begin around nine, with the onset of puberty, and gradual pubescent changes occur over a four- to five-year period. In boys, puberty begins around 11 to 12, and dramatic growth changes occur over the four- to five-year pubertal period. However, noticeable laryngeal growth and the dramatic change in vocal fundamental frequency occur in the last year of puberty: The "average time from onset to completion of adolescent voice change is three to six months, one year at most" (Aronson, 1990, p. 45). By age 17, adolescents of both sexes have usually reached their full adult development (Offer, 1980). As we discuss elsewhere in this text (see Chapters 2 and 8), the voice pitch levels of males and females drop dramatically after puberty (the male voice drops at least a full octave; the female voice drops almost half an octave). Laryngeal and airway growth does not happen overnight. Although the changes are gradual, over a four-year period, marked laryngeal growth (particularly in boys) occurs in the last six months of change. During this time of rapid laryngeal growth, boys may experience temporary dysphonia and occasional pitch breaks that are not cause for parental or clinical concern. Because these mass changes in puberty tend to thwart any serious attempts at singing or other vocal arts, middle school is often a poor environment for choral music. A boy who is a soprano in September may well be the choir baritone by June. Until children experience some stability in laryngeal and airway growth, the demands of singing might well be inappropriate for their rapidly changing mechanisms. Even though it has become common to involve young singers in more sophisticated musical tasks, the fact still remains that adolescents are particularly susceptible to vocal fatigue while singing. Many adolescents are not trained in the proper technique of singing and are not cognizant of the physical limits of their voice (Jamison, 1996). Because of the rapid changes, attempting to develop optimum pitch or modal-pitch levels in adolescents should be avoided. We present pubertal voice changes in more detail in Chapter 8, and outline Voice Facilitating Approaches in Chapter 7.

SULCUS VOCALIS

Sulcus vocalis may be either congenital or acquired and is of unknown etiology, although vocal abuse and laryngopharyngeal reflux may play a role in the acquired form (Belafsky and colleagues, 2002). A study by Xu and colleagues (2007) suggested 5% sulcus vocalis among children referred for voice disorders. Although Ford and colleagues (1996) cite the earliest mention of sulcus vocalis in the literature (Giacomini in 1892), there has been a lot of clinical confusion over the years about both the etiology and description of the disorder. *Sulcus* is a generic term that means "furrow" or "indentation." In sulcus vocalis, on endoscopy or stroboscopy, we see a furrowed medial edge of the vocal fold, usually bilaterally symmetrical. The spindle configuration may involve all or any segment of the edge of the fold. The furrow may be confined to the superficial layer of the mucosa or penetrate into the vocal ligament and muscle (Giovanni and colleagues, 2007). The patient presents clinically with some degree of dysphonia, often referred with a confusing array of previous diagnoses such as bowing, presbylaryngis, paralysis, or thyroarytenoid atrophy (Hirano and colleagues, 1990).

The SLP today sees more patients with sulcus vocalis than in former years. With mirror examination, many of these abnormalities were missed. However, videostroboscopy permits close examination of vocal fold cover abnormalities. With sulcus vocalis, when the folds are abducted, we can often identify the fold furrow; on adduction with phonation, we can see the compromised mucosal wave produced by the stiff, compromised lamina propria and glottal incompetence, with air leakage through the midline of the anterior two-thirds of the folds. Vocal quality reveals a strained quality with little pitch change and low intensity with difficulty speaking loudly without fatigue. Individuals may experience periods of aphonia and increased tension in the laryngeal muscles (Giovanni and colleagues, 2007).

Treatment for sulcus vocalis is determined by a number of factors, including the anatomic and physiological severity of the sulcus and the patient's response to behavioral probing by the clinician. Often, when we introduce techniques that seek to adjust the balance among proper glottal closure, pitch, and loudness, vocal quality improves and the need for medical intervention is obviated. When the sulcus is severe, however, treatment for the sulcus vocalis will often be a combination of medical and behavioral approaches. One surgical approach is described by Hirano and Bless (1993) as a sulcusectomy, in which an incision is made on each fold above the sulcus, usually for the length of each fold; the upper and lower borders of the sulcus are then sutured together, securing a mechanical coupling of the two parts as healing progresses. A second surgical approach for correcting sulcus vocalis is a mucosal slicing technique, making many microvertical slices across the sulcus, as described by Pontes and Behlau (1993). Others have attempted to reduce the sulcus by injecting collagen, fat, or fascia into the sulcus, usually in the middle of the offended vocal fold (Sulica, 2009; Dursun and colleagues, 2008). Collagen is one of the components of Reinke's space and it can be injected in the deep layers of the lamina propria. Kishimoto and colleagues (2009) suggested that the replacement of scar tissue with an implant might lead to regeneration of the vocal fold mucosa and its tissue properties. Six patients were implanted with atelocollagen sheets into the lamina propria. The authors reported that postoperative changes in aerodynamic and acoustic properties were variable among patients; however, gradual improvements in those measures were seen in most cases within a year. Medialization thyroplasties (Isshiki and colleagues, 1996) and strap muscle transposition (Su and colleagues, 2004) have also been suggested to reduce glottal incompetence.

After medical intervention, glottal function needs reassessment by the SLP. Improved function may still require that old habits of the patient need to be identified and corrected, particularly in reducing vocal hyperfunction. Although voice therapy after surgery for sulcus vocalis is highly individualized, Voice Facilitating Approaches (VFAs) that have been productive include pitch shifts, loudness changes, lateral digital pressure, and experimentation with firmer glottal closure. Auditory feedback with real-time amplification has been found useful in establishing easy-onset phonation after surgery with this patient group.

WEBBING

A laryngeal web growing across the glottis between the two vocal folds inhibits normal fold vibration, often producing a high-pitched, rough sound during vibration and seriously compromising the open glottis. Webs may be congenital or acquired. A congenital web, which is detected at the time of birth, is the result of the glottal membrane failing to separate in embryonic development. Depending on the size of the web, the baby will produce stridor (inhalation noises), shortness of breath, and often a different high-pitched (squeal) cry. Approximately three-fourths of all laryngeal webs cross the glottis (Strome, 1982). Testing for chromosome 22q deletion is suggested because this may be associated with velocardiofacial syndrome (Miyamoto and colleagues, 2004). The presence of a congenital web requires immediate surgery, often followed by a temporary tracheostomy; usually, an infant larynx will recover over a period of four to six weeks.

Acquired webs result from some kind of bilateral trauma of the medial edges of the vocal folds. Anything that might serve as an irritant to the mucosal surface of the folds may be the initial cause of the webbing. Because the two vocal folds are so close together at the anterior commissure, any surface irritation due to prolonged infection or trauma may cause the inner margins of the two fold surfaces to grow together. To explain further, one principle of plastic surgery is that, when approximated together, offended tissue surfaces tend to grow and fuse together. This same principle explains why webbing occurs. The offended surface of the two approximated folds tends to grow together, in this case forming a thin membrane across the glottis. Webbing grows across the glottis in an anterior to posterior fashion, usually ceasing about one-third of the distance from the anterior commissure, where the distance between the two folds becomes too great. Severe laryngeal infections sometimes cause enough glottal irritation to precipitate web formation. Bilateral surgery of the folds, perhaps for papilloma or nodules, can also be followed by a web (Wetmore and colleagues, 1985). External trauma to the folds, such as a direct hit on the thyroid cartilage that causes it to fracture, may damage the folds behind it, thus creating enough glottal irritation for a web to develop. Laryngeal or tracheal surgery is the most frequent event producing the postsurgical acquired web. As an abnormal healing process, both folds grow together anteriorly, forming a glottal web sometimes called a synechia.

A laryngeal web may cause severe dysphonia as well as shortness of breath depending on how extensively the webbing crosses the glottis. The treatment for the formation of a web is surgery. The webbing is cut, freeing the two folds. To prevent the surgically removed web from growing again, a vertical keel is placed between the two folds and kept there until complete healing has been achieved. The laryngologist fixates the keel, which is shaped very much like a boat rudder and is about the size of a fingernail, between the folds, preventing them from approximating. The patient is then on voice rest as long as the keel is in place because its presence inhibits normal fold vibration. When the keel is removed, often in six to eight weeks, the patient generally requires some voice therapy to restore normal phonation. If there was extensive damage to the larynx from the trauma, it may well be impossible after healing and voice therapy to develop the same kind of normal voice the patient had before the accident. The prognosis for voice recovery after webbing and its surgical treatment is highly individualized and depends on the extent of the trauma and the size of the resulting web. We have had patients who were able to speak and sing with a normal voice following surgical reduction of the web and a course of voice therapy.

LARYNGEAL CANCER

Cancer or carcinoma in the vocal tract is a life-threatening disease that requires comprehensive medical–surgical management. Lip and intraoral cancers rarely contribute to changes in voice, but they may have obvious negative effects on articulation. Extensive oral lesions involving the tongue, perhaps even requiring partial or total surgical removal of the tongue (glossectomy), or palatal and velar cancer can seriously affect articulation, vocal resonance, and, of course, swallowing. The American Cancer Society estimated 52,000 new cases of head and neck cancer in 2011 (American Cancer Society, 2011). Head and neck cancers are among the fifteen most common cancers and account for nearly 3% of all new cancers each year, according to the National Cancer Institute (Siegel and colleagues, 2011). In terms of costs, head and neck cancers are responsible for $3.2 billion in healthcare expenditures and approximately 4.4% of all cancer treatment expenditures each year (Jemal and colleagues, 2010).

Some of the identified causes of oral cancer include smoking (particularly pipe smoking), use of smokeless tobacco, chronic infections, herpes, repeated trauma to the irritated site, and leukoplakia (whitish plaque). Often patients first experience chronic lesions in the mouth or on the tongue that do not seem to heal. Usually continuous pain near the lesion site brings the patient to the physician. The majority of these oral lesions are treated successfully with microsurgery (removal of small lesions) and radiation therapy. The primary goal of surgery–radiation therapy is to eradicate the primary lesion so that it does not spread (metastasize) to another adjacent or remote body site. Sometimes carcinoma is detected in the nasal sinuses and at sites within the pharynx, although such lesions are relatively rare. The most serious vocal tract malignancies, however, are those that involve the larynx. Malignancies involving the larynx, by their position in the airway, present a serious potential threat to airway adequacy. Laryngeal cancer comprises approximately 6% of all malignancies diagnosed annually in the United States (American Cancer Society, 2011).

In general, laryngeal cancers can be classified into three groups, depending on the site of the lesion: (1) supraglottal, involving structures such as the ventricular and aryepiglottic folds, the epiglottis, the arytenoid cartilages, and the walls of the hypopharynx; (2) glottal, from the anterior commissure to the vocal process ends of the arytenoids; and (3) subglottal, involving the cricoid cartilage and trachea. The treatment combines radiation therapy and surgery for small to moderate lesions; extensive cancer requires perhaps a hemilaryngectomy, a supraglottal laryngectomy, or total laryngectomy. We consider laryngeal cancer, rehabilitation after laryngectomy, and the role of the SLP in detail in Chapter 9.

SUMMARY

Organic voice disorders may result from various laryngeal conditions, such as papilloma, granuloma, webbing, and reflux. For each of the various organic voice disorders, we discussed medical management and the role of the SLP in evaluation and therapy. It is the responsibility of the SLP to be familiar with each voice disorder, its sequelae (e.g., signs and symptoms), and management. By being familiar with the pathology of the voice disorder, we can better counsel our clients and provide efficacious behavioral intervention. In many cases, we are the first professional to detect an organic-related voice disorder and the first professional to make the critical referral to the ENT physician.

CLINICAL CONCEPTS

The following clinical concepts correspond with many of the objectives at the beginning of this chapter:

1. Long ago Van Riper and Irwin (1958) said that speech is defective if it interferes with communication, draws undue attention to itself, or causes the speaker to be somehow maladjusted. The same may be said for voice (see Chapter 1).

2. Hoarseness that persists longer than several days is often identified by the laryngologist as a possible symptom of serious laryngeal disease, and it may be. Reflux, laryngeal cancer, and recurrent respiratory papillomatosis are examples of organic disease processes that require immediate attention and referral.

3. Contact granulomas (ulcers) are multifactorial in nature and are considered a chronic inflammatory disease of the larynx. They seem to result from one of three causes or a combination of these: hard glottal attack along with throat clearing and coughing, laryngopharyngeal reflux, and endotracheal intubation. Behavioral voice therapy in combination with medical intervention is a powerful approach (see Chapter 7).

4. Cysts may masquerade as space-occupying lesions of a functional nature, such as vocal nodules or polyps, because they are associated with hoarseness and breathiness. Due to their etiology, however, they normally require surgical intervention followed by voice therapy to eliminate any maladaptive vocal behaviors the speaker may have adopted (see Chapter 7).

5. Acid reflux can contribute to respiratory compromise, sinusitis, contact ulcers, and other pathologies of the upper aerodigestive tract and airway. The symptoms of acid reflux vary considerably among voice patients, ranging from no symptoms to mild heartburn, to extreme burning or choking in the larynx, awakening the patient from a deep sleep. It is imperative that the SLP be aware of the symptoms of GERD and LPRD, and make appropriate referrals.

GUIDED READING

Read the following articles.

Gupta, R., & Sataloff, R. T. (2009). Laryngopharyngeal reflux: Current concepts and questions. *Current Opinion in Otolaryngology & Head and Neck Surgery, 17*(3), 143–148.

Karkos, P. D., Leong, S. C., Apostolidou, M. T., & Apostolidis, T. (2006). Laryngeal manifestations and pediatric laryngopharyngeal reflux. *American Journal of Otolaryngology—Head and Neck Medicine and Surgery, 27*(Suppl. 1), 200–203.

Discuss the authors' findings with respect to upper airway changes related to GERD and LPRD.

Read the following article.

Harris, A. T., Atkinson, H., Vaughan, C., & Knight, L. C. (2012). Presentation of laryngeal papilloma in childhood: The Leeds experience. *The International Journal of Clinical Practice, 66*(2), 183–184.

Discuss the authors' take-home message with respect to children who present with hoarse voice quality and shortness of breath.

PREPARING FOR THE PRAXIS™

Directions: Please read the case study and answer the five questions that follow. (Please see page 319 for the answer key.)

> *A 38-year-old music salesman presented to the clinic with pain in the laryngeal area following a bout of bronchitis and extensive coughing and throat clearing. He reported occasionally coughing up small amounts of blood. He said he lifts weights but reported the healthy strategy of exhaling while flexing. He does not smoke and he reports minimal water intake. Vocal quality was normal in pitch and quality. He coughed and throat-cleared throughout the assessment. The salesman was overheard chastising an employee on his cell phone using hard glottal attack. He said he was recently prescribed anti-reflux medication by his physician. The patient's F0 for a sustained /a/ revealed 161Hz with a RAP of .236% and shimmer of 1.56%. Transglottal airflow was 138 ml/s.*

1. This client most likely presents with:
   A. Adult-onset papilloma
   B. Contact granuloma
   C. Laryngomalacia
   D. A laryngeal cyst

2. The near normal acoustic measures are likely due to the fact that the lesions are:
   A. Located on the nonvibrational portion of the glottis
   B. Soft and pliable
   C. Located lateral to the glottal margin
   D. Pedunculated

3. Laryngostroboscopic examination will most likely reveal:
   A. An anterior web
   B. Vocal nodules
   C. Granulated tissue at the posterior aspect of the glottis
   D. Bowed vocal folds

4. This hyperplastic laryngeal abnormality is most likely secondary to:
   A. Laryngopharyngeal reflux
   B. Chronic laryngeal collisional forces of coughing and throat clearing
   C. Hard glottal attack
   D. All of these

5. The most comprehensive approach to this vocal fold pathology is:
   A. Surgical removal of the abnormality
   B. Continued anti-reflux regimen and intervention for reduced hard glottal attack
   C. Vocal hygiene only
   D. Voice rest

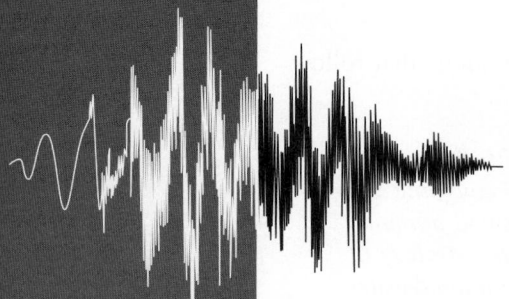

Neurogenic Voice Disorders

In Chapter 2, we reviewed the normal anatomy and physiology required for voice. We considered the causes and treatment of a number of non-neurogenic voice disorders in Chapters 3 and 4. In this chapter, we review the neurological structures and processes that must function in coordinated balance to produce normal voice. By gaining an appreciation of the neurophysiological bases of voice, we can then begin to recognize and pinpoint the causes of neurogenic dysphonia, the focus of this chapter. As Duffy (2005) suggests, speech changes can be the first or only a manifestation of neurogenic disease. Recognition of speech changes can have a significant impact on medical diagnosis and care. Indeed, on numerous occasions, the speech-language pathologist (SLP) has been the first to identify the salient features of myasthenia gravis (MG), Parkinson's disease (PD), amyotrophic lateral sclerosis (ALS), and even progressive supranuclear palsy (PSP). Only through early detection and differential diagnosis are the SLP and others on the patient's healthcare team able to generate an intervention program that directly addresses the patient's deficits and long-term communication options.

To understand the complexities of neurogenic dysphonia, it is necessary to have an understanding of the innervation of the larynx and resonators from the central and peripheral nervous system. Note that a comprehensive discussion of the neuroanatomical and neurophysiological bases of phonation is beyond the scope of this text. Readers are directed to textbooks by Brookshire (2007), Duffy (2005), Yorkston and colleagues (2010), and the classic textbook by Darley and colleagues (1975). In this chapter, however, we do offer a working view of the central nervous system, the peripheral nervous system, and innervation of the muscles necessary for voice.

A WORKING VIEW OF THE NERVOUS SYSTEM

The central nervous system (CNS) and the peripheral nervous system (PNS) coordinate all laryngeal operations, from the elevation of the larynx for swallowing, to the tri-level valve closure required for a cough, to the nuanced vocal fold vibrations of the operatic lyric soprano. We know far less about the neural controls required for human singing and talking than we do about the neural governing of laryngeal vegetative functions such as breathing, coughing, or swallowing. The human not only has all the sensory-motor structures and functions of most mammals, but also has added abilities to subdue or augment response (for example, suppress crying when the situation is not appropriate), or to use the voice for emotional or artistic expression. The expanded cerebral cortex unique to humans enables one to use voicing cues (for example, pitch and loudness inflections) for speaking, singing, and other forms of verbal communication.

THE CENTRAL NERVOUS SYSTEM, THE CORTEX, AND ITS PROJECTIONS

The CNS is composed of the brain and spinal cord, and is located within the bony, protective structures of the cranium and vertebral column. Sensory and motor areas within the cerebral cortex, cerebellum, and basal ganglia contribute to production of voice (Loucks and colleagues, 2007; Simonyan and Horwitz, 2011). Researchers suggest that both the frontal and left temporal lobes are primarily, though not exclusively, involved with the motor aspects of voice production, while the bilateral parietal lobes provide important sensory feedback about voice production (Dronkers, 1996; Baldo and colleagues, 2010). Initiation of voice begins in the inferior and lateral aspects of the primary motor cortex (Brown and colleagues, 2008; Parkinson and colleagues, 2012). Nerve impulses are sent then primarily via the corticobulbar tract to brainstem nuclei, in particular, the nucleus ambiguus. Other cortical areas, such as the premotor cortex, the supplemental motor cortex, and Broca's area, contribute to planning and programming phonation, relying on input from the cerebellum and basal ganglia (Ferrand, 2012).

Normal voice also depends on one's ability to hear and process ongoing voice production. The temporal lobes provide cortical input for audition. Heschl's gyrus, the primary auditory cortex, bilaterally receives tonotopic frequency input from the medial geniculate bodies of the thalamus. Other auditory areas, such as the auditory association area and Wernicke's area, may also play a role in processing one's own voice production (Friederici, 2011).

Pyramidal and Extrapyramidal Tracts

The pyramidal and extrapyramidal tracts are part of the CNS. The pyramidal tract is composed of long axons that extend from the cortical neurons located in the primary motor strip and travel uninterrupted until they reach their corresponding cranial nerve nuclei in the brainstem. As illustrated in Figure 5.1, the pyramidal tract is composed of white-matter nerve fibers (corticobulbar and corticospinal) that pass in a bundle between the basal ganglia and the thalamus, which is called the internal capsule.

One way to think of the pyramidal tract is that it functions like a neural turnpike, permitting the transmission of impulses from the cortex to the cranial nerve nuclei without interruption of local neural traffic. Conversely, the extrapyramidal tract (Figure 5.2) is similar to a country road, with fibers stopping in many locations, bringing neural transmissions to synapses with the basal ganglia, across to the thalamus and the subthalamus, and to the cerebellum, among other structures. The extrapyramidal tract enables extensive checking and balancing of sensory and motor information with its many interconnections among the cortex, thalamus, and the basal ganglia. The many checks and balances afforded by the extrapyramidal system are crucial for maintaining posture, tone, and associated activities that provide a foundation for skilled movements executed by the pyramidal tract.

FIGURE 5.1 Schematic View of the Pyramidal Tract

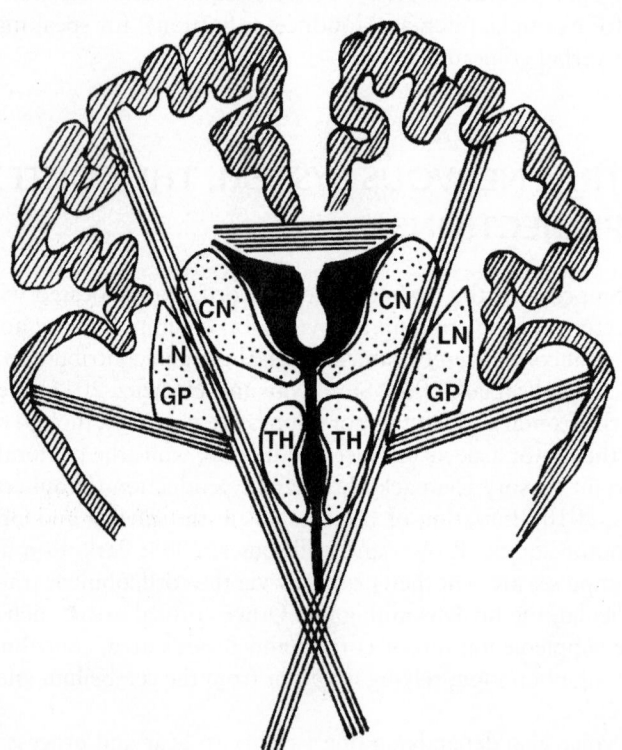

The pyramidal tract is like a neural turnpike with fibers descending uninterrupted via the internal capsule from their cortical origins to their terminations at cranial nerve nuclei in the brain stem. This line drawing shows basal ganglia (including CN, caudate nucleus; LN, lenticular nucleus; GP, globus pallidus), and TH, thalamus. Pyramidal fibers are depicted as ▤▤.

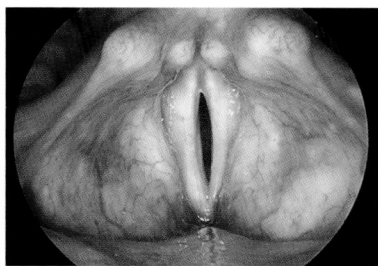

Normal vocal folds

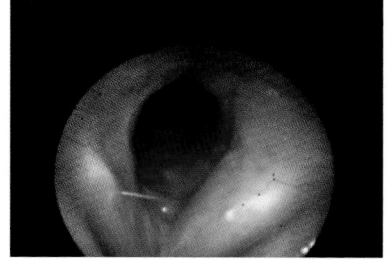

Amyloid deposits

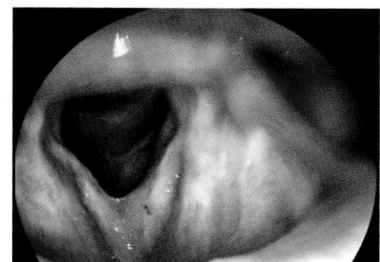

Anterior web

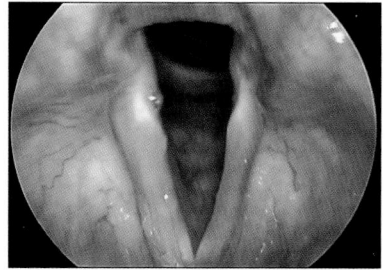

Atrophy abducted

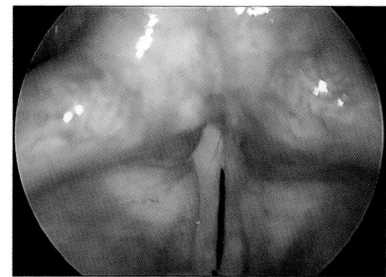

Atrophy adducted

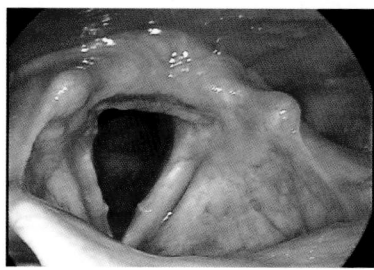

Bilateral nodules 1 abducted

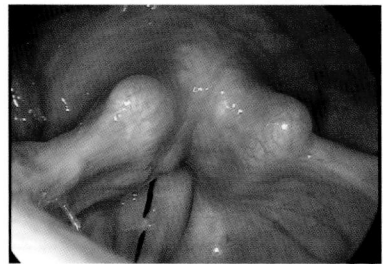

Bilateral nodules 1 adducted

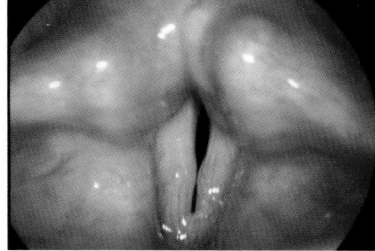

Bilateral nodules 2 adducted

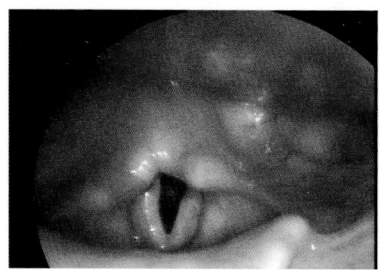

Bilateral adductor paralysis

Photos courtesy of Ozlem Tulunay-Ugur, M.D., UAMS Voice and Swallowing Center
(http://www.uamshealth.com/seniorvoiceandswallowing).

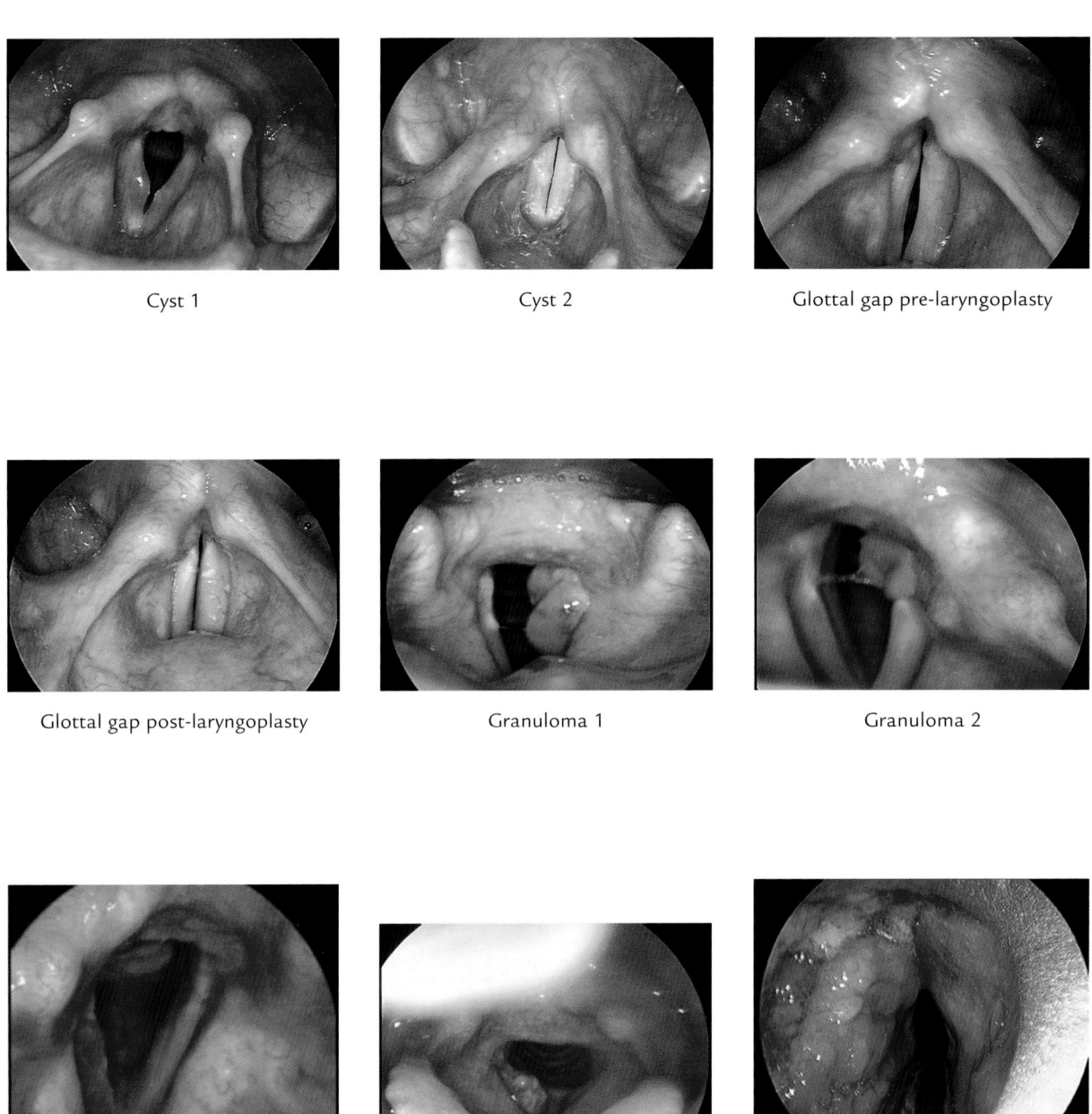

Cyst 1

Cyst 2

Glottal gap pre-laryngoplasty

Glottal gap post-laryngoplasty

Granuloma 1

Granuloma 2

Hemorrhage

Laryngeal cancer 1

Laryngeal cancer 2

Photos courtesy of Ozlem Tulunay-Ugur, M.D., UAMS Voice and Swallowing Center
(http://www.uamshealth.com/seniorvoiceandswallowing).

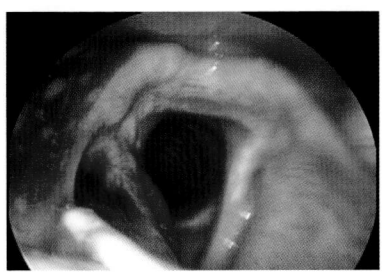

Laryngeal fracture

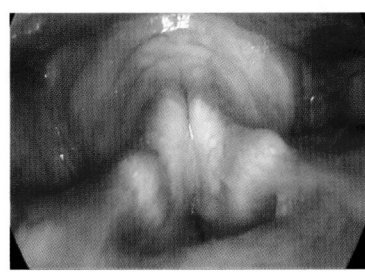

Laryngeal muscle tension 1

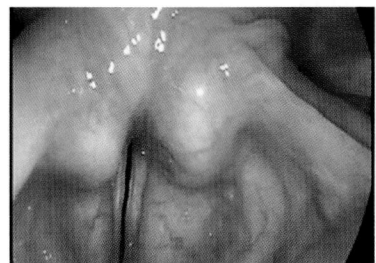

Laryngeal muscle tension 2

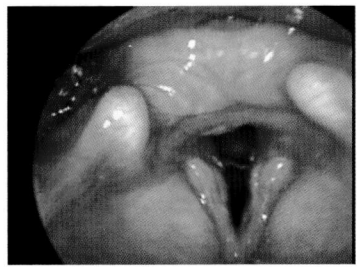

Laryngitis

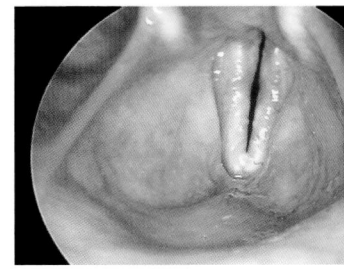

Laryngitis, post-voice rest

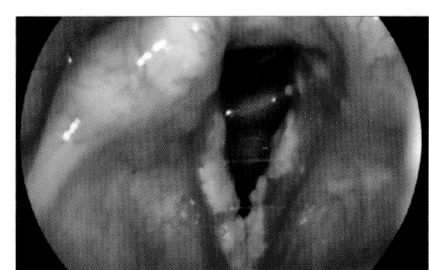

Leukoplakia

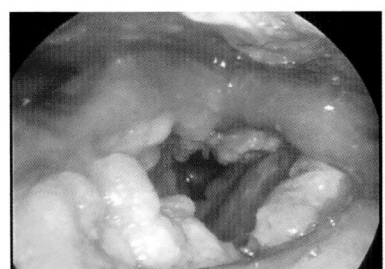

Papilloma

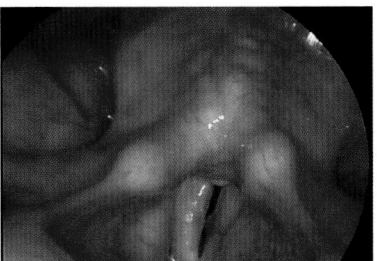

Polyp 1

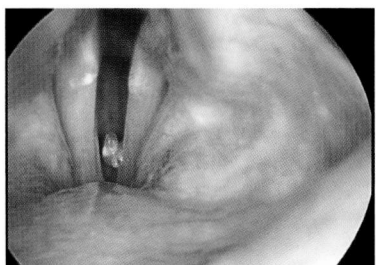

Polyp 2

Photos courtesy of Ozlem Tulunay-Ugur, M.D., UAMS Voice and Swallowing Center
(http://www.uamshealth.com/seniorvoiceandswallowing).

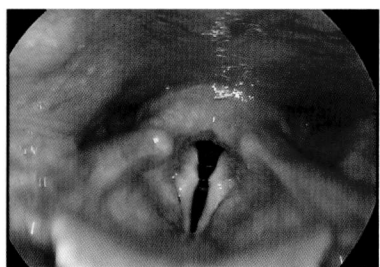

Presbylaryngis

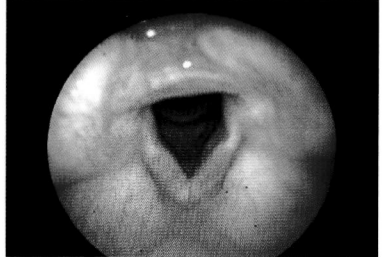

Pseudosulcus

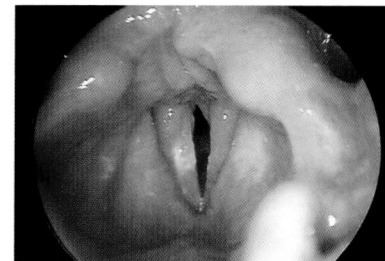

Reflux pre-PPI

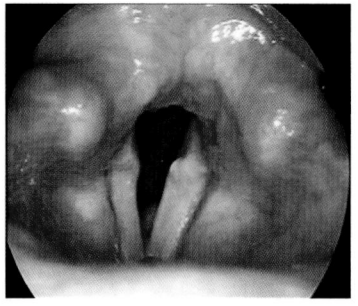

Reflux post-PPI

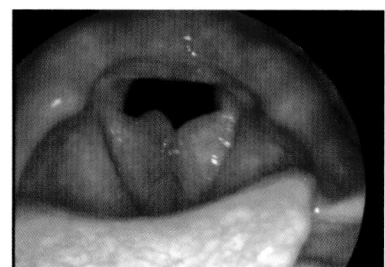

Reinke's edema

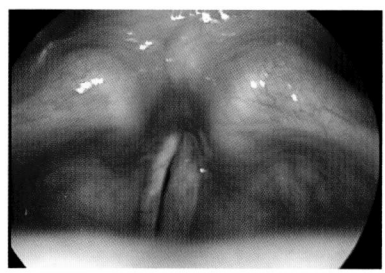

Scar

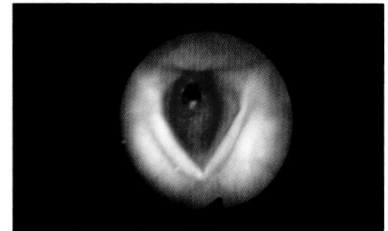

Subglottic stenosis

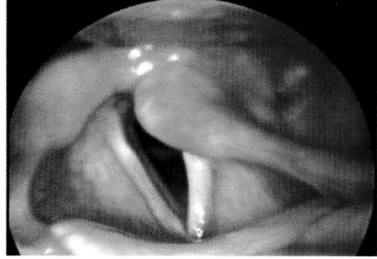

Unilateral paralysis

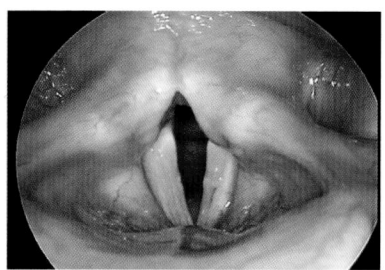

Varix-ecstasia

Photos courtesy of Ozlem Tulunay-Ugur, M.D., UAMS Voice and Swallowing Center
(http://www.uamshealth.com/seniorvoiceandswallowing).

FIGURE 5.2 Schematic View of the Extrapyramidal Tract

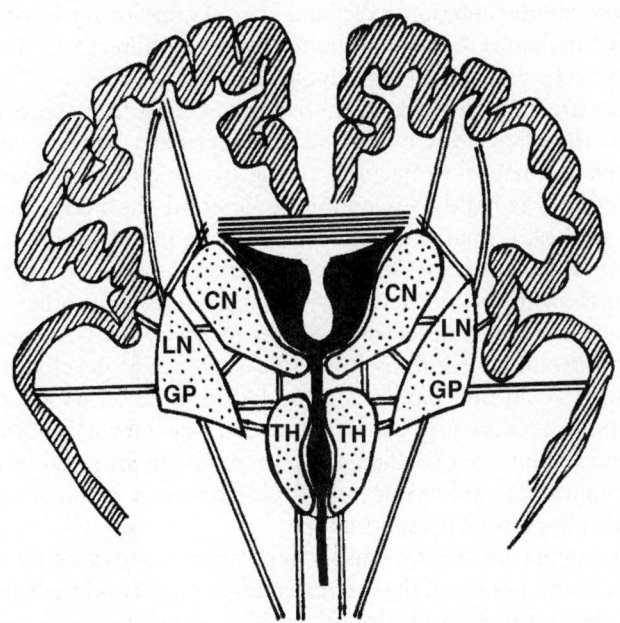

The line drawing of the extrapyramidal tract depicts its neural fibers like a neural country road, starting and stopping at various cortical, basal ganglia, and thalamic sites and ending (or starting) at lower brain stem sites. These extrapyramidal fibers are depicted as ══════. This line drawing shows the basal ganglia (including CN, caudate nucleus; LN, lenticular nucleus; GP, globus pallidus); and TH, thalamus.

Thalamus, Internal Capsule, and the Basal Ganglia

The subcortical areas occupied by the thalamus, which is medial in the hemisphere; the internal capsule that runs laterally adjacent to it; and the more lateral basal ganglia are known collectively as the corpus striatum, which gets its name from the contrast of the gray matter nuclei and the white-matter projections between them. The corpus striatum is the site of most of the sensory–motor integrations of the cerebrum. The thalamus is to sensation what the basal ganglia are to motor behavior.

Even the thalamus has its posterior (pure sensory) and anterior (sensory-influenced motor) divisions. The posterior thalamus is known as the pulvinar body and receives neural impulses from the auditory tract via the medial geniculates, the most inferior–posterior of the pulvinar. From the medial geniculates and after some central mixing within the thalamus, the auditory fibers radiate in a bundle superiorly to the primary auditory cortex, Heschl's gyrus. Similarly, the visual fibers come into the lateral geniculate bodies of the pulvinar section of the thalamus, undergo central mixing, exit in a bundle, and go directly to the primary visual cortex in the occipital lobes.

There is also some speculation (Boone, 1997, 1998; Minckler, 1972) that afferent–efferent fibers between the lateral wall of the pulvinar body and the temporale planum play an important role in auditory comprehension of the spoken word and have some control in producing vocal response. Within the main thalamic body, there appears to be much integration of sensory information occurring, getting organized for some kind of motor response via the anterior nuclei and ventral anterior nuclei of the thalamus. From the anterior thalamus, sensory projections go either directly to the sensory cerebral cortex or to nuclei within the basal ganglia.

While there are some basal ganglia–thalamic connections crossing within the internal capsule, the main body of the internal capsule is largely composed of the descending–ascending neural projections of the pyramidal tract. The internal capsule area of the brain is highly susceptible to cerebral vascular accidents (CVAs), also known as strokes, primarily because much of its blood supply is furnished by an artery known as the lenticular striata (often called the artery of apoplexy), which for some reason seems to be blocked by thrombosis more than other cerebral arteries. Such blockage of blood causes white-matter projections to die, resulting in contra-unilateral symptoms of paralysis (note that such a high-level lesion would not cause contralateral vocal fold paralysis). Any lesion (disease, stroke, or trauma) to the internal capsule could cause contralateral sensory–motor symptoms of skeletal muscles; these lesions are classified as upper motor neuron lesions. Sensory loss could include hypothesia, and motor loss would be seen in hemiparesis or hemiplegia (paralysis with hypertonicity/spasticity).

The basal ganglia utilize the sensory information provided by the thalamus. The main nuclei of the basal ganglia are the caudate nuclei and the lenticular nuclei, which include the putamen and globus pallidus. Bilateral innervations of both smooth and striated muscle occur within both the caudate and lenticular nuclei and, at this level, we first see bilateral innervation of velar, pharyngeal, and laryngeal muscles. The basal ganglia utilize the continuous, multiple sensory information from the thalamus in organizing appropriate motor responses (including vocalization).

Neurotransmitters

It should be acknowledged at this point that the transmission of neural impulse among various nuclei via white-matter nerves is facilitated by several enzymes known as neurotransmitters. At the termination of nerves within the cerebrum, where neural synapses occur, serotonin functions as a nervous system neurotransmitter. The sympathetic nervous system employs epinephrine and norepinephrine to aid in the transmission of neural impulses for innervation of smooth muscle, glands, and viscera. The basal ganglia depend on dopamine as the primary neurotransmitter. The facial, neck, and skeletal muscles depend on acetylcholine as the chemical mediator between the muscle's nerve nucleus and the muscle body itself. While neural transmission can be altered or stopped by isolated lesions to the gray body or its nerve connections, many of the diseases of the CNS cause inhibition or overproduction of neurotransmitters. For example, it is well known that degenerative changes in the substantia nigra cause a deficiency in a chemical neural transmitter known as dopamine in the caudate nucleus and putamen. The disturbed basal ganglia and extrapyramidal control circuit results in a hypokinetic dysarthria observed in PD (this is discussed later in this chapter). The symptoms of PD are vastly minimized by Levodopa, a synthetic dopamine.

The Brainstem and the Cerebellum

The projection fibers from both the pyramidal and extrapyramidal tracts extend anteriorly into the pons and posteriorly via the cerebral peduncle terminating into the medulla oblongata. This cortical to lower center tract includes both afferent and efferent fibers. There are neural connections from the midbrain to the pons and then to the cerebellum, and connections from the peduncle area into the cerebellum. The medial hypothalamus is the lowest structure of the midbrain; under it are the lesser (in number) gray bodies and myelinated nerve tracts (innumerable) that comprise the brainstem. The hypothalamus forms the lateral walls of the central third ventricle. Connected to it are some gray bodies hugging the third ventricle aqueduct; these gray bodies contain an important vegetative respiratory area known as the periaqueductal gray (Davis and colleagues, 1996). Hypothalamic fibers and pyramidal and extrapyramidal projections communicate anteriorly in the brainstem to the pons, while posterior fibers form the cerebral peduncle, which extends down, forming the medulla. The medulla extends from the lowermost portion of the pons, with its upper portion forming the floor of the fourth ventricle.

The cerebellum wraps around the pons and cerebral peduncle, and has many interconnections with the pons, cerebral peduncle, medulla, and spinal cord. The cerebellum functions as the great regulator of the extrapyramidal tract, coordinating sensory information (proprioceptive, kinesthetic, tactile, auditory, and visual) with coordinated motor response. Lesions to the cerebellum from trauma or disease cause speech symptoms of incoordination, known as ataxic dysarthria. The voice–speech symptoms of cerebellar lesions are prosodic slowdown (scanning speech); abrupt and unpredictable changes in resonance, pitch, and loudness; and reduced articulatory accuracy for speech, all sounding like the speech of someone highly intoxicated.

Eighty percent of the descending projection fibers coming from the cerebral peduncle cross over (decussate) to the other side in the medulla just below the brainstem; 20% remain ipsilateral (on the same side). Of great importance to voice is the nucleus ambiguus in the superior medulla, located just below the pyramidal decussation. As the medulla extends downward, it begins to narrow into the spinal column. The same posterior–sensory/anterior–motor organization continues in the medulla and down into the spinal cord. Posterior nerve tracts and gray nuclei (left and right) are sensory in nature, while the anterior white-matter tracts and anterior horn nuclei (left and right) execute motor function.

Let us consider briefly what constitutes an upper motor neuron (UMN) lesion or a lower motor neuron (LMN) lesion. Functionally, a bilateral UMN lesion produces symptoms of hypertonity, such as in a CVA (stroke) in which the patient may experience hemiparesis or hemiplegia (one-sided weakness or full paralysis of extremities, respectively). Functionally, an LMN lesion results in flaccidity and muscle atrophy, such as when the cutting of the recurrent laryngeal nerve (RLN) during surgery causes unilateral vocal fold paralysis. UMNs begin at the cerebral cortex and end at the nucleus ambiguus; LMNs begin at the nucleus ambiguus and travel down the spinal cord, ending at the lowest spinal nucleus. Also included as LMNs are the nerves exiting from the pons and medulla (such as the cranial nerves), and the nerves that carry sensory and motor impulses to and from the various spinal nuclei for their particular muscles. The autonomic motor system and these cerebrospinal nerves, including their associated sensory receptors, constitute the PNS.

THE PERIPHERAL NERVOUS SYSTEM (PNS)

We will limit our discussion of the PNS primarily to the cranial nerves that have a direct impact on voice, and in particular to two branches of cranial nerve X (Vagus)—the superior and recurrent laryngeal nerves—which innervate the larynx.

Cranial nerves V, VII, and VIII have a direct impact on speech, but they do not appear primary in the production of voice. Cranial nerve V, trigeminal, emerges from the pons with its primary motor fibers innervating the muscles of mastication; the sensory components that might influence voice are the tactile sensations of the nose and oral mucosa. Cranial nerve VII, facial, leaves the lower portion of the pons and terminates in its motor innervation of facial muscles; its sensory components include taste in the anterior two-thirds of the tongue and sensation to the soft palate. Cranial nerve VIII, acoustic, has its cochlear division ending in the dorsal and ventral cochlear nuclei in the superior medulla; leaving the cochlear nuclei, the auditory pathways begin and continue to various neural stations, ending in Heschl's gyrus in the temporal lobe. As mentioned earlier in this chapter and throughout the text, the auditory system appears to play a primary role in voice production and control.

Cranial Nerves (IX, X, XI, XII)

We give special attention to cranial nerves IX, X, XI, and XII because each has some role in phonation and voice resonance. For each nerve, we will look at origin and insertion with a brief statement relative to nerve function, especially as it relates to voice.

Cranial Nerve IX, Glossopharyngeal. Originating laterally in the medulla, the nerve passes through the jugular foramen coursing between the internal carotid artery and the external jugular vein and subdivides into its numerous branches that go to various innervation sites. Its functions include taste in the posterior third of the tongue and sensation to the fauces, tonsils, pharynx, and soft palate. Its primary motor innervation is to the superior pharyngeal constrictor in the pharynx and to the stylopharyngeus muscle.

Cranial Nerve X, Vagus. The Vagus nerve, in addition to its many functions of control of the autonomic nervous system involving thoracic and abdominal viscera, has two important branches that innervate the larynx: the superior laryngeal nerve (SLN) and the recurrent laryngeal nerve (RLN) (see Figure 5.3). In the next section of this chapter, we will present in detail the origins and functions of the SLN and the RLN. The Vagus nerve originates in the nucleus ambiguus in the medulla, from which it emerges laterally and courses its way, continually branching along the way, with particular branches terminating at the various innervation sites from the pharynx to the abdominal viscera (Ardito and colleagues, 2004). Affecting voice are the sensory components of the Vagus, with sensory innervation of the pharynx and larynx. Motor aspects affecting voice include innervation of the velum; the base of the tongue; superior, middle, and inferior pharyngeal constrictors; larynx; and autonomic ganglia of the thorax (affecting the respiratory aspects of phonation).

As the Vagus nerve leaves the nucleus ambiguus and exits laterally from the superior medulla and descends, it soon begins a series of branches (see Figure 5.3). The first and most superior nerve branch off the Vagus is the pharyngeal branch, which contains both sensory and motor branches that supply the mucous membrane and selected muscles of the pharynx and soft palate (see Chapter 10). The second branch is the SLN, which transmits sensory information from the base of the tongue and the mucous membrane of the supraglottis; it also transmits motor innervation to part of the lower pharyngeal constrictor and to the cricothyroid muscles. The third branch is the RLN, which transmits sensory

FIGURE 5.3 The Vagus Nerve

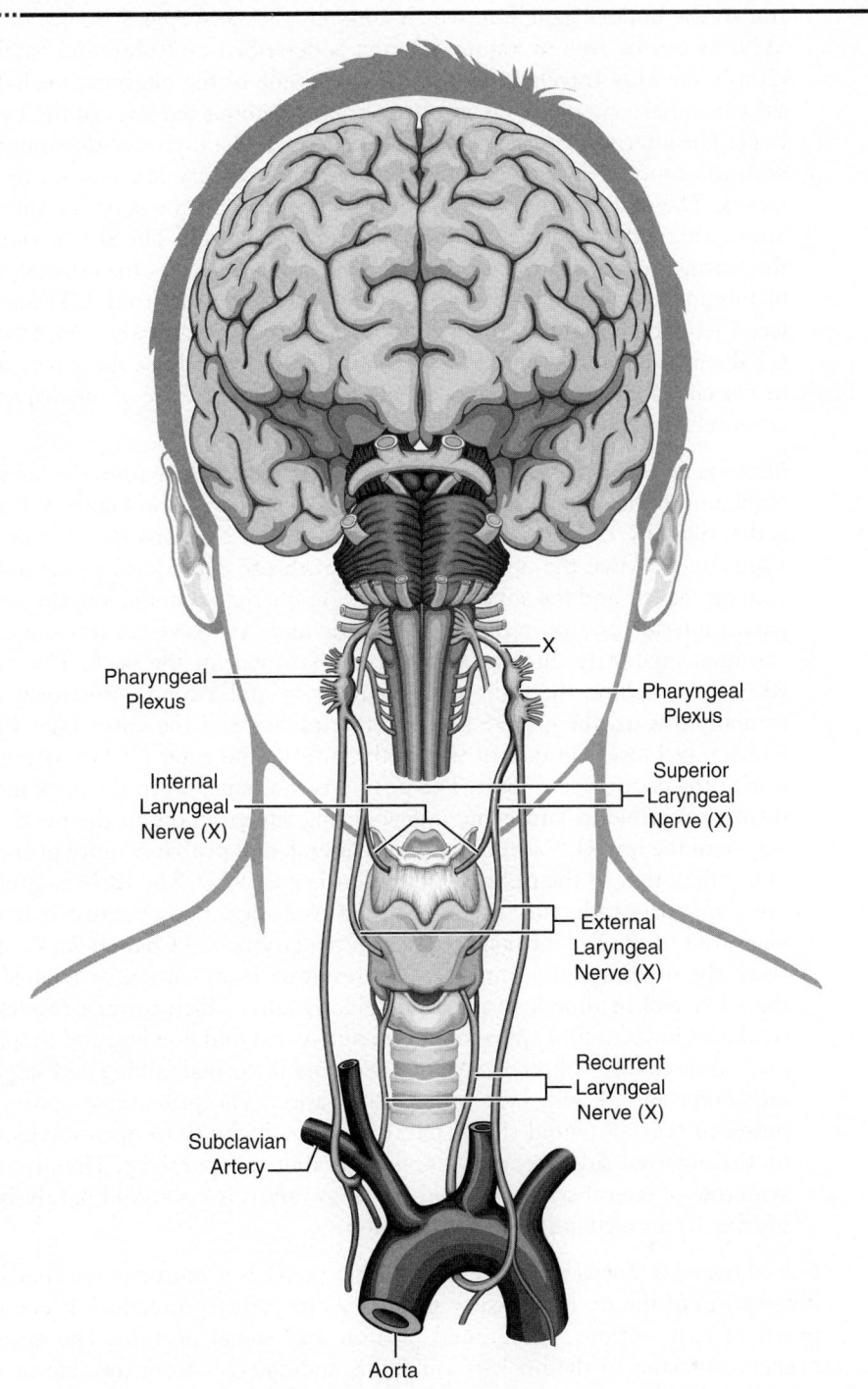

Pharyngeal Plexus

Pharyngeal Plexus

X

Internal Laryngeal Nerve (X)

Superior Laryngeal Nerve (X)

External Laryngeal Nerve (X)

Recurrent Laryngeal Nerve (X)

Subclavian Artery

Aorta

information from the subglottis; it also transmits motor innervation to all the intrinsic laryngeal muscles except the cricothyroid. In the list below, we review the anatomy and physiology of the SLN and the RLN (see also Chapter 2) and we summarize the major laryngeal and voice findings with paresis or paralysis of these nerves.

Superior Laryngeal Nerve. The SLN branches from the vagus nerve just inferior to the nodose ganglion, which contains the sensory cell bodies of the SLN. As can be seen in Figure 5.3, and is described by Rubin and Sataloff (2007), the SLN travels inferiorly along the side of the pharynx, medial to the carotid artery, and splits into two branches about the level of the hyoid bone. The internal division of the SLN penetrates the thyrohyoid membrane with the superior laryngeal artery and supplies sensory innervation to the larynx. The external division of the SLN lies close to the superior thyroid artery, although its exact relation to the artery is variable. The SLN is vital to the tensing–relaxing of the true vocal folds, as it penetrates the cricothyroid membrane and provides motor innervation to the cricothyroid (CT) muscle (see Chapter 2). Inability to elevate vocal pitch is the primary symptom of CT disease or trauma; in the case of unilateral CT paralysis, there may also be extreme hoarseness and occasional diplophonia (because of the disparate tension between the two vocal folds).

Recurrent Laryngeal Nerve. The nuclei of the RLN axons lie within the nucleus ambiguus in the medulla of the brainstem. As can be seen in Figure 5.3, and is described by Rubin and Sataloff (2007), the RLN axons travel with the Vagus nerve down the neck until they branch off at the level of the aortic arch on the left and the subclavian artery on the right. On the left, the nerve passes inferior and posterior to the aortic arch and reverses its course to continue superiorly into the visceral compartment of the neck. The right RLN loops behind the right subclavian artery and ascends superiorly and medially toward the groove between the trachea and the esophagus. Both RLNs travel just lateral to or within this groove and enter the larynx posterior to the cricothyroid joint. The positions of the nerves in the neck make them susceptible to iatrogenic injury during surgery. Low in the neck, the course of the left RLN is more oblique, lateral, and probably more prone to injury than that of the right RLN (Hollinshead, 1982). The RLN is vital to the abductory–adductory function of the true vocal folds because it innervates four of the five intrinsic muscles of the larynx (see Chapter 2). Paralysis of the thyroarytenoid muscle (TA) resulting from cutting or trauma to the RLN will in time lead to vocal fold atrophy, which in turn results in weakness in vocal fold approximation, mid–vocal fold bowing, and dysphonia. Subtle changes of pitch variation required in normal talking and singing are compromised with lack of TA innervation. The primary symptom of posterior cricoarytenoid (PCA) paralysis is the inability to open the glottis on the involved side, creating a unilateral abductor paralysis. The primary symptom of lateral cricoarytenoid (LCA) paralysis is vocal fold paralysis in the fixed, paramedian, abducted position.

Cranial Nerve XI, Spinal Accessory. Cranial nerve XI is a motor nerve that has innervation of the neck accessory muscles as its primary function. It is composed of two sections, the cranial portion and spinal portion. The cranial branch originates in the nucleus ambiguus and emerges from the side of the medulla with five successive small rootlets. Some fibers are distributed to the superior branches of the Vagus nerve, innervating the levator veli palatini and uvula. Fibers from the spinal portion of the nerve originate from the anterior horn of the spinal cord and merge with lower spinal portion fibers to innervate the major muscles of the neck, such as the sternocleidomastoid and the trapezius muscles. Lesions to cranial XI can cause obvious problems of resonance and in the contribution of neck accessory muscles to respiration.

Cranial Nerve XII, Hypoglossal. The hypoglossal nerve is a motor nerve innervating (as the name suggests) the extrinsic and intrinsic muscles of the tongue as well as some of the neck strap muscles. The nerve originates in its own nucleus, the hypoglossus nucleus, in the lower medulla, exiting laterally and entering the hypoglossal canal in the occipital bone, descending and then moving laterally into its many innervation sites. The muscles it innervates are the omohyoid, sternothyroid, styloglossus, hyoglossus, genioglossus, geniohyoid, sternohyoid, and all of the intrinsic muscles of the tongue. Cranial nerve XII has much to do with positioning of the larynx, that is, depression or elevation of the total laryngeal body, and is essential for all intrinsic movements of the tongue. Its primary impact on voice is on resonance and quality.

CHECK YOUR KNOWLEDGE

1. Which voice and resonance changes would one observe with a lesion high in the Vagus nerve? With a lesion in the SLN? With a lesion in the RLN?
2. Which branch of the Vagus nerve is more susceptible to injury from trauma or surgery? Explain.

CONDITIONS LEADING TO NEUROGENIC DYSPHONIA

Medical diagnoses associated with neurogenic dysphonia include vocal fold paralysis, laryngeal dystonia, essential tremor, Parkinson's disease, Huntington's disease, myasthenia gravis, multiple sclerosis, amyotrophic lateral sclerosis, progressive supranuclear palsy, multiple systems atrophy, and acquired brain injury (traumatic brain injury [TBI], CVA), to name just a few. A complete review of all medical conditions leading to dysphonia is beyond the scope of this text. The interested reader may refer to excellent textbooks about neurogenic speech disorders written by Duffy (2005) and Yorkston and colleagues (2010) for detailed information. For quick reference see Table 5.1, which summarizes the differential features in each dysarthria subtype.

In the following sections, we will review the identification and management of the neurogenic voice disorders most commonly seen by ENTs and SLPs in the voice clinic (Cohen and colleagues, 2012): vocal fold paralysis (unilateral and bilateral); laryngeal dystonia, for example, spasmodic dysphonia; essential tremor; Parkinson's disease; and acquired brain injury. Management of each requires cooperation among ENTs, neurologists, and SLPs, and the synthesis of each discipline's expertise becomes the genesis for innovative treatment approaches (McFarlane and Von Berg, 1998).

VOCAL FOLD PARALYSIS

Patients who suffer damage to cranial nerve X anywhere along its path, from the medulla to the larynx, have voice difficulties because of vocal fold paralysis. The roles of the ENT and SLP are to confirm the diagnosis and to be certain that

TABLE 5.1 Dysarthria Differential Features

Dysarthria Type	Site of Lesion	Neurophysiologic Impairment	Associated Neurologic Signs	Prominent Auditory-Perceptual Speech Characteristics
Flaccid	Lower motor neurons for speech (CNs V, VII, IX, X, XI, XII), cervical and thoracic spinal nerves.	Weakness.	Diminished reflexes (hyporeflexia), decreased muscle tone (i.e., flaccidity), muscle atrophy, fasciculations, (spontaneous, localized visible twitch in resting muscle).	Indistinct and labored articulation, hypernasality, breathy voice quality.
Spastic	Upper motor neuron (bilateral).	Spasticity.	Loss of skilled movement; hypertonia, manifested as spasticity; hyperreflexia; clonus; Babinski sign; Hoffman sign.	Slow, imprecise articulation; harsh voice quality; monopitch and monoloudness; short phrases.
Hypokinetic	Extrapyramidal (substantia nigra).	Rigidity, reduced range of movement, resting tremor.	Rigidity, bradykinesia, akinesia, resting tremor, postural abnormalities.	Reduced loudness, monopitch and monoloudness, reduced syllable stress, accelerated rate and short rushes of speech, palilalia, inappropriate silences.
Hyperkinetic	Extrapyramidal (basal ganglia).	Quick-to-slow, regular or irregular involuntary movements.	One or more of: chorea, dystonia, athetosis, dyskinesia, myoclonus, tics, tremor.	Highly variable, affecting one or more components of speech production, often with rate and prosodic abnormalities. Speech features consistent with nature of involuntary movements.
Ataxic	Cerebellum.	Dyscoordination; possible intention tremor.	Dyscoordination	Excess and equal stress; irregular articulatory breakdown; rhythm disturbances; sound prolongations; excess loudness.
Unilateral upper motor neuron	Upper motor neuron (unilateral)	Weakness, spasticity, lack of coordination, singly or in combination.	Hemiparesis/hemiplegia, unilateral central face and tongue weakness.	Imprecise articulation, irregular articulatory breakdowns, slow rate, harsh-strained or breathy-hoarse voice, reduced loudness.
Mixed	Two or more of above	Combinations of above	Combinations of above	Combinations of above

Note: From source material in Duffy (2005) and Weismer (2007).

the movement deficit is not a result of mechanical causes, such as arytenoid cartilage dislocation or subluxation, cricoarytenoid arthritis or ankylosis, or a tumor (Rubin and Sataloff, 2007). The type and extent of dysphonia largely depends on the lesion site, and whether damage is unilateral or bilateral, and partial or complete.

Unilateral Vocal Fold Paralysis (UVFP)

The etiology of UVFP can be broadly divided into four categories: neoplastic (compression or infiltration of the Vagus or RLN), traumatic (surgical and nonsurgical), secondary to medical disease, and idiopathic (Tucker, 1980). There is glottic incompetence due to the inability of the affected true vocal fold to adduct completely and meet the normally mobile opposing true vocal fold. The paralyzed vocal fold is fixed in the paramedian position, that is, neither fully abducted nor adducted. The vocal fold remains at the paramedian position for both inspiration and expiration (including attempts at phonation). The voice in UVFP is markedly dysphonic or aphonic. Perceptual characteristics include breathy, hoarse vocal quality; reduced phonation time; decreased loudness and monoloudness; diplophonia; and pitch breaks. The breathy vocal quality, reduced loudness, and short phonation times result from air escape through an open glottis during phonation. Hoarseness, pitch breaks, and diplophonia result from the reduced ability to adjust the internal tension of the paralyzed vocal fold. Secondary muscle tension may contribute to the perception of hoarseness.

Disease or trauma to the RLN on one side is the most common form of vocal fold paralysis (Case, 2002; Rubin and Sataloff, 2007). Because of the extended course of the left RLN, it appears to be more prone to traumatic or surgical injury than the right RLN. Bhattacharyya and colleagues (2002) reported that, of 64 patients presenting with UVFP, 53 cases were left-sided. In a retrospective review of patient cases, Hughes and colleagues (2000) reported that isolated right vocal fold paralysis comprised only about 3% of laryngeal evaluation cases. Surgical trauma predominated as an etiology, followed by viral and idiopathic causes. In a study by Heman-Ackah and colleagues (2011), undiagnosed thyroid disease was discovered in about 50% of patients presenting to the ENT with UVFP and dysphonia. Geography may also influence etiologies of UVFP. Researchers in Scotland found a high rate of UVFP secondary to bronchogenic carcinoma, likely, the authors speculate, associated with the high levels of smoking in Scotland (Loughran and colleagues, 2002).

Because many traumatic vocal fold paralyses have spontaneous recovery within the first 9 to 12 months post-onset, permanent corrective procedures are usually delayed until voice therapy has been tried. In many cases, strengthening the vocal muscles and improving voicing technique result in very good voice quality, and surgery is unnecessary (Mattioli and colleagues, 2011; Schindler and colleagues, 2008; Dworkin and Treadway, 2009). Behavioral voice therapy may be the only treatment required or it may suffice as a temporary measure until medical intervention is feasible. One study found that voice therapy reduced mean airflow rate in 16 patients with UVFP by nearly 50% (McFarlane and colleagues, 1998). The Voice Facilitating Approaches we normally introduce in clinic are focus, half-swallow boom, head positioning, tuck-chin, digital manipulation, tongue protrusion /i/, yawn-sigh, pitch shift up, and inhalation phonation (see Chapter 7). Each approach affords an anatomical and physiological rationale for improving voice in individuals with UVFP.

Medical Management of UVFP

The two main surgical options for patients who have UVFP are vocal fold medialization and vocal fold reinnervation (Ruben and Sataloff, 2008). Medialization procedures include injection laryngoplasty and laryngeal framework surgery. Several injectable materials have been used to medialize the vocal fold and improve glottic competence. These include autologous fat, gelatin sponge, micronized cadaveric dermis, calcium

Phonation in this **video** example reveals a longitudinal gap, diplophonia, and extensive air escape. Grand Rounds: Describe three behavioral approaches you would probe to reduce air escape and supraglottal interference and increase vocal quality.

Parkinson's Disease
Note in this **video** the increases in respiratory support, articulation accuracy, and phonatory volume for the reading passage pre- and post-voice intervention. Grand Rounds: Describe the changes in physiology for three subsystems of speech (respiration, phonation and articulation) that underlie these changes.

hydroxylapatite, sodium carboxymethylcellulose aqueous gel, hyaluronic acid, and collagen. Teflon has long been abandoned due to the risk of granuloma formation (Dedo, 1992). Most ENTs agree that the use of injectable materials appears to be (1) a temporary step for patients with UVFP who require immediate medialization, but in whom some recovery is likely, or (2) a minimally invasive option for those patients whose medical–surgical status precludes a procedure such as thyroplasty.

Sulica and colleagues (2010) performed a retrospective review of patients who underwent injection laryngoplasty at seven university medical centers from July 2007 to June 2008. They found that the most popular mode of injection delivery was by transcricothyroid, peroral, and transthyroid membrane. Five-year data showed that injections in patients who were awake rose from 11% to 43%. Readers are encouraged to explore the latest literature to learn of the long-term effects and voice outcomes of the various injection fillers and methods (Arviso and colleagues, 2011; Carroll and Rosen, 2011; Rudolph and Sibylle, 2012; Rosen and colleagues, 2009; Umeno and colleagues, 2012; Yung and colleagues, 2011). It appears that injections are a safe and largely durable treatment option for the management of glottal insufficiency in both children and adults (Cohen and colleagues, 2011; Lakhani and colleagues, 2011), although suboptimal results are sometimes observed (Ting and colleagues, 2012).

Thyroplasty type I, first described by Isshiki and colleagues (1975), is a surgical approach to medialization of the paralyzed vocal fold, using a free-moving wedge to move the vocal fold to midline (Dursun and colleagues, 2008). The surgeon cuts a rectangular window out of the thyroid cartilage on the side of the paralyzed vocal fold. The patient is conscious during the procedure and produces voice when the surgeon places the wedge at various sites against the paralyzed vocal fold. When it is confirmed that a certain site produces the best phonation, the wedge is fixed surgically at that point. Thyroplasty in the hands of a competent surgeon produces excellent results, and patients should expect "voice improvement as early as 1 month postoperatively and should remain stable with slight fluctuations for at least 6 months" (p. 576). Dean and colleagues (2001) introduced a modification of the thyroplasty technique by introducing a titanium implant with a micrometric screw that allows for secondary adjustment of medialization, if necessary. Titanium is MRI safe.

There are numerous reports on the long-term results of both injection and medialization thyroplasty. One notable study by Morgan and colleagues (2007) reported a retrospective study of 19 patients with UVFP who received either vocal fold injection with Radiesse or Type I thyroplasty. Outcome measures were laryngostroboscopy, perceptual analysis, and patients' subjective voice handicap assessment. Results revealed that both approaches were comparable in their improvements of subjective and objective voice outcomes at 3 months. In a follow-up study from the same institution, Vinson and colleagues (2010) retrospectively assessed outcomes for 34 patients with UVFP at 6 months, and reported that both approaches were comparable in terms of voice outcomes. A retrospective study by Sipp and colleagues (2007) compared outcomes for three procedures (injection laryngoplasty, thyroplasty, and laryngeal nerve reinnervation) and reported successful surgical and quality-of-life outcomes with all three procedures.

While injection laryngoplasty, medialization thyroplasty, and arytenoid adduction (Su and colleagues, 2005) are effective in improving voice quality, they cannot prevent vocal fold atrophy. As a result, some researchers have explored a variety of vocal fold reinnervation approaches, including primary neurorrhaphy (nerve suture), ansa cervicalis to RLN anastomosis, Vagus nerve to RLN anastomosis, and free nerve grafting (Grover and Bhattacharyya, 2012). Recent studies (Marcum and colleagues, 2010; Rohde and colleagues, 2012; Smith and colleagues, 2008) suggest that each approach can result in positive laryngeal and voice outcomes for children, adolescents, and adults.

Some patients, after injection or surgery, continue to display the hyperfunctional vocal behaviors they were using before treatment. Direct symptom modification can usually reduce problems such as squeezing the words out, using pushing behaviors, and using excessive glottal attack. Following injection or medialization, the SLP may help the patient reestablish a normal voice, giving some attention to adequate breath support and focused phonation free of effort.

CHECK YOUR KNOWLEDGE

1. Many SLPs and ENTs recommend that corrective procedures for UVFP be delayed for at least nine months. Explain why.
2. Describe three behavioral approaches to UVFP and their rationales.

Bilateral Vocal Fold Paralysis (BVFP)

The pathophysiology of BVFP includes two major categories: neurogenic paralysis and mechanical fixation (Woodson, 2011). BVFP is usually the result of lesions high in the trunk of the Vagus nerve or at the nuclei of origin in the medulla (see Figure 5.3). If the lesion is above the nodose ganglion, other muscles innervated by the Vagus, as well as muscles supplied by other cranial nerves, will be affected as well. These high lesions include tumors at the base of the skull, carcinoma, or trauma. In the case of children, BVFP is a common cause of neonatal stridor (Smith and Sauder, 2009; Baker and colleagues, 2003). Most cases are associated with intracranial pathology such as meningomyelocoele, hydrocephalus, or Arnold-Chiari malformation. Other reports of rare etiologies are motor axonal neuropathy (Marchant and colleagues, 2003) and familial clustering with autosomal recessive mode of inheritance (Raza and colleagues, 2002).

BVFP may be of the abductory or adductory type; both are life threatening. Voice per se is of secondary concern to respiratory survival and feeding. In bilateral adductor paralysis, neither vocal fold is capable of moving to the midline, thus making phonation impossible and placing the individual at risk for aspiration. In abductor paralysis, the vocal folds remain at the midline, causing serious respiratory problems for which most patients will need a tracheostomy. In 2011, Belafsky and other leading experts in the surgical management of BVFP arrived at a number of conclusions regarding current practice. Among those conclusions are that laryngeal electromyography EMG is necessary to distinguish among the vocal fold paralysis and vocal fold fixation; surgical procedures to open the posterior glottis airway remain the current gold standard for treatment of BVFP; and novel treatment such as laryngeal pacing (Zealer and colleagues, 2003; Mueller, 2011), bilateral selective reinnervation (Marina and colleagues, 2011; Woodson, 2011), and BTX-A™ injections (Ongkasuwana and Courey, 2011) hold great promise. Continued BVFP may require surgery to improve greater airway competence in both children and adults. Surgical reinnervation of the muscles of the vocal folds has been successfully reported by Su and colleagues (2007). An alternative to surgery for some patients with abductor vocal fold paralysis may be inspiratory pressure threshold training. Baker and colleagues (2003) reported reductions in dyspnea during speech and exercise for a six-year-old child with congenital bilateral abductor paralysis after eight months of respiratory muscle strength training.

Andrews and Summers (2002), Hoffman and colleagues (2008), and Harvey-Woodnorth (2004) offer specific procedures for the SLP to use in working with young children with BVFP—that is, how to manage the tracheostomy, the use of tracheal valves, and the need for minimizing the negative effects of the vocal fold dysfunction on the child's expressive language and speech development.

SPASMODIC DYSPHONIA (SD)

Spasmodic dysphonia (SD) is a relatively rare voice disorder that results from laryngeal dystonia. Dystonia is a neurological dysfunction of motor movements, either more generalized to major body movements or seen in focal disorders, such as in the eyelids (blepharospasm), in the neck (spasmodic torticollis), or in the larynx (SD). As such, it is a hyperkinetic movement disorder. The site in the brain where a lesion might occur that in turn would result in SD is still not definitively known. One of the first studies using magnetic resonance imaging (MRI), single-photon emission computed tomography (SPECT), or brain electrical activity mapping (BEAM) for identifying possible SD lesion sites was reported by Finitzo and Freeman (1989), who concluded that "SD is a supranuclear movement disorder primarily, but not exclusively, affecting the larynx. Fully half of our subjects had evidence of isolated functional cortical lesions" (p. 553).

The patient with SD exhibits a strain-strangled and harsh voice with observable effort in pushing the air out during most voicing attempts. Endoscopic examination shows that this voice results from hyperadduction of the true vocal folds, often accompanied by tight closure of the false vocal folds with supraglottal constriction of the aryepiglottic vocal folds and contraction of the lower pharyngeal constrictors. The total laryngeal and lower pharyngeal airway appears to close down. No wonder we hear a strained, strangled voice in such patients. Hirano and Bless (1993) nevertheless caution that the voice clinician should not anticipate seeing one particular laryngeal pattern. They suggest that SD presentation can be heterogeneous, ranging from spasmodic hyperfunction to hypofunction, to irregular twitching of the true vocal folds. Kendall and Leonard (2011) have reported that approximately one-third of patients presenting with adductor SD have an associated vocal tremor.

In addition to the problem of voicing, patients with SD complain about the difficulties they experience trying to force expiratory air out whenever they desire to phonate. Aronson (1990) comments that the tight voice during adductor SD "occurs only during voluntary phonation for communication purposes and not during singing, vowel prolongation, laughing, or crying" (p. 161). However, in patients who have carried the diagnosis of SD for some period and whose symptoms are more severe, we see symptoms of this disorder in prolonged vowels as well. The patients soon learn to expect phonation difficulties whenever they attempt to speak. Most patients with SD experience some normal voice in certain situations. Case histories of these patients reveal that, in situations such as "talking to my cat" or "speaking to others in a pool while I tread water," patients have experienced normal voice.

The most common type of SD appears to be related to tight laryngeal adduction, known as adductor SD. Aronson (1990), however, also described a second form of the disorder, known as abductor spastic dysphonia (ABSD), in which patients exhibit normal or dysphonic voices that are suddenly interrupted by temporary abduction of the vocal folds, resulting in fleeting aphonia. After such momentary aphonia, the patients' voice patterns are restored again (until the next aphonic break). Endoscopy shows that the vocal folds of such patients abduct suddenly, "exposing an extremely wide glottic chink" (Aronson, 1990, p. 185). In our clinical experiences, more often than not, the abductor spasms appear to be triggered by unvoiced consonant sounds. The abductor-type disorder is a much rarer form of SD. For example, Davis and colleagues (1988) reported that, of 25 successive cases of SD observed in a Sydney, Australia, hospital, 24 were adductor type and one was an abductor type. Mixed abductor and adductor SD is seen sometimes in the clinic. The abductor spasms are often treated as a phonation break. We encourage the patient to blend the abductor aphonic event into the next vowel or voiced consonant by gently easing into phonation. Additional symptoms and treatment for the sudden abductory spasms described by Aronson (1990) are discussed as phonation breaks in this text. Because the symptoms and the treatment of adductor and abductor SD are so different, we will confine further comments about SD to the adductor type.

Schweinfurth and colleagues (2002) attempted to identify risk factors and demographics in patients with adductor SD. Results of a retrospective survey of 168 patients revealed that there "appears to be no significant environmental or hereditary patterns in the etiology of SD" (p. 220). The authors did identify some trends, however. The majority of patients were females (79%). A significantly higher incidence of childhood viral illness was found in the patients with SD (65%). Patients with SD had a significant incidence of both essential tremor (26%) and writer's cramp (11%), but no history of major illness or other neurological disorder. Tanner and colleagues (2012) also conducted an epidemiological study that examined risk factors associated with SD and reported that factors included (1) a personal history of cervical dystonia, sinus and throat illnesses, mumps, rubella, dust exposure, and frequent volunteer voice use; (2) a family history of voice disorders; (3) an immediate family history of vocal tremor and meningitis; and (4) an extended family history of head and neck tremor, ocular disease, and meningitis. Vocal tremor coexisted with SD in 29% of cases. Tanner and colleagues concluded that SD is likely associated with several factors that may contribute to the onset of SD later in life.

Kaptein and colleagues (2010) examined psychosocial concomitants, illness perceptions, and treatment perceptions in 49 patients with adductor SD by comparing their responses from a battery of psychometric assessment instruments to those from a matched control group. Scores on psychosocial measures were elevated in male patients especially, indicating levels of psychological morbidity significantly above those seen in the general population. Assessments of illness perceptions and treatment perceptions indicated that patients perceive that they have a very low degree of control over the disorder, and they experience a high emotional impact from it. Voice Handicap Index (see Chapter 6) scores illustrated substantial degrees of perceived handicap. These researchers suggested that future research should be conducted in order to improve self-management and enhance quality of life of persons with adductor SD.

Judgment Scales for SD

The description and quantification of the symptoms of SD require administration of perceptual judgment scales and instrumental measures. Because SD is a rare disorder, the less-experienced SLP may not recognize it. Barkmeier and colleagues (2001) discovered that SD could be misinterpreted as essential voice tremor or muscle tension dysphonia (see Table 5.2). These clinical researchers investigated whether voice clinicians with infrequent exposure to SD patients could learn to identify speech symptoms of adductor SD and abductor SD compared to voice clinicians having extensive experience with these disorders. Results revealed that while the nonexpert judges tended toward false positive judgments for the speech symptoms of interest, the overall speech symptom profiles for each type of voice disorder appeared comparable to those obtained from the expert judges. Readers are encouraged to review this study to become familiar with the identification scale used.

Another excellent judgment scale developed by Stewart and colleagues (1997) for assessing the SD patient is known as the Unified SD Rating Scale (USDRS). The scale offers the SLP a standardized way of asking for speech–voice responses and a seven-point rating scale for evaluating SD-voice parameters such as overall severity, aspects of voice quality, abrupt voice initiation, voice arrests, loudness variations, tremor, expiratory effort, speech rate, speech intelligibility, and related movements and grimaces (p. 100). The administration of the perceptual rating scale should precede instrumental assessments such as airflow and pressure data, fundamental frequency values, perturbation measures, and intensity documentation (see Chapter 6).

What treatment options are available today for reducing the hypertonic approximation of the vocal folds during SD voicing attempts? Let us consider separately several treatment options for the SD patient: voice therapy, surgical resection of the RLN, injection of botulinum toxin type A (BTX-A), and surgical modification of the vocal folds.

Voice Therapy for SD

Throughout our clinical careers, each of us has encountered each new SD patient with the optimism that the strangled-sounding, harsh voice could be modified by voice therapy, only to find repeatedly with each new patient that apparent success in producing an easy normal voice temporarily in the voice clinic seemed to have no carryover outside the clinic. Case (2002) wrote of similar poor outcomes of traditional voice therapy, noting that many patients made slight improvements when

TABLE 5.2 Differences Among Essential Tremor, Spasmodic Dysphonia, and Muscle Tension Dysphonia

Disorder	Age of Onset	Gender	Suspected Etiology	Presentation	Intervention
Essential tremor	Any age	Predominantly females	CNS neurogenic	Regular rhythmic vocal arrest; may involve supraglottal structures	Behavioral; Botox® not recommended due to numerous supraglottal structures involved
Vocal hyperfunction	Any age	Predominantly male children and adolescent and adult females	Functional	Various: anteroposterior and medial squeezing of supraglottal structures	Behavioral
Adductor SD	Two-thirds of onset between 40 and 60	Predominantly adult females	CNS neurogenic	Irregular vocal arrests involving TA muscle	Botox injection, surgery, behavioral

speech was produced in small units, such as monosyllabic utterances, but rarely in contextual speech. "Historically, the poor prognosis is one of the most significant symptoms of this disorder and has been pathognomonic and diagnostic to it" (p. 189). There have been few reported positive outcomes for SD patients receiving voice therapy, such as Cooper's (1990) "direct voice rehabilitation" and the more conventional voice therapy. Our role with the SD patient is a careful, meticulous assessment to permit evaluation of treatment outcomes and to combine voice therapy efforts with pharmacological or surgical treatment, before and after intervention.

Some trial voice therapy should follow assessment, used at least as diagnostic probes. Many SD patients experience an easier voice with less effort "pushing voice out" through working on an easy breath cycle, employing Yawn-Sigh relaxation methods coupled with hierarchy analysis. Boone (1998) has found real-time amplification, Auditory Feedback, and Masking to be facilitative for some SD patients. Speaking on inhalation is reported as less likely to reduce the symptoms of longstanding adductor SD (Harrison and colleagues, 1992). Roy and colleagues (1996) have employed the musculoskeletal tension reduction techniques recommended by Aronson (1990) with over 150 cases of muscle tension dysphonia, described under laryngeal massage in Chapter 7 of this text. Included in the group of muscle tension dysphonia patients were some SD patients (the number was not specified in the article) who received the manual lowering of their larynx but experienced only "transient improvements in voice that could not be stabilized or generalized" (Roy and colleagues, 1996, p. 855).

In summary, from long clinical experience and in reviewing the literature, there are scarce efficacy data to show that the struggling of SD patients to get air out while producing harsh, strangled voice is resolved solely with voice therapy. Rather, those patients who do respond positively to voice therapy may likely have originally presented with muscle tension dysphonia, which often masquerades as SD. It would appear that voice therapy coupled with surgery or BTX-A injections offers the best therapeutic management of SD. These interventions are described in the following sections.

Recurrent Laryngeal Nerve (RLN) Sectioning

Introduced by Dedo (1976), the RLN section (Izdebski and colleagues, 1984) was the first widely used surgical procedure for SD. Patients are selected for RLN section after a thorough diagnostic evaluation by both the surgeon and the SLP, which includes an injection of Lidocaine into the RLN to produce a temporary unilateral adductor paralysis (Smith and colleagues, 2006). The patient's airflow, relative ease of phonation, and change of voice quality are assessed. If there is marked improvement in airflow (greater flow rates with less glottal resistance), and in both ease and quality of phonation, the decision may be made to cut the RLN permanently. Postoperatively, then, the patient usually has an easily produced but breathy voice, similar in sound to the patient with unilateral adductor paralysis. Voice therapy focusing on a slight elevation of pitch, some ear training, head positioning, and digital manipulation have all been effective in developing a better-sounding voice.

The long-term results of RLN resection are mixed. Wilson and colleagues (1980) reported a woman who had received RLN cut 13 months previously and then experienced a regeneration of the severed RLN and a return of SD; a second RLN resection again produced immediate relief from her phonatory struggle. Over three years Aronson and DeSanto (1983) followed 33 patients with SD who had each received RLN cut. Although all experienced improved voice and ease of air-flow immediately after surgery, three years later, 21 of them, or 64%, had failed to maintain their gains and were considered failures. Much different results were reported by Dedo and Izdebski (1983) on over 306 patients who had received RLN cut for SD; they reported that 92% of the patients maintained voice improvement and required less effort to phonate.

The arguments over the long-term effectiveness of RLN section as posed by Aronson and DeSanto (1983) versus Dedo and Izdebski (1983) contributed to a significant reduction in the use of RLN sectioning as a treatment for SD. Regeneration of the severed RLN appears to be the primary factor in symptoms of tight voice coming back a few months or years after RLN section. To meet this regeneration problem, Weed and others (1996) recommended the use of avulsion (tearing out or entire removal) of as much of the RLN as is surgically possible. In the Weed study, long-term follow-up of RLN avulsion patients revealed that "72 to 78 percent of patients retained clear benefit from the procedure beyond 3 years" (p. 600).

Berke and colleagues (1999) described a surgical technique for adductor SD that paralyzes the thyroarytenoid and lateral cricoarytenoid muscles bilaterally by denervating the RLN branches to these muscles. To prevent unwanted reinnervation and to preserve muscle tone, the TA nerve branch is reinnervated with a branch of the ansa cervicalis. The procedure, the authors note, obviates the breathy voice and other typical sequelae of unilateral vocal fold paralysis. The long-term results of 21 sequential cases were reported, with 19 patients judged to have an "absent to mild" dysphonia following the procedure and one patient requiring further BTX-A treatments. The opposite vocal behaviors were reported by one patient presenting to our clinic for voice therapy. Twenty months earlier, he underwent bilateral laryngeal adductor denervation with ansa cervicalis reinnervation. He reported that, although he no longer had to worry about strained and strangled phonation, he now had to worry about a soft voice that was insufficient for many social and professional activities of daily living. This patient responded well to Voice Facilitating Approaches for unilateral vocal fold paralysis (digital manipulation, focus, head positioning) (see Chapter 7).

A study by Smith and colleagues (2006) assessed the phonatory effects of RLN lidocaine block in adductor SD. Twenty-one consecutive patients with suspected adductor SD underwent unilateral RLN block, causing temporary ipsilateral vocal fold paralysis. Voices were recorded before and during the block. Patients completed self-ratings of overall level of dysphonia severity, vocal effort, and laryngeal tightness. Listeners completed auditory-perceptual ratings, and the frequency of phonatory breaks was acoustically analyzed. Although individuals varied in their outcomes, group results suggest that response to RLN lidocaine block warrants further study as a possible diagnostic tool in adductor SD.

Botulinum Toxin Type A (BTX-A) Injections

The gold standard for treating SD is the injection of BTX-A in one or both vocal folds or interarytenoid muscles, or a combination thereof (Kendall and Leonard, 2011; Birkent and colleagues, 2009). Physicians who are members of the National SD Association database were polled about their BTX-A delivery method; the majority who responded reported that they use electromyographic guidance (Chang and colleagues, 2009).

The largest treatment series to date in the literature (as reported in Blitzer, 2010) spanned the years from 1984 to 2007 and included over 1,300 patients. Of these, 82% are of the adductor type, 63% were female, 12% had a positive family history, and 82.4% had a focal distribution. All of the patients were managed with varying degrees of success with individualized dosing of BTX-A injected into the laryngeal musculature under EMG guidance. Most typically, BTX-A was injected bilaterally into the thyroarytenoid muscle. The average onset of action was reported to be 2.4 days; the average peak effect was 9 days; the average duration of benefit was15.1 weeks; and the average benefit was 91.2% of normal function, as rated by the patient. The side effects of the adductor injections were 25% with mild, transient breathy voice; 10% with mild, transient cough on drinking fluids; and less than 1% with local pain, bruising, or itch. Birkent and colleagues (2009) followed 55 patients for BTX-A injections over approximately 12 years, for an average of 20 doses per patient. They found that they were able to reduce BTX-A dosages over time with no negative effects on voice.

It is commonly observed in patients who have received BTX-A injection in the TA muscle that they experience for a short time (10 to 14 days) some mild symptoms of aspiration, coughing, and breathiness (Novakovic and colleagues, 2011). Instead of tight phonation with low airflow rates and high subglottal pressures, the SD patient now displays temporarily the symptoms of a patient with unilateral vocal fold paralysis, that is, high flow rate, low pressure, and a breathy voice. The patient at this time requires counsel from the SLP that the aspiration and breathiness are temporary. About three weeks after injection, the patient should return to the SLP for voice therapy. Murry and Woodson (1995) found in 27 patients that those who received both injection plus voice therapy had significantly better flow rates and acoustic improvement than patients who received only BTX-A without follow-up voice therapy. Typically, those patients who received both BTX-A and follow-up voice therapy maintain good, functional voice from four to six months. As the patient experiences increasing adductory tightness while phonating, reinjection of BTX-A is required.

Murry and Woodson (1995) usually begin with "five voice-therapy sessions planned for each patient" (p. 462). Some patients may require less therapy and some may need more. Beginning therapy is designed to reduce continued vocal hyperfunction. The typical SD patient has used for many years hyperfunctional behaviors in an attempt to push voice out. Even though such excessive effort is no longer needed after injection, the patient's habit set of vocal hyperfunction continues. Counseling, showing the patient differential airflow rates, and listening to pre- and postinjection recordings can be utilized to help the patient recognize that effort for voicing is no longer required. A useful task is to model in front of a mirror or on a digital recorder the saying of "ah" with no discernible effort and no visible neck muscle activity, resulting in a slightly easy, breathy voice. Stay with this task until the patient can demonstrate taking the work out of voicing. Therapy then follows with learning to find the optimal breath for saying a series of syllables on one expiration, perhaps reducing voice production in the beginning to saying only six to eight syllables per breath. If the patient is observed to squeeze out the last syllable or two, the syllable target per breath should be reduced further. Practice should be given to developing the number of syllables that can be comfortably voiced on one exhalation. When breath volume gets low, the patient should pause; during the pause, breath will renew without the patient doing anything consciously but pausing (Boone, 1997).

We have established a therapy plan that monitors the patient's vocal behaviors post-BTX-A injection. Each patient's program is individualized, beginning with several follow-up telephone calls. We ask the patient whether the postinjection aspiration has resolved; we can hear any latent vocal hyperfunction, which would necessitate a follow-up visit to the clinic. Several weeks after injection, we listen for spasmodic vocal behaviors, which would also necessitate a return to the clinic. If we detect the return of the dystonia, we ask the patient to return for acoustic and airflow assessment and possible reinjection.

ESSENTIAL VOICE TREMOR

Organic or essential voice tremor is often viewed as a disorder separate from the other dysarthrias, yet it can be classified as a hyperkinetic dysarthria of tremor (Duffy, 2005). Essential tremor is the most common of the movement disorders and is considered a benign autosomal dominant condition with variable penetrance (Jankovic, 1986). The tremor may appear present in tongue, velar, pharyngeal, and laryngeal structures, producing a vocal tremor in the 4- to 7-per-second range. Other patients with voice tremor may show similar tremulous movements in the hands, arms, neck, and face. Familial tremor is a common form of essential tremor (approximately 50% of all cases), often beginning in early adulthood. The patient shows exaggerated tremor behavior, more than the normal tremor that may be observed in people who are overworking particular muscles, such as may be felt or seen while carrying a heavy weight, "like carrying a case of twenty-four quarts of milk." Another form of essential tremor appears related to aging (Benito-Leon and colleagues, 2005).

Voice tremor is a feature of many neurological conditions, such as SD and PD. Such tremors must be differentiated from a diagnosis of essential tremor, which is intention tremor that appears to exist independently of other neurogenic conditions. It should be noted that vocal tremor has been found to co-exist with SD in approximately 30% of cases (Tanner and colleagues, 2012; Kendall and Leonard, 2011). The diagnosis of essential tremor is best made by eliminating contextual speech, asking the patient to sustain the production of vowels in isolation. Lederle and colleagues (2012) found that vocal tremor is perceived as significantly more severe during sustained phonation than during connected speech, and perceived tremor is greater the longer the vowel is sustained. On prolonged vowel production, the tremor is well isolated, permitting a frequency count and an acoustic evaluation of the tremulous voice. Endoscopic examination of the vocal folds while prolonging the vowel shows a structurally normal larynx with the vocal folds producing the alternate tension changes that are part of the overall tremor production. Flexible endoscopy can also reveal velar, pharyngeal, and tongue movements in absolute tremulous synchrony with one another, all contributing to the acoustic observation of voice tremor (Gillivan-Murphy and Miller, 2011).

There is a growing body of literature that suggests BTX-A injection into the thyroarytenoid muscle may reduce tremor, as measured by patient responses on a tremor rating scale and acoustic changes (Adler and colleagues, 2004). Other researchers are exploring the effects of deep brain stimulation on reducing the periodic modulations in fundamental frequency and intensity (Deuschl and colleagues, 2011).

The SLP who first encounters an essential tremor patient, either of the familial or aging type, should make a referral to a consulting neurologist who might offer some medication control, reducing the severity (amplitude) of the tremor (but not its frequency). Professional meeting papers and anecdotal reports by voice clinicians offer three therapy approaches that seem to minimize voice symptoms: (1) reducing voice intensity levels appears to minimize tremor identification, (2) elevating voice pitch a half note seems to change the tension level of the vocal folds sufficiently to reduce severity of the tremor, and (3) attempting to shorten vowel duration while speaking minimizes the identification of voice tremor (we are less likely to hear it).

When clients understand the nature of voiced versus nonvoiced phonemes, they discover that, by abbreviating the vowels and overarticulating the nonvoiced phonemes, the tremor is less noticeable. We often refer these patients to the Iowa Phonetics website, which offers robust animations of the anatomy and physiology of sound production. In addition, we encourage the client to produce an "easy" /h/ at the beginnings of vowel initial words, such as /h/apples, to reduce the amplitude of tremor. This technique worked well for a young client who worked as a telephone receptionist at Andressen Towing. Prior to intervention, when announcing her company's name on the telephone, she produced the initial /a/ with extended vowel duration, which only served to announce the tremor. With intervention, she softened and abbreviated the /a/ by making the voice breathy, devoiced the /d/, and anticipated the production of the nonvoiced /ss/. Using these strategies, there was an attenuation of the perceptual features of the tremor.

DIFFERENCES AMONG SD, ESSENTIAL VOICE TREMOR, AND MUSCLE TENSION DYSPHONIA

SD can easily be misinterpreted as an essential tremor or vocal hyperfunction. This should come as no surprise because the three conditions may present very similarly (Barkmeier and colleagues, 2001). In Table 5.2, we have attempted to identify some of the differences among the disorders, although it should be noted that the disorders may, and do, overlap. For example, a patient with severe adductor SD may attempt to control the capricious vocal fold movements by squeezing down on the supraglottal structures. SD is only differentially identified when the individual undergoes trial voice therapy that eliminates the hyperfunctional posturing.

CHECK YOUR KNOWLEDGE

1. Describe the differences and similarities among adductor SD, essential tremor, and muscle tension dysphonia.
2. Describe the evidence-based approaches for adductor SD, essential tremor, and muscle tension dyphonia.

PARKINSON'S DISEASE (PD)

The patient with PD exhibits a hypokinetic dysarthria, characterized by reduced loudness, breathy voice, monotony of pitch, intermittent and rapid rushes of speech, and reduced articulatory contacts (Duffy 2005). Some investigators of PD have found diminished function in one or more components of speech–voice. For example, De Letter and colleagues (2007) found significant respiratory difficulties as possibly contributing to the PD patient's voice symptoms. Ramig and colleagues (1994) found that 35 of 40 PD subjects had bowed vocal folds. Duffy (2005) and Yorkston and colleagues (2004) write that many of these abnormalities can be related to the underlying neuromuscular deficits of rigidity, reduced range of movement, and slowness of movement in the laryngeal muscles. Resting tremor is also considered a neuromuscular deficit and can be attributed to the reduction of dopamine to the basal ganglia. See Fahr and colleagues (1987) for the Unified Parkinson Disease Rating Scale (UPDRS), a comprehensive and widely used rating scale to document levels of motor behavior and activities of daily living for individuals with PD (see Zraick and colleagues [2003] for a report on the use of this scale by SLPs). Fortunately, the most effective voice therapy approach is a holistic one, finding that to exaggerate one component helps improve function in all other components.

When patients attempt to speak in a quick conversational pattern, speech is often unintelligible due to the rapid and accelerated movement of the articulators. When they speak with intent, however, their speech can be slower and louder, and can have better voice quality and better articulation. Following the model of intention used in physical therapy for gait training (thinking where you are going to place each foot as you walk makes walking easier), the same model of intent works to improve speech. Using intention with these patients, the writers have asked PD patients to speak with an accent, or to use a different pitch, or to speak louder (Boone and Plante, 1993). Taking the automatic motor set out of speaking by speaking intentionally different seems to help the patient's speech in all parameters: loudness, voice quality, appropriate pitch, and rate. We have also found that instructing patients to deliberately pronounce the final sound of each word results in increases in vocal loudness and intelligibility.

Ramig and colleagues (2001) and Spielman and colleagues (2011) have studied the model of intention in a formal voice and speech improvement program that is driven by a number of perceptual features of phonation in PD. The main goal of the Lee Silverman Voice Treatment (LSVT®/LOUD) program is to increase vocal fold adduction and respiratory effort, which in turn is intended to increase loudness, vocal quality, and subsequently intelligibility.

Sapir and colleagues (2002) investigated whether increased loudness is maintained over several months after conclusion of the LSVT program. Judges listened to reading samples produced by two groups: one that had undergone LSVT and one that had undergone a high-effort respiratory treatment program. Of the two groups, the speech samples in the LSVT group were significantly more likely to be perceived as louder and of better quality at follow-up. Tindall and colleagues (2008) compared the efficacy of LSVT/LOUD using a videophone versus conventional administration. Similar results were obtained, suggesting both methods result in an overall increase in loudness. Researchers in the Netherlands suggested that increased respiratory–phonatory effort raises vocal pitch and laryngeal muscle tension (de Swart and colleagues, 2003). These researchers generated an intervention program called Pitch Limiting Voice Treatment (PLVT), which instructs patients to increase respiratory support but to phonate at a low pitch. A study by these researchers comparing LSVT and PLVT revealed the same increases in loudness for both groups, but the authors suggested that PLVT limited increases in vocal pitch, thus preventing strained and pressed voicing.

For patients who are initially stimulable for behavioral voice programs but who experience difficulty generalizing the gains beyond the clinic, we have offered delayed auditory feedback (DAF), with mixed results. DAF is an instrumental procedure that feeds an individual's speech trace back to the individual's auditory system via earphones at a delayed rate. The effect of the delay is to slow speech rate, increase vocal loudness, and increase articulatory accuracy. Several case studies in our clinics and reports in the literature have suggested improved speech using DAF for individuals presenting with hypokinetic dysarthria (Downie and colleagues, 1981; Hanson and Metter, 1983; Yorkston and colleagues, 2004). These authors suggest that the benefits included marked reduction in speech rate, increased loudness, reduced phonetic errors, and increased acoustic distinctiveness.

DAF intervention produced remarkable results in the vocal intensity, rate, and intelligibility of an individual seen at our clinic with PD. This patient, a former physician, had received a thalamic (deep brain) stimulator four years earlier to reduce tremors and was taking Sinemet (combined levodopa and carbidopa). Nevertheless, speech was rapid and blurred, and the voice was hypophonic. Various clinic probes of speaking with intent, speaking to a metronome, pacing, respiratory–phonatory training, and hyperarticulation were not effective. He was fitted with the Facilitator™ (KayPENTAX® Corp., Montvale, New Jersey) set at the 170-ms feedback mode and the effect was dramatic. He increased vocal intensity, extended the vowels, and increased articulatory contacts, thus increasing intelligibility. He subsequently purchased a pocket-sized DAF unit that he wore at all times. He said the system was so innocuous that people thought he was listening to the ballgame. Even though he did not return to his former practice, he did begin to deliver lectures at the medical school and spoke at PD support group meetings. This success with DAF has been supplemented by frequency-altered feedback (FAF) at our clinics. FAF, along with babble noise feedback, works along the same principles as DAF. A number of applications exist for DAF, FAF, and babble noise.

The diagnosis of PD and its medical management belongs to the neurologist, although we and many other voice clinicians have been instrumental in alerting health professionals to patients who present to our clinics with hypokinetic features that may have previously gone undetected. We have found that an interdisciplinary healthcare team, consisting of the SLP, physician, nurse, nutritionist, and various rehabilitation experts, comprises the best medical care for patients with this complex disorder. Over time, the period of relief from continued dopaminergic administration becomes shorter, requiring new medication protocols and possible neurosurgical approaches to reduce tremor, such as stereotactic surgery deep-brain stimulation (DBS). In deep-brain stimulation, a thin stimulator is surgically placed in the thalamus, the part of the brain that is believed to activate tremors. The stimulator is powered by a tiny generator implanted in the patient's chest. Different researchers have identified different areas of the thalamus that are most receptive to stimulation, resulting in reduced tremors. Hamel and colleagues (2003) suggest that stimulation of the subthalamic nucleus results in marked improvement in levodopa-sensitive Parkinsonian symptoms and levodopa-induced dyskinesias. With respect to the influence of DBS on voice and speech, researchers cite mixed results. Putzer and colleagues (2008) and Mate and colleagues (2011) noted improvement, while others, such as Klostermann and colleagues (2008) did not. Spielman and colleagues (2011) conducted a small-group study to evaluate voice and speech in individuals with and without DBS of the subthalamic nucleus (STN-DBS) before and after LSVT/LOUD, to determine whether outcomes for surgical subjects were comparable to nonsurgical cohorts. It was reported that both treated groups showed significant increases in sound pressure level from pre- to post- and six-month follow-up.

CHECK YOUR KNOWLEDGE

1. Describe the underlying deficits of PD.
2. Why is a holistic approach to PD advocated by the authors? What is meant by the term *holistic*?

Intervention for spastic dysarthria may appear counterintuitive. Many patients think that if they only work harder, the voice will become stronger and better in quality. The reverse is true. Note in this **video** how a reduction in vocal effort and attention to resonance in the facial mask yield improvements in all four subsystems of speech. Grand Rounds: Explain why reduced effort at the level of the vocal folds may result in improved vocal quality and pitch and amplitude flexibility.

CEREBROVASCULAR ACCIDENT (CVA)

Cerebrovascular accident (commonly referred to as stroke) is the third leading cause of death in the United States, behind heart disease and cancer (American Heart Association, 2012). It affects as many as 5% of the population over 65 years old, and this number is growing annually due to the aging population. A significant portion of stroke patients that initially survive are faced with the risk of aspiration, as well as quality-of-life issues relating to impaired communication (Feigin and colleagues, 2003).

Voice and connected speech changes in CVA are complex and highly dependent on the nature and site of lesion. Vocal fold paralysis as a direct result of stroke is rare and is most commonly associated with brainstem stroke, lateral medullary syndrome, Wallenberg syndrome, and Horner syndrome (Rigueiro-Veloso and colleagues, 1997). In the absence of vocal fold paralysis, voice quality is characterized principally as either spastic or flaccid. Spastic voice changes are common with upper motor neuron lesions, as seen in bilateral CVAs. Speech is characterized by slowed articulation, strained voiced quality, and hypernasality. In contrast, flaccid voice changes result from a lower motor neuron lesion in the brainstem, principally from loss of muscle tone and reflexes. Speech is characterized by a breathy voice quality with diminished loudness and air wastage (Aronson, 1995). A stroke to the cerebellum may result in an ataxic dysarthria, described earlier in this chapter.

Laryngeal stroboscopy is a key procedure in the diagnosis of laryngeal dysfunction in CVA. Stroboscopy provides an assessment of the mucosal wave, which is abnormal in subtle paresis or atrophy of the vocal folds (Altman and colleagues, 2007). Sensation can also be tested by touching the endoscope tip to the arytenoids bilaterally, where a strong vocal fold closure should be elicited. Pooling of secretions in the hypopharynx suggests impairment of sensation or secretion management. Though not as commonly used, laryngeal electromyography (LEMG) is helpful in the assessment of immobility of one or both vocal folds (Munin and colleagues, 2003).

Treatment of laryngeal dysfunction in stroke encompasses four major areas: (1) tracheotomy/airway management, (2) dysphagia/aspiration, (3) secretion management, and (4) dysphonia. Review of the first three areas is beyond the scope of this text; the interested reader is referred to Altman and colleagues (2007) for an overview. Treatment of dysphonia involves managing glottic incompetency due to vocal fold paralysis, a topic covered earlier in this chapter.

TRAUMATIC BRAIN INJURY

Traumatic brain injury (TBI) is the result of external forces acting on the head. Most TBIs are caused by motor vehicle accidents; falls; assaults; and, more recently, explosion injuries experienced by members of the armed forces (Shively and Perl, 2012). These injuries can cause focal or diffuse lesions, axonal shearing, and hypoxia, all of which can be secondary to vascular or tissue damage.

Dysarthria associated with TBI may be temporary or chronic, mild or severe, and accompanied or not by other language and cognitive disorders. Most dysarthrias are of the mixed type, and variability in the nature and severity of the physiological impairment calls for custom treatment programs based on a clear appreciation for the subsystems of respiration, phonation, resonance, articulation, and prosody. For example, patients presenting primarily with pontocerebellar axonal injuries may demonstrate ataxic symptoms of paradoxical breathing patterns and velar mistiming. For these patients we emphasize the Voice Facilitating Approaches of auditory feedback, counseling, and respiratory training (see Chapter 7). Other patients with more involved injuries of the motor system bilaterally may present with spastic dysarthria and have lower vital capacities than nondisabled speakers (Murdoch and colleagues, 1994). Kinematics of the same group revealed that the speakers with TBI have problems coordinating the actions of the rib cage and abdomen during speech. This lack of coordination is apparent in patients with TBI, many of whom take replenishing breaths at inappropriate phrase junctures during conversational speaking and oral reading tasks. For these patients, we advise intervention focusing on altering the pitch (usually slightly upward) and reducing vowel duration within words. Auditory and visual biofeedback is critical for this population to increase meta-awareness of speaking deficits and strategies that increase naturalness of conversational speech.

SUMMARY

At the beginning of this chapter, we looked at the neurological bases of human laryngeal function. We reviewed the latest research in behavioral, pharmacological, and surgical management of neurogenic voice disorders and listed a number of Voice Facilitating Approaches that have been effective for many patients presenting with dysarthria (see Chapter 7). The key to effective behavior-based intervention for patients presenting with static or progressive neurogenic dysphonia is an understanding of the nature of deficits in the subsystems of speech and knowing how to address them.

CLINICAL CONCEPTS

The following clinical concepts correspond with the objectives at the beginning of this chapter.

1. Changes in speech can be the first or only manifestation of neurogenic disease. Recognition of these changes can have a significant impact on medical diagnosis and care. The SLP may be the first professional to recognize the breakdown of a single system, such as in idiopathic UVFP, or multiple subsystems, such as amyotrophic lateral sclerosis.
2. In many cases, strengthening the vocal muscles and improving voicing technique in UVFP result in very good voice quality. The Voice Facilitating Approaches of head positioning, establishing a new pitch, focus, and auditory feedback (see Chapter 7) should be explored in patients with UVFP.
3. Holistic approaches to the hypokinetic reductions in many of those with Parkinson's disease are effective in increasing respiration, phonation, and articulatory range of motion and accuracy. Auditory feedback and visual feedback are effective strategies for helping to maintain these improvements.
4. Adductor SD and vocal tremor originate from neurogenic etiologies, whereas muscle tension dysphonia is of a functional nature. SLPs are skilled in the differential diagnosis of each of these disorders and often work collaboratively with ENTs to identify and manage these patients.
5. Voice and speech problems originating from TBI are multifactorial in nature and call for custom treatment programs based on a clear appreciation of the subsystems of respiration, phonation, resonance, articulation, and prosody.

GUIDED READING

Read the following articles.

> Sulica, L, Rosen, C. A., Postma, G. N., Simpson, B., Amin, M., Courey, M., & Merati, A. (2010). Current practice in injection augmentation of the vocal folds: Indications, treatment principles, techniques, and complications. *Laryngoscope, 120,* 319–325.

> Paniello, R. C., Edgar, J. D., Kallogeri, D., & Piccirillo, J. F. (2011). Medialization versus reinnervation for unilateral vocal fold paralysis: A multicenter randomized clinical trial. *Laryngoscope, 121,* 2172–2179.

Using the information reported in the two articles, identify current approaches to vocal fold augmentation and the considerations for vocal fold medialization versus laryngeal reinnervation for UVFP.

PREPARING FOR THE PRAXIS™

Directions: Please read the case study and answer the five questions that follow. (Please see page 319 for the answer key.)

> *John is a 60-year-old high school teacher who presented to our clinic with a 14-month history of a progressive dysphonia following removal of his thyroid gland. A suspected vocal fold paralysis had been ruled out by his ENT. We performed a follow-up rigid endoscopy at our clinic and observed normal vocal fold mobility. Our endoscopic findings further revealed that the ventricular vocal folds tended to move toward the midline upon phonation, thus damping the vibration of the true vocal folds and interrupting the mucosal wave. Thick, sticky mucus was seen throughout the laryngeal vestibule, and pachydermia was observed at the posterior commissure. The patient presented with a strained voice that was occasionally choked off during the clinical interview. He reported that at times the voice improved, during singing or whistling, but otherwise, it was becoming harder and harder to force the voice out. The dysphonia was threatening his job as a teacher and coach, and he could no longer enjoy normal outings with his family. Voice Facilitating Approaches of focus and inhalation phonation resulted in easier vocal quality for a few phonatory attempts, but the strained quality and vocal arrests soon returned.*

1. Based on the patient's history and perceptual findings, respond to the following: A unilateral vocal fold paralysis was originally suspected in this case because of surgical intervention in the vicinity of cranial nerve:
   A. IV
   B. X
   C. XII
   D. IX

2. The involvement of the ventricular vocal folds during voicing attempts is most likely associated with a(n):
   A. Ataxic dysarthria
   B. Result of laryngopharyngeal reflux

    C. Maladaptive behavior adopted to try to compensate for the irregular vocal fold arrests

    D. Precursor to hypokinetic dysarthria

3. The Voice Facilitating Approach of focus was probed in an attempt to:

    A. Increase vocal fold closure

    B. Increase vocal amplitude

    C. Increase F⁰

    D. Move voiced energy from the larynx to the face

4. This patient is most likely presenting with:

    A. A primary muscle tension dysphonia

    B. Myasthenia gravis

    C. Adductor SD

    D. Essential tremor

5. The gold standard medical approach to this disorder calls for:

    A. BTX-A injections

    B. Vocal fold augmentation

    C. Medialization thyroplasty

    D. Laryngeal massage

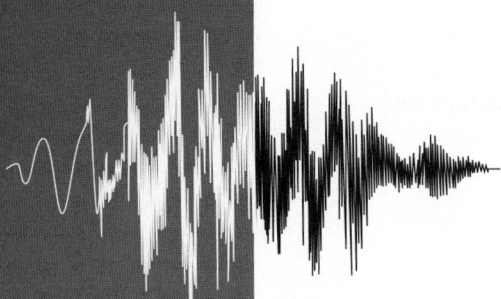

CHAPTER 6

Evaluation of the Voice

When encountering a patient presenting with a voice disorder, the clinician begins a systematic process of assessment, evaluation, and diagnosis. *Assessment* is the process of collecting relevant data for clinical decision making. *Evaluation* is an appraisal of the implications and significance of the assessment. *Diagnosis* calls for the clinician to make a decision about whether a problem exists and, if so, differentiating it from other, similar problems. In a medical model, diagnostic emphasis is on identification of possible causes and maintaining factors (Paul, 2002).

The results of the voice evaluation serve as the foundation for a sound treatment plan. As such, the voice evaluation must be a carefully and scientifically validated procedure performed by a competent clinician. Ideally, the voice assessment should follow examination of the patient by a laryngologist (an ENT physician with special knowledge of the larynx and voice). In instances where a patient is assessed prior to examination by the laryngologist, the speech-language pathologist ("clinician") should reserve diagnosis and treatment planning until results of the medical assessment can be evaluated. While it is the province of the laryngologist to make a laryngeal diagnosis, and to establish and oversee a medical management plan, it is the province of the clinician to make a voice diagnosis and to establish and carry out a voice therapy plan.

Although we present the comprehensive voice evaluation here as a separate chapter, it is important for the reader to appreciate that effective voice therapy requires continuous assessment and evaluation. While we believe in the value of using appropriate instrumentation for assessment, the knowledgeable and skilled clinician is the one who is of ultimate value in the evaluation, diagnosis, and treatment of the patient with a disordered voice.

We begin this chapter with a brief discussion about screening individuals for voice disorders. An overview of the laryngologist's evaluation of the larynx follows. We then present detailed information about the comprehensive voice evaluation, emphasizing the role of the SLP clinician. We conclude with three case studies that will help the reader put the information in this chapter into clinical context.

SCREENING FOR VOICE DISORDERS

As discussed in Chapter 1, the actual prevalence of voice disorders in children is difficult to determine. A number of researchers have concluded conservatively that between 6% and 9% of school-age children may have a voice disorder (Andrews, 2002; Carding and colleagues, 2006; Cornut and Troillet-Cornut, 1995). Kahane and Mayo (1989) suggest that the majority of children with voice disorders are not seen by a clinician. Reports from Davis and Harris (1992) and from Broomfield and Dodd (2004) estimate that children with voice disorders make up less than 5% of any given school-based clinician's caseload.

Individuals other than the school clinician often identify the majority of children with voice problems (Davis and Harris, 1992). Typically, the child's teacher, nurse, or family member first notices a vocal feature such as harsh quality. The ability of such individuals to make accurate judgments about the normalcy of voice is not quite as good, however, as that of an experienced clinician (McFarlane and colleagues, 1991). Therefore, rather than relying on other well-meaning individuals to refer children for therapy, the clinician should develop screening procedures for the early identification of children with voice problems.

Most public and private schools have screening programs to identify speech and language disorders in new students and those in certain grades at specified times of the year. By using some kind of voice screening form, clinicians are better able to identify and document those children in need of voice assessment and potential treatment. With very little additional testing time per child (5 minutes or so), a voice screening can be added to existing speech and language screening protocols. The importance of identifying and managing voice disorders in children cannot be overemphasized because dysphonia can have an impact on a child's educational and psychosocial development, as well as his or her physical and emotional health (Connor and colleagues, 2008).

Clinicians in various settings have developed different voice screening forms. The items on the screening form usually represent the aspects of voice that the clinician considers important for identifying children who may be having voice problems. The screening form helps clinicians focus, organize, and report their listening observations. Two easy-to-administer screening protocols are the Voice Screening form in the *Boone Voice Program for Children* (Boone, 1993) and the *Quick Screen for Voice* (Lee and colleagues, 2004, 2005).

The Quick Screen for Voice addresses respiration, phonation, and resonance. It takes about 10 minutes to administer and is appropriate to use with students from preschool through high school. The clinician responds to a checklist of observations made during spontaneous conversation, picture description, imitated sentences, recited passages, counting, and other natural samples of voice and speech. The student fails the screening if there are one or more disorders in production in any section. Lee and colleagues report in the manual accompanying this instrument that approximately 10% of preschool students in a field test failed the voice screening, a prevalence rate in line with that reported in the literature by others (e.g., Boyle, 2000).

The *Boone Voice Program for Children* Voice Screening form also addresses respiration, phonation, and resonance. It is relatively quick and easy to administer and is appropriate for students in all grades. The clinician listens to natural samples of voice and speech and, for each of the scale judgments (pitch, loudness, quality, nasal resonance, oral resonance), notes whether the child's voice sounds like the voices of peers of the same age, gender, and race. To facilitate scoring, the clinician records his or her perceptual judgments using a simple three-point system. For example, if a child's voice appears lower in pitch than that of his or her peers, a minus sign (−) is circled; if pitch appears normal, the neutral symbol (N) is circled; if the pitch level is higher than the child's peers, the plus sign (+) is circled. If the child receives either a (−) or (+) on any of the five clinical parameters, he or she should be rechecked within a few weeks. Those individuals who, on follow-up, continue to demonstrate some departures in voice from their peers should receive full medical and voice evaluations (Boone, 1993).

MEDICAL EVALUATION OF THE VOICE-DISORDERED PATIENT

Sataloff and colleagues (2003) have written extensively about the history taking and physical examination of patients with voice disorders. They suggest the use of a history questionnaire (often completed in advance) to help the patient document all the necessary information, sort out and articulate his or her problems, and save office time in recording information (p. 138). Figure 6.1 lists the essential items covered in such a questionnaire. Depending on the nature of the patient's chief complaint and symptoms, the clinician may pursue additional areas of questioning.

A detailed history and interview often suggests the cause of a voice disorder; however, a comprehensive physical examination is still necessary to confirm or rule out certain medical conditions that may require the laryngologist to consult with specialists such as neurologists, pulmonologists, endocrinologists, psychiatrists, internists, physiatrists, and others with special knowledge of, and interest in, voice disorders. Physical examination should include an assessment of general physical condition, and a thorough ear, nose, and throat evaluation. Depending on the patient's age and observed signs, additional areas of examination may be pursued (McMurray, 2003; Pontes and colleagues, 2006).

Visual inspection of the larynx is perhaps the most important in terms of understanding the cause of a voice disorder and its potential for treatment. There is a rich history of research supporting the importance of laryngoscopy in the diagnosis of voice disorders (see Kendall and Leonard [2012] for both a historical perspective and the current state of the art). Office-based visual examination of the larynx traditionally takes one of two forms: mirror laryngoscopy or endoscopic laryngoscopy (more commonly referred to as laryngeal endoscopy). In mirror laryngoscopy, a small laryngeal mirror is placed at the back of the patient's mouth and light is shone on the mirror from the physician's headset. If the mirror is angled properly, a reflected view of the hypopharynx can be seen. In laryngeal endoscopy, either a rigid fiberoptic

FIGURE 6.1 Sample Medical History Questions

How old are you?

What is your voice problem?

Do you have any pressing voice commitments?

How much voice training have you had?

Under what kinds of conditions do you use your voice?

Are you aware of misusing or abusing your voice during singing?

Are you aware of misusing or abusing your voice during speaking?

Do you have pain when you talk or sing?

What kind of physical condition are you in?

Have you noted voice or bodily weakness, tremor, fatigue, or loss of control?

Do you have allergy or cold symptoms?

Do you have any breathing problems, especially after exercise?

Have you been exposed to environmental irritants?

Do you smoke, live with a smoker, or work around smoke?

Do any foods seem to affect your voice?

Do you have morning hoarseness, bad breath, excessive phlegm, a lump in your throat, or heartburn?

Do you have trouble with your bowels or your belly?

Are you under particular stress or in therapy?

Do you have problems controlling your weight; are you excessively tired; are you cold when other people are warm?

Do you have menstrual irregularity, cyclical voice changes associated with menses, recent menopause, or other hormonal changes or problems?

Do you have jaw joint or other dental problems?

Do you or others living with you have hearing loss?

Have you suffered whiplash or other bodily injury?

Did you undergo any surgery prior to the onset of your voice problems?

What medications and other substances do you use?

scope is placed in the mouth or a flexible fiberoptic scope is passed through one of the nasal passages. The rigid laryngoscope has a prism at the end that directs light and receives images at an angle of either 70° or 90°, permitting optimum visualization of the normal inverted-V position of the vocal folds. Figure 6.2 lists the advantages and disadvantages of these indirect laryngeal examination methods.

The information gained from laryngoscopic visualization of the larynx has often been the most important information gained during the diagnostic assessment

FIGURE 6.2 Advantages and Disadvantages of Laryngeal Examination Methods

I. Mirror laryngoscopy
  A. Advantages
    1. Quick overview of laryngeal anatomy and physiology
    2. Prognostic for either rigid or flexible laryngoscopy
  B. Disadvantages
    1. Poorly tolerated by some patients
    2. Can only assess sustained vowels and not connected speech or singing
    3. Alters typical laryngeal behavior
II. Rigid (oral) laryngoscopy
  A. Advantages
    1. Excellent lighting, contributing to good photography
    2. Excellent magnification, contributing to good videography
  B. Disadvantages
    1. Poorly tolerated by some patients
    2. Can only assess sustained vowels and not connected speech or singing
    3. Cannot assess the entire vocal tract
    4. Alters typical laryngeal behavior
III. Flexible (nasal) laryngoscopy
  A. Advantages
    1. Well-tolerated by almost all patients
    2. Minimal alteration of typical laryngeal behavior
    3. Can assess connected speech and singing across the vocal range
    4. Can assess the entire vocal tract
  B. Disadvantages
    1. Optics and magnification inferior to that of rigid (oral) laryngoscopy
IV. Stroboscopy (coupled to rigid or flexible laryngoscopy)
  A. Advantages
    1. Allows for examination of vocal fold vibratory behavior
  B. Disadvantages
    1. Requires that patient produce a steady fundamental frequency
    2. Requires additional technical skills of the examiner

Source: Modified from Koufman (2003).

(McFarlane and Watterson, 1990; McFarlane and colleagues, 1990). When coupled with the other information, visualization of the larynx has greatly improved our accuracy of diagnosis, and set the foundation for successful voice therapy plans.

The Roles of the SLP and Physician and the Need for a Medical Evaluation

The American Speech-Language-Hearing Association (ASHA) Preferred Practice Patterns for the Profession of Speech-Language Pathology (2004d) states:

> A physician, preferably in a discipline appropriate to the presenting complaint, must examine all patients/clients with voice disorders. The physician's examination may occur before or after the voice evaluation by the clinician (p. 99).

If a patient arrives for treatment for dysphonia but has not had a previous medical examination, the clinician should wait to make treatment recommendations until he or she has obtained all necessary medical information. The voice evaluation by the speech-language pathologist may begin, however, even in the absence of all the medical information. A case history can be taken, and assessment of respiration, phonation, and resonance can be conducted—only the decision about whether to begin voice therapy need be deferred until all medical information is obtained. This deferment is necessary because a patient's voice may sound a particular way for a number of reasons, some more serious and complicated than others. For example, a particular patient's vocal symptoms may include decreased speaking pitch, pitch variability, and pitch range; decreased loudness, loudness variability, and loudness range; increased breathiness; voice breaks; and vocal fatigue. Such complaints are common when there is an additive vocal fold mass. However, such a mass lesion may take the form of a nodule, for example, which is benign, or it may take the form of an invasive malignant tumor. Without a complete medical examination, including imaging, the clinician does not know the etiology of the voice disorder.

The roles of the laryngologist and clinician differ in regard to evaluation of the voice-disordered patient, although the assessments conducted by each may overlap. In general, the laryngologist's primary role is to identify and manage those conditions or diseases that interfere with normal voice production, while the clinician's primary role is to evaluate and facilitate voice production given the known medical status of the patient. Optimally, both professionals work together in evaluating and managing the patient.

In larger urban cities, patients may have ready access to a voice care team in settings such as local hospitals and clinics, private otolaryngology practices, or academic medical centers. In smaller cities or rural areas, however, access may be quite limited. In such cases, patients may have to travel a considerable distance to see a laryngologist. In such cases, it is important for patients to understand why they need to see the laryngologist. A brief written note from the referring clinician can often help facilitate communication between the patient and laryngologist. If the patient is a child who failed a voice screening, for example, inclusion of the voice screening form may help the parents to discuss their child with the laryngologist and help focus the child's examination. Upon completion of his or her medical examination, it is equally important for the laryngologist to communicate the findings to both the patient (or parent, where applicable) and the referring clinician. Depending on the nature of the medical examination, a variety of written forms may be used. These written forms may include a narrative/descriptive note stating the medical diagnosis and findings, record forms for specific types of assessment (such as laryngoscopy), and copies of photos or videos of the laryngeal and related findings.

Evaluation of the Voice-Disordered Patient by the SLP

In an interview with Thibeault (2007), Bless describes the SLP's role in the evaluation of persons with voice disorders as follows:

> The clinician's role is to describe the structure and function of the larynx and make recommendations regarding further testing needed to understand the etiology or maintenance of the voice problem and to make recommendations for treatment. (p. 4)

The American Speech-Language-Hearing Association (ASHA) has published a comprehensive document titled *Preferred Practice Patterns for Speech-Language*

FIGURE 6.3 Components of the Comprehensive Voice Evaluation

- Review of auditory and visual status.
- Case history.
- Behavioral observation.
- Auditory-perceptual ratings.
- Voice-related quality of life.
- Oral-peripheral examination.
- Laryngoscopy/phonoscopy.
- Acoustic analysis.
- Electroglottographic analysis.
- Aerodynamic analysis.
- Phonatory-respiratory efficiency.
- Voice dosage (e.g., typical daily use of the voice, both professionally and socially).

Pathology (American Speech-Language-Hearing Association, 2004a). Based on this document, and our many decades of clinical experience, we present in Figure 6.3 a list of the major components in the evaluation of the voice. We recognize that not every patient will need to undergo all the assessments listed in Figure 6.3, and we recognize that not every clinician will have access to, and be comfortable with, the equipment needed to conduct all the assessments. It is our intent here to provide sufficient breadth and depth, knowing that the individual clinician will have the final "voice" in evaluating any given patient.

REVIEW OF AUDITORY AND VISUAL STATUS

Hearing acuity is important in monitoring and regulating one's own voice production (Lee and colleagues, 2007). Thus, hearing loss has the potential to alter respiration, phonation, resonance, and prosody (Boone, 1966; Higgins and colleagues, 2005; Horga and Liker, 2006). For example, an elderly patient may have a hearing loss and/or his or her spouse may have a hearing loss. In this clinical scenario, there is potential for the patient to develop a functional dysphonia characterized by the use of inappropriate pitch and/or loudness and/or glottal attack. Other clinical scenarios include a child with a congenital hearing loss or a teen or adult with noise-induced hearing loss. About 8% of persons in the United States have hearing loss, which may vary from mild loss of sensitivity to total loss of hearing (Liu and Yan, 2007). The prevalence of hearing loss accelerates dramatically with age. It is estimated that 5% of children under the age of 17 years have hearing loss. The percentages increase throughout the years: 23% of those age 18 to 44 years have hearing loss, 29% of those age 45 to 60 years, and 43% of those 65 years or older (Davis and colleagues, 1997; National Academy on an Aging Society, 1999). Self-reported hearing loss can be identified in half of those aged 85 years and older (Mulrow and Lichtenstein, 1991). These numbers are expected to rise with the rapidly increasing number of elderly people (Hobbs and Stoops, 2002). When evaluating the patient with a voice disorder, a hearing screening should be conducted by the clinician when hearing difficulty is suspected (either by patient self-report or behavioral observation of others) (Bogardus and colleagues, 2003). Conducting hearing screenings in such a situation is within the American Speech-Language-Hearing Association (2007) *Scope of Practice for Clinicians* and is addressed in the American Speech-Language-Hearing

Association (2004) *Preferred Practice Patterns for Speech-Language Pathology.* Cohen and Turley (2009) investigated the co-prevalence of voice problems and hearing loss in 248 elderly residents living independently in two retirement communities, and reported that nearly 20% had dysphonia, 50% had hearing loss, and just over 10% had both. Persons with hearing loss were more likely to have dysphonia than those without hearing loss, and persons with both dysphonia and hearing loss had greater depression scores than those with neither symptom (p. 1987). What remains unknown in the literature is whether there is a relationship between hearing loss and dysphonia in nonelderly adults or children. However, there is a wealth of literature that suggests a relationship between hearing loss and resonance disorders (see Chapters 8 and 10).

Visual acuity is also an important consideration when assessing the person with a voice disorder. Decreased visual acuity may lead a patient to misjudge his or her distance from the listener and to alter his or her voice in ways that are detrimental. If visual feedback is provided by a mirror reflecting the patient's head and body posture, or a computer monitor showing a voice tracing, it is important that the patient be able to see well. In the case of the alaryngeal speaker who is learning to use an electrolarynx, visual acuity is important in learning to place the electrolarynx in the right location. More than 38 million Americans age 40 and older are estimated to experience blindness, low vision, or an age-related eye disease, with persons older than age 65 being the most affected (Congdon and colleagues, 2004).

CASE HISTORY

During the case history, the clinician must establish rapport with the patient so that there is an open and honest sharing of information, and so that the patient will ultimately feel empowered to change his or her behavior if called upon to do so (van Leer and colleagues, 2008). Behrman (2006) has written recently about the concept of motivational interviewing (MI), which centers on eliciting the patient's motivation to adhere to behavioral change in a nonthreatening manner. Behrman also describes certain clinical considerations that may affect resistance, and therefore adherence, to voice therapy. Such considerations may include a history of controlling interactions with medical professionals; previous exposure to exaggerated vocal hygiene messages; confusion regarding vocal identity; failure of other treatment modalities, including voice rest and medical management; prior experience with nonadherence in voice therapy; and lack of support from individuals in the patient's life, including business colleagues, friends, and family members (p. 216). The clinically astute clinician monitors his or her own verbal and nonverbal behaviors during the case history interview in order to elicit clinically relevant information from the patient in a supportive and motivating manner.

In the following sections, we provide an overview of the key areas in the case history and interview. Depending on the particular clinical scenario, one may pursue other areas.

Description of the Problem and Cause

It is valuable to ask patients directly what they feel are the problems and what might have caused them. It is often effective to ask the same questions of family members, a spouse, or teachers. The different views about what the problem may be and the various guesses about probable causation may offer tips for management. Patients' descriptions often reveal much about their own conceptualization of the problem. What a patient feels the problem is may not be consistent with the opinions of the referring physician or the clinician, a discrepancy that may be due to what we call the patient's reality distance. This distance may be the result of the patient's lay background and inability to understand adequately what had been explained. Often we hear highly discrepant reports of "what the doctor said" as a patient recounts the diagnoses of previous clinicians. More often than not, this distance is primarily the result of the patient's reluctance to accept and cope with the real problem. An individual's defenses may force him or her to describe the problem in a way that is not consistent with the perceptions of others. What a patient says about a problem, however, may provide the clinician with insights that no amount of observation or testing can match.

Onset and Duration of the Problem

How long patients believe they have had the voice problem is important. A problem of acute and sudden onset of a dysphonia usually poses a severe threat to a patient. That is, it keeps the patient from carrying out his or her customary activities (playing, singing, acting, selling, preaching, teaching, campaigning). Sudden onset of aphonia or dysphonia deserves thorough exploration by both the laryngologist and the clinician. Sometimes dysphonia develops very gradually. Such a gradual, fluctuating dysphonia is often related to varying situations in which patients may find themselves; sometimes it occurs only during moments of stress or after fatigue. A history of slow onset sometimes suggests a gradually developing pathology, such as the development of Reinke's edema or dysphonia that is an early developing symptom of some kind of progressive neurological disease. Voice therapy, like other forms of remedial therapy, is usually more successful with those patients who are motivated to overcome their problems. Patients with a long history of indifference toward their dysphonia usually present an additional challenge to the clinician and a more unfavorable prognosis than the patients who have recently acquired the disorder, depending, of course, on the type and etiology and relative extent of the pathology involved.

Variability of the Problem

Most voice patients can provide rather accurate timetables of the consistency of their problem. If the severity of a voice problem is variable, a clinician may be able to identify those vocal situations in which the patient experiences the best voice and the worst voice. The typical patient with vocal hyperfunction reports a better voice earlier in the day, with increasing dysphonia later in the day after more voice use. For example, a high school social studies teacher reported a normal-sounding voice at the beginning of the day; toward the end of a day, after six hours of lecturing, he reported increasing hoarseness and a feeling of fullness and dryness in the throat. Voice rest and then dinner at the end of the day usually restored his voice to its normal pitch and quality. Obviously, such fluctuation in the daily quality of the voice enables the clinician to identify easily the situations contributing to the patient's vocal abuse. Another patient, whose dysphonia was related closely to allergy and postnasal drip experienced during sleep, presented this variation in hoarseness: severity in the morning on awakening, decrease in severity with use of the voice, complete disappearance by late afternoon, and severity again the next morning. This pattern is also closely associated with night-time laryngopharyngeal reflux.

The variation of the voice problem can reveal which situations tend to aggravate the disorder. A heavy metal rock band singer reported that she had no voice problem during the day in conversational situations or while practicing with her band. She developed hoarseness only on those nights she performed. Observation of her performances revealed that the adverse factors were the cigarette smoke around her, to which she was unusually sensitive, and the noise of the crowd, above which she had to increase her volume in order to be heard by the audience. Her singing technique was satisfactory. Adherence to a strict vocal hygiene program that included voice use reduction on the days of her performances (Zraick and colleagues, 2009) provided her with immediate relief. She was also encouraged to invest in a more sophisticated and powerful sound system.

Description of Vocal Demands

Abuse, misuse, and overuse of the voice cause most functional voice problems. It is important for clinicians to determine how voice patients are using their larynges in most life situations. The voice a child or adult exhibits in the clinician's office may not represent the voice used on the playground, in the classroom, or in other settings. Sometimes patients can re-create some of their aversive laryngeal behaviors as a demonstration for the clinician, but more often, a valid search for aversive vocal behaviors requires the clinician to visit the environment where the abuse-misuse occurs. Successful voice clinicians must thus build into their schedules actual visits to playgrounds, theaters, churches, courtrooms, or offices. Case (2002), for instance, has demonstrated the effects of cheerleading on the larynges of teenagers, comparing laryngoscopic examinations before and after two weeks of attendance at a cheerleading camp. His data strongly suggest that continued cheerleading has a direct adverse effect on the larynges of the majority of the adolescents studied. It is obviously important for the clinician to identify the vocal use pattern of the patient.

Additional Case History Information

It is important to determine at the time of the voice evaluation if the patient has ever had previous voice therapy. If the patient has, what type of past therapy would have obvious relevance to present management? When previous voice therapy attempts have failed to improve the vocal quality or have been unsuccessful in reducing a vocal pathology, the knowledge of previous therapy is important. We must make every effort, however, to present the appearance of a fresh and different approach to the patient who has experienced failure in previous voice therapy; even if we use the same goals of therapy as before, we must redirect the new approach to voice therapy in a manner that appears to the patient to be headed down a completely different road. Determining whether other members of the family have similar voice problems is helpful. We have had particular patients present a certain voice problem, only to interview members of the family and find that all or many of them have the same voicing patterns. Once a patient is comfortable with an examiner, or perhaps after voice therapy has begun, a social history should be taken to provide the clinician with useful information about the patient as a person. One patient spoke with two completely different voices, constantly shifting between one voice and the other. When we asked why she used these two voices, she said her first voice was "my voice before I died." Further case history questioning revealed that she had been a patient in a mental hospital on two occasions. It became clear as the interview progressed that she was still having psychological problems and that her voice disorder was a symptom of a more serious unresolved disorder. She was convinced that she had died and that she was now a channel for another person who had also died. The different voices represented different people.

BEHAVIORAL OBSERVATION

One should keep in mind that observation of our patients often tells us more about them than their histories and assessment data. Clinicians must become critical observers, attempting to describe behavior they see rather than merely labeling it. Writing observations about a patient is one of the few ways clinicians can note what they observe (audio and video recordings are two other means). Even here, however, it is important for clinicians to minimize any subjectivity by describing only what they see and hear, and not adding interpretation to the observation.

Because voice difficulties are often symptomatic of the inability to have satisfactory interpersonal relationships, it is imperative that the clinician consider the patient's degree of adequacy as a social being. Patients who exhibit extremely sweaty palms; who avoid eye contact with people to whom they are speaking; who speak through clenched teeth; who use excessive postural changes or demonstrate facial tics; who sit with a masked, nonaffective facial expression; or who exhibit obvious shortness of breath may be displaying behaviors frequently considered as symptomatic of anxiety. The struggle to phonate may reflect a struggle to maintain a conversational relationship. Such observed behavior in the voice patient may be highly significant to the voice clinician planning a course of voice remediation. The decision about whether to treat a problem symptomatically (that is, by voice therapy) or by improving the patient's potential for interpersonal adjustment (perhaps by psychotherapy) is often aided by a review of the observations of the patient. A patient who demonstrates friendly, normal affect is telling the clinician, at least superficially, that he or she functions well in a two-person relationship; such information may well have clinical relevance. Such observations are extremely valuable to clinicians planning treatment approaches. Note, however, that in our experience very few voice patients require referral for psychotherapy.

AUDITORY-PERCEPTUAL RATINGS

Clinicians appear to prefer auditory-perceptual measures to instrumental measures when assessing dysphonia and documenting therapy progress (Bassich and Ludlow, 1986; Carding and colleagues, 2000). Behrman (2005) surveyed voice clinicians regarding common diagnostic practices in patients referred for therapy with the diagnosis of muscle tension dysphonia. Each respondent reported that perceptual assessment of voice quality was very important for therapy tasks such as defining overall therapy goals, defining specific therapy session goals, helping the patient to achieve a target production, providing reinforcement to the patient, and measuring treatment outcome. The clinician's perceptual assessment of voice quality occurred significantly more commonly than stroboscopic, acoustic, aerodynamic, and electroglottographic assessments. Behrman concluded that "efforts to make voice quality assessment standard and strengthen perceptual scaling methods appear well justified, given its dominant role in voice evaluations" (p. 468).

When performing an auditory-perceptual evaluation of voice quality, clinicians should consider a number of factors that might influence their resulting judgments (Kent, 1996). According to a seminal paper by Kreiman and colleagues (1993), these factors include the nature of the speaking task (Law and colleagues, 2012; Zraick and colleagues, 2005), listener experience and training (Chan and Yiu, 2006; Eadie and Baylor, 2006; Eadie and colleagues, 2010), the use of anchors (Awan and Lawson, 2009; Chan and Yiu, 2002), and the type of rating method used (Patel and colleagues, 2010). A number of different voice perceptual scales are available for clinical use, but two seem to be used most in current clinical practice. The first is the GRBAS Scale (Hirano, 1981), and the second is the Consensus Auditory Perceptual Evaluation of Voice (CAPE-V) (Kempster and colleagues, 2009).

The GRBAS Scale was developed by the Committee for Phonatory Function Tests of the Japanese Society of Logopedics and Phoniatrics. Each parameter on the GRBAS scale represents a dimension of phonation: G (grade) represents the overall severity of voice abnormality, R represents roughness, B represents breathiness, A represents aesthenic (weak), and S represents strain. The GRBAS uses a four-point, equal-appearing rating scale of 0 (normal) to 3 (extreme) for all five parameters.

The CAPE-V was drafted following the Consensus Conference on Auditory-Perceptual Evaluation of Voice held at the University of Pittsburgh in June 2002. The conference, sponsored by ASHA's Special Interest Group 3 (Voice and Voice Disorders), brought together researchers and clinicians interested in the problem of measuring voice quality. A working group drafted the instrument known as the CAPE-V following the conference (Kempster and colleagues, 2009). The CAPE-V shares several of the parameters of the GRBAS scale. Judges rate six aspects of voice (Overall Severity, Roughness, Breathiness, Strain, Pitch, and Loudness) by placing a tick mark on a 100 mm horizontal line. The instrument includes two unlabeled scales in the event a voice includes other significant features (e.g., tremor).

Zraick and colleagues (2007, 2010) validated the CAPE-V for use with adults in a national, multicenter study sponsored by ASHA. This study examined agreement for expert clinicians' ratings of dysphonia using the CAPE-V and the GRBAS. There was also an assessment of inter-rater and intra-rater reliability across both scales. It was reported that expert clinicians' perceptions of dysphonia appeared to be reliable and unaffected by rating instrument, and that the CAPE-V appeared to be more sensitive than the GRBAS to small differences within and among patients. Additional studies have further validated the use of the CAPE-V (Helou and colleagues, 2010; Karnell and colleagues, 2007; Kelchner and colleagues, 2010; Solomon and colleagues, 2011). Figure 6.4 shows a CAPE-V form completed for a 37-year-old woman with primary muscle tension dysphonia.

FIGURE 6.4 Sample CAPE-V Form

Consensus Auditory-Perceptual Evaluation of Voice (CAPE-V)

Name: **T.J.**   Date: **4/5/12**

The following parameters of voice quality will be rated upon completion of the following tasks:
1. Sustained vowels, /a/ and /i/ for 3-5 seconds duration each.
2. Sentence production:
   a. The blue spot is on the key again.   d. We eat eggs every Easter.
   b. How hard did he hit him?   e. My mama makes lemon muffins.
   c. We were away a year ago.   f. Peter will keep at the peak.
3. Spontaneous speech in response to: "Tell me about your voice problem." or "Tell me how your voice is functioning."

Legend: C = Consistent   I = Intermittent
MI = Mildly Deviant
MO =Moderately Deviant
SE = Severely Deviant

SCORE

Overall Severity _____ X ____   C   I **75**/100

Roughness _____ X _____   C   I **50**/100

Breathiness X _____   C   I **0**/100

Strain _____ X ____   C   I **75**/100

Pitch   (Indicate the nature of the abnormality): **HIGH**
_____ X _____   C   I **15**/100

Loudness (Indicate the nature of the abnormality): **LOW**
_____ X _____   C   I **15**/100

_____   C   I ___/100

_____   C   I ___/100

COMMENTS ABOUT RESONANCE: (NORMAL)   OTHER (Provide description):_____

ADDITIONAL FEATURES (for example, diplophonia, fry, falsetto, asthenia, aphonia, pitch instability, tremor, wet/gurgly, or other relevant terms):

Clinician: **ZRAICK**

Source: Reprinted with permission from Consensus Auditory-Perceptual Evaluation of Voice: Development of a Standardized Clinical Protocol by G. B. Kempster, B. R. Gerratt, K. Verdolini Abbott, J. Barkmeier-Kraemer, and R. E. Hillman. *American Journal of Speech-Language Pathology, 18*(2), 124–132. Copyright 2009 by the American Speech-Language-Hearing Association. All rights reserved.

VOICE-RELATED QUALITY OF LIFE

Two basic approaches to quality-of-life measurement in persons with voice disorders are available: generic assessments that provide a summary of overall health-related quality of life, and specific assessments that focus on specific communication-related quality of life. In a recent survey of diagnostic practices of experienced voice clinicians

(Behrman, 2005), 94% responded that communication-related quality-of-life instruments are important for assessment of treatment outcomes, and 81% considered the data from such instruments important in defining overall therapy goals (p. 460).

In general, voice-disordered patients report poor overall health-related quality of life and communication-related quality of life (Cohen and colleagues, 2006). The choice of which instrument to administer is often driven by the clinician's personal preference and the dynamics of clinical practice. Regardless of which instrument is used, the clinician should be aware that variables such as life events and experiences, personality factors, and the effects of adaptation may influence reported subjective well-being (O'Connor, 2004).

Zraick and Risner (2008) provide a comprehensive review of instruments for assessing communication-related quality of life in persons with voice disorders. Table 6.1 lists some of the instruments currently available to clinicians, most of which are psychometrically sound (Agency for Healthcare Research and Quality, 2002; Branski and colleagues, 2010; Franic and colleagues, 2004). Review of Table 6.1 indicates that the available scales can be grouped and categorized using criteria such as patient age (e.g., adult versus child), rater (e.g., patient versus parent or other proxy), and patient population (e.g., singer versus nonsinger). One important consideration in choosing an instrument is the ability of the patient to read and comprehend its contents. A recent analysis by Zraick and Atcherson (2011) of the readability of the scales listed in Table 6.1 revealed that all are at a reading grade level too high for the average adult to read with ease and to comprehend.

Of the instruments listed in Table 6.1, the *Voice Handicap Index* (VHI) (Jacobson and colleagues, 2007) is the one used most commonly in clinical practice. Figure 6.5 shows a pre-therapy VHI scale completed by the patient in Case Study 1 at the end

TABLE 6.1 Major Voice-Disordered Quality-of-Life Instruments

Instrument Name and Acronym	Developers
Voice Handicap Index (VHI)	Jacobson and colleagues (1997)
Voice Handicap Index–10 (VHI-10)	Rosen and colleagues (2004)
Voice Handicap Index–Partner (VHI-P)	Zraick and colleagues (2007)
Pediatric Voice Handicap Index (pVHI)	Zur and colleagues (2007)
Singing Voice Handicap Index (SVHI)	Cohen and colleagues (2007)
Vocal Performance Questionnaire (VPQ)	Carding and colleagues (1999)
Voice Disability Coping Questionnaire (VDCQ)	Epstein and colleagues (2009)
Voice Symptom Scale (VoiSS)	Deary and colleagues (2003)
Voice Activity and Participation Profile (VAPP)	Ma and Yiu (2001)
Voice-Related Quality of Life (V-RQOL)	Hogikyan and Sethuraman (1999)
Pediatric Voice-Related Quality of Life (PVRQOL)	Boseley and colleagues (2006)
Voice Outcomes Survey (VOS)	Glicklich and colleagues (1999)
Pediatric Voice Outcomes Survey (PVOS)	Hartnick (2002)

FIGURE 6.5 Voice Handicap Index (VHI) Form for Case Study 1

Voice Handicap Index (VHI)
(Jacobson, Johnson, Grywalski, et al.)
Henry Ford Hospital

Instructions: These are statements that many people have used to describe their voices and the effects of their voices on their lives. Check the response that indicates how frequently you have the same experience. (Never = 0 points; Almost Never = 1 point; Sometimes = 2 points; Almost Always = 3 points; Always = 4 points)

	Never	Almost Never	Sometimes	Almost Always	Always
F1. My voice makes it difficult for people to hear me.				✔	
P2. I run out of air when I talk.				✔	
F3. People have difficulty understanding me in a noisy room.				✔	
P4. The sound of my voice varies throughout the day.		✔			
F5. My family has difficulty hearing me when I call them throughout the house.				✔	
F6. I use the phone less often than I would like.			✔		
E7. I'm tense when talking with others because of my voice.			✔		
F8. I tend to avoid groups of people because of my voice.				✔	
E9. People seem irritated with my voice.			✔		
P10. People ask, "What's wrong with your voice?"				✔	
F11. I speak with friends, neighbors, or relatives less often because of my voice.					✔
F12. People ask me to repeat myself when speaking fact-to-face.				✔	
P13. My voice sounds creaky and dry.				✔	
P14. I feel as though I have to strain to produce voice.				✔	
E15. I find other people don't understand my voice problem.				✔	
F16. My voice difficulties restrict my personal and social life.				✔	
P17. The clarity of my voice is unpredictable.				✔	
P18. I try to change my voice to sound different.			✔		
F19. I feel left out of conversations because of my voice.			✔		
		(1)	(10)	(36)	(4) = 51

	Never	Almost Never	Sometimes	Almost Always	Always
P20. I use a great deal of effort to speak.				✔	
P21. My voice difficulties restrict my personal and social life.				✔	
F22. My voice problem causes me to lose income			✔		
E23. My voice problem upsets me.				✔	
E24. I am less outgoing because of my voice problem.			✔		
E25. My voice makes me feel handicapped.				✔	
P26. My voice "gives out" on me in the middle of speaking.				✔	
E27. I feel annoyed when people ask me to repeat.			✔		
E28. I feel embarrassed when people ask me to repeat.			✔		
E29. My voice makes me feel incompetent.			✔		
E30. I'm ashamed of my voice problem.				✔	

Note: The letter preceding each item number corresponds to the subscale (E = emotional subscale, F = functional subscale, P = physical subscale).

(10) (18) = 28
       + 51
Total: 79
→ E = 24
Sub scales   F = 28
             P = 27

of this chapter. In the development study for the VHI, patients self-rated their voice handicap as either mild, moderate, or severe, and researchers correlated those ratings with the total VHI scores. Table 6.2 presents the mean and standard deviation for each category of perceived voice handicap. A self-perceived reduction in voice handicap correlates with a lowering of the total VHI score by 18 points or more, and/or a lowering of any VHI subscale score by 8 points or more (Jacobson and colleagues, 1997). To date, there is no published literature reporting VHI scores for individuals without voice disorders, but it is likely that such individuals would not have a total score of zero.

After completing a thorough records review and patient interview, the next step for the clinician is to assess each aspect of voice production, with an eye toward determining a differential diagnosis, determining prognosis for change,

TABLE 6.2 Mean Values (SD) for VHI Subscale and Total Scale Scores as a Function of Self-Perceived Severity

	Patient Group		
Scale	Mild	Moderate	Severe
Functional	10.07 (1.99)	12.41 (1.38)	18.30 (1.50)
Physical	15.54 (1.97)	18.63 (1.37)	22.78 (1.48)
Emotional	8.08 (2.31)	13.33 (1.61)	20.30 (1.74)
Total	33.69 (5.60)	44.37 (3.88)	61.39 (4.21)

Source: Reprinted with permission from The Voice Handicap Index: Development and Validation by B. H. Jacobson, A. Johnson, C. Grywalski, A. Silbergleit, G. Jacobson, & M. S. Benninger. *American Journal of Speech-Language Pathology, 6,* 66–70. Copyright 1997 by the American Speech-Language-Hearing Association. All rights reserved.

and formulating a treatment plan. The clinician may use instrumental or noninstrumental approaches to assess the voice. In the noninstrumental approach, one relies on behavioral observation of the patient, examination of the patient's oral-peripheral mechanisms, auditory-perceptual judgments about various aspects of the voice (e.g., pitch, loudness, quality, respiratory-phonatory control, resonance, effort, etc.), and the patient's voice-disordered quality of life. In the instrumental approach, one obtains indirect measures of voice production (e.g., visualization of the larynx, acoustic measures of the voice signal, aerodynamic measures of pressure and flow, physiological measurement of laryngeal muscle function, etc.). Each approach has its advantages and limitations, and the clinician must be skilled at using both approaches and must have a clear purpose in using each.

While it may seem that the instrumental approach is less subjective than the noninstrumental approach, it should be noted that a skilled voice clinician could conduct a valid assessment of voice with or without instrumentation. The use of instrumentation does not ensure that results will be more accurate. In the hands of a well-trained clinician, the use of instrumentation does add important elements of documentation and quantification, which may or may not otherwise be available. Nevertheless, one should not rely on instrumentation to strengthen weak powers of observation, modest clinical skills, or lack of knowledge about voice production. If one has mediocre skills, instrumentation alone does *not* compensate for this weakness. The most important skills are to be able to listen critically and carefully, and to analyze objectively.

THE ORAL-PERIPHERAL MECHANISM EXAMINATION

Careful assessment of the oral-peripheral mechanism is part of the voice assessment. Although we focus on assessment of the larynx and respiratory systems, examination of the face, oral and nasal cavities, and pharynx is also required.

Beyond observing obvious problems in breathing, the clinician should note the amount of neck tension. The accessory neck muscles and the supralaryngeal strap muscles in some patients literally stick out like bands as the patient speaks (this is also observed in untrained singers). Often, mandibular restriction is closely

Clinicians with expertise in voice disorders and with specialized training in laryngoscopy are qualified to use laryngoscopy for the purpose of assessing voice production and vocal function. In this **video**, we appreciate that videolaryngoscopy, combined with the clinician's eyes and ears, helps form the differential diagnosis of the voice disorder. Grand Rounds: Describe how videolaryngoscopy assisted with the differential diagnosis of Adductor Spasmodic Dysphonia.

associated with neck tension; affected patients speak with clenched teeth, with little or no mandibular movement. Such restricted jaw movement places most of the burden of speech articulation on the tongue, which must make fantastic adjustments to produce the various vowels and diphthongs in connected speech if no cavity-shaping assistance from the mandible is forthcoming. Any excessive elevation or lowering of the larynx, as well as the tipping forward of the thyroid cartilage in the production of high pitches, should be noted as possible hyperfunctional behavior (Lowell and colleagues, 2012). The angle of the thyroid cartilage may be digitally palpated as the patient sings a number of varying pitches; typically the fingertips feel little discernible change in the thyroid angle as the patient sings up and down a scale. Sometimes, however, the thyroid cartilage can be felt to rock forward slightly in the production of high pitches, as it sweeps upward to a higher position toward the hyoid bone. One should gently move the larynx manually from side to side to note the degree of tension with which the strap muscles of the neck hold the larynx in place. We also ask patients to move their larynx manually from side to side and to observe how fixed it appears compared with the clinician's own larynx.

The majority of hyperfunctional behaviors associated with voice problems are probably not directly observable from examination of the oral-peripheral mechanism. For example, to determine the extent of the tongue's impinging on the oropharyngeal space, we would need to rely on oral or nasal laryngoscopy.

Laryngoscopy/Phonoscopy

It is worth noting that indirect laryngoscopy is not the sole province of the physician. Clinicians may employ indirect laryngoscopy (and other laryngeal visualization techniques) in accordance with American Speech-Language-Hearing Association's (2007) *Scope of Practice for Clinicians*. The American Academy of Otolaryngology Voice and Swallow Committee and ASHA's Special Interest Group 3 (Voice and Voice Disorders) have published a joint statement regarding the use of laryngoscopy. It states in part that "[c]linicians with expertise in voice disorders and with specialized training in laryngoscopy are professionals qualified to use this procedure for the purpose of assessing voice production and vocal function. . . ." (American Speech-Language-Hearing Association, 1998a).

The American Speech-Language-Hearing Association (2004b) has also published a position statement regarding laryngeal stroboscopy, a technical report on laryngeal stroboscopy (American Speech-Language-Hearing Association, 2004c), and a knowledge and skills document for clinicians with respect to vocal tract visualization and imaging (American Speech-Language-Hearing Association, 2004d). Figure 6.6 presents the laryngostroboscopic findings in an 11-year-old female cheerleader with small bilateral vocal fold nodules. To document findings, forms such as the Stroboscopy Evaluation Rating Form (Poburka, 1999) and the Stroboscopy Rating Instrument (Rosen, 2005) are sometimes used.

Kendall and Leonard (2012, p. 69) uses the term *phonoscopic* examination to describe the flexible endoscopic examination of dysphonic patients performed by the voice clinician. This term emphasizes the focus of the exam on understanding the relationship between laryngeal behaviors and the voice. The phonoscopic examination allows the clinician to both see and hear voice production. Figure 6.7 lists the speaking tasks typically observed during a phonoscopic examination.

High-speed digital imaging (HSDI) of the larynx is undergoing evaluation for its clinical value compared to traditional laryngostroboscopy (Kendall, 2009; Patel

In addition to being a powerful diagnostic tool, videolaryngoscopy can serve as a powerful biofeedback therapy tool. In this **video**, the patient observes the anatomy and physiology of his own larynx, and is able to reiterate why certain approaches facilitate better voice. This leads to greater compliance with the therapeutic process. Grand Rounds: Cite two reasons why this patient might sense a fullness at the level of the larynx.

FIGURE 6.6 Laryngostroboscopic Findings in a Patient with Bilateral Vocal Fold Nodules

Parameter	Description	Finding
Glottic closure	Degree and pattern of closure during a cycle of vibration.	Moderate posterior gap (low frequencies) and hourglass (high frequencies).
Supraglottic activity	Degree of medial or anteroposterior compression of the ventricular/false folds.	Mild mediolateral compression; normal anteroposterior compression.
Extent of opening	Degree of vocal fold opening when maximally adducted.	Normal.
Vertical level approximation	Degree to which both vocal folds are on the same plane.	Normal.
Vocal fold edge	Smoothness and straightness of medial margins of the vocal folds.	Small "kissing" nodules at the anterior one-third–posterior two-thirds junction.
Vocal fold mobility	Ability of vocal fold to abduct and adduct.	Normal.
Amplitude of vibration	Extent of lateral excursion of the vocal folds.	Mild to moderately decreased bilaterally.
Mucosal wave	Should travel from inferior to superior margins of the folds and spread bilaterally.	Mild to moderately decreased bilaterally.
Nonvibrating portion	Any portion of the vocal fold(s) that does not participate in vibration.	Mild at location of the nodules.
Phase closure	Open and closed phases should be roughly equal.	Closed phase mildly dominant.
Phase symmetry	Degree to which both vocal folds adduct/abduct at the same time.	Normal.
Periodicity/regularity	Degree of similarity of successive cycles of vibration.	Normal.
Overall laryngeal function		Mild hyperfunction.
Other	Anything other than the above.	Moderate erythema and edema in the interarytenoid area; thick persistent mucus at site of nodules.

FIGURE 6.7 Elements of the Phonoscopic Examination

Observation of:
- Respiratory behavior.
- Vegetative voicing.
- Fundamental frequency range.
- Intensity range at different frequencies.
- Different phonatory modes (i.e., whisper, falsetto).
- Different phonetic contexts (i.e., single sounds, connected speech).
- Voicing of variable duration (i.e., sustained vowels, repetition of voiced syllables).

Source: Information from Leonard (2012).

and colleagues, 2008, 2012; Zhang and colleagues, 2010). Laryngostroboscopy works by synchronizing the flash of the stroboscopic light with the fundamental frequency of the vocal fold vibration, revealing an average pattern of vibration across multiple cycles. It requires a periodic voice signal and is of somewhat limited value with severely dysphonic patients. HSDI captures several thousand frames per second, providing a true view of vocal fold movement that does not require periodic phonation, and is able to visualize vocal fold vibration regardless of the degree of aperiodicity and level of dysphonia. Patel and colleagues conclude that HSDI has value for evaluating grade II (moderate hoarseness) and grade IV (severe hoarseness) voice qualities and patients with neuromuscular conditions. In addition, HSDI provides valuable information on vocal fold movement that is not available via laryngostroboscopy, including the observation of phonatory onset, very short voicing segments, and spasms. Limitations of HSDI (compared to laryngostroboscopy) include the lack of audio, the inability to use a flexible endoscope with the procedure, and a limited sample of phonation (usually 2 seconds).

Many times the information gained from the laryngoscopic and/or phonoscopic examination has been the most important information gained during the diagnostic assessment (McFarlane and Watterson, 1990; McFarlane and colleagues, 1990). When coupled with the other information, visualization of the larynx has greatly improved our accuracy of diagnosis and set the foundation for successful voice therapy plans.

THE CLINICAL VOICE LABORATORY

Instrumental analysis of voice, as described in this chapter, is common in many voice clinics and other settings. Due to advances in microprocessor technology, computer-based hardware and software systems are becoming more affordable and automated. However, clinical instrumentation, no matter how sophisticated, cannot replace the mind, eyes, and ears of a well-trained clinician. That is, instrumental data must be paired with clinical impressions and auditory-perceptual judgments of voice to be used meaningfully.

When instrumentation is utilized, there are principles of calibration, standardization of measurement technique, data interpretation, reliability, hygiene, and examiner training that are fundamental to valid outcomes (Brown and colleagues, 1996; Klein and colleagues, 2000). At a minimum, the clinician should be mindful of the following equipment considerations when obtaining voice recordings for clinical purposes: (1) sound isolation and ambient room noise, (2) microphone choice, (3) sound level meter choice, (4) cable choice, (5) computer specifications, (6) recording software, and (7) choice of video recorder and monitor (Spielman and colleagues, 2007).

Stemple and colleagues (2000, p. 180) suggest that the clinical utility of instrumental measures can be assessed on four levels of clinical application. Specifically, does the instrumentation (1) identify the existence of a voice problem; (2) assess the severity or stage of progression of the voice problem; (3) identify the differential source of the voice problem; and (4) serve as a primary treatment tool for behavioral modification, biofeedback, or patient education? These questions often guide the choice of instruments used and the recording protocols followed. In the following sections, we describe the types of voice analyses the clinician can conduct using relatively affordable and easy-to-use equipment.

ACOUSTIC ANALYSES AND INSTRUMENTATION

Due to advances in technology and an increase in affordability of equipment, acoustic analysis of the voice is becoming increasingly more common in clinical practice. For acoustic measurements to be valid, they must be able to (a) discriminate the normal from dysphonic voice, (b) correlate positively with the clinician's auditory-perceptual judgments of the voice, and (c) be sufficiently stable to assess change across time (Stemple and colleagues, 2010). The clinician can conduct the following acoustic analyses of the frequency, intensity, and quality of the voice: (1) sound spectrography, (2) frequency-related parameters, (3) intensity-related parameters, (4) vocal perturbation-related parameters, and (5) vocal noise-related parameters. We will now describe each of these.

Sound Spectrography

When conducting acoustic analysis of the voice, it is generally a good idea to begin by carefully examining its spectrogram. A sound spectrogram is a visual representation of the frequency and intensity of the sound wave as a function of time. The resulting graphic, known as a spectrogram, reflects the harmonic structure of the glottal sound source and the resonant characteristics of the vocal tract. Frequency is represented on the vertical axis, time is represented on the horizontal axis, and intensity is represented by the darkness of the trace on the screen (see Figure 6.8). The lowest energy band represents the fundamental frequency, with energy in the higher frequencies in the bands above. When grayscale is used, darker gray bands represent greater energy. When obtaining a spectrogram, the clinician needs to decide how he or she wants the spectrograph to filter and then display the sound signal. Two choices are possible: narrow-band filtering and wide-band filtering. The bandwidth refers to the analysis window around the fundamental frequency. With narrow-band filtering, there is good frequency resolution but poor time resolution. In wide-band filtering, there is good time resolution but poor frequency resolution. That is, the narrow-band spectrogram displays individual harmonics well, while the wide-band spectrogram displays a number of harmonics at once. Narrow-band spectrograms are particularly well suited to inspecting the vocal acoustic signal in persons with dysphonia. By inspecting changes in the harmonic structure of the voice, the clinician can observe the stability of the patient's vocal fold vibration (Sapienza and Ruddy, 2009). Figure 6.9 shows a spectrogram of an 18-year-old female with bilateral vocal fold nodules. Figure 6.10 shows a spectrogram of a 70-year-old male with unilateral vocal fold paralysis. Note that, in both Figures 6.9 and 6.10, the harmonics are not clear or strong, and there is "noise" between the harmonics. The speaker and listener would likely perceive these voices as having an abnormal vocal quality.

Fundamental Frequency

Average fundamental frequency (average F_0) is the rate of vibration of the vocal folds. It is expressed in hertz (Hz)—the number of cycles of vocal fold vibration per second. Speaking tasks for determining average F_0 include isolated vowels, and reading or connected speech. When reported from connected speech, average F_0 is often called speaking fundamental frequency (SFF).

FIGURE 6.8 Narrow-Band Spectrogram of a Voice with Normal Quality

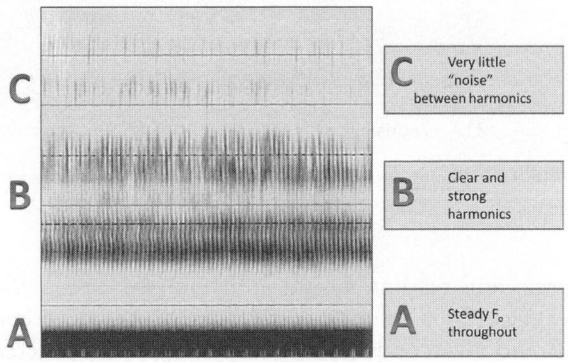

FIGURE 6.9 Narrow-Band Spectrogram of a Patient with Vocal Fold Nodules

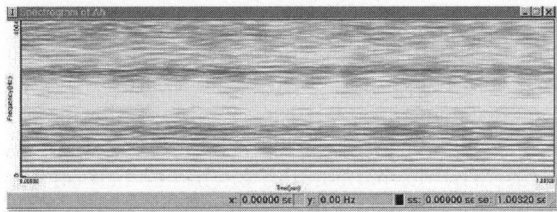

Source: Courtesy of KayPENTAX®.

FIGURE 6.10 Narrow-Band Spectrogram of a Patient with Vocal Fold Paralysis

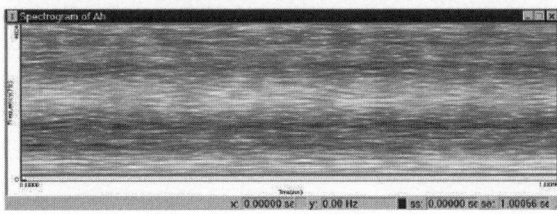

Source: Courtesy of KayPENTAX®.

An individual's habitual pitch depends on age, gender, and race. Average F_0 and SFF norms for a variety of speaker groups have been published, and the clinician should use these norms when making a clinical judgment about the suitability of a particular patient's habitual pitch. For quick reference, Table 6.3 presents average SFF data for adults and children (Siupsinskiene and Hugo Lycke, 2011). There is a clear relationship between habitual pitch and a speaker's age and gender. There are marked differences in habitual pitch between males and females after puberty; both experience a lowering of habitual pitch, with the change much more noticeable in males. There are also changes in habitual pitch with advancing age. A slight increase in habitual pitch can occur in elderly men due to vocal fold atrophy. In women, there can be a slight decrease in habitual pitch postmenopause.

There are various methods for eliciting SFF. Zraick and colleagues (2000) compared SFF across four different speaking tasks (automatic speech, elicited speech,

TABLE 6.3 Average Speaking Fundamental Frequency (SFF) for Adults and Children

	Adult Males		Adult Females		Children	
	Mean	Range*	Mean	Range*	Mean	Range*
Average SFF (Hz)	112.4 (nonsingers)	89.0–175.0	212.4 (nonsingers)	164.5–260.0	251.9 (nonsingers)	201.8–302.0
	130.5 (singers)	98.0–175.0	223.6 (singers)	181.0–269.0	244.8 (singers)	196.0–322.4

*Plus or minus two (±2) standard deviations.

spontaneous speech, and reading aloud) and reported no significant differences. Zraick and colleagues (2005) compared SFF across five different speaking durations (1, 5, 15, 30, and 60 seconds) and reported significant differences between the 30- and 60-second samples. Zraick and colleagues (2006) compared SFF across six different social contexts (speaking during a voice evaluation, speaking in public, speaking to a peer, speaking to a superior, speaking to a subordinate, and speaking to a parent or spouse) and reported that SFF differed depending on who was the patient's communication partner. Results of these studies (and others) indicate that SFF should be interpreted in light of how it was elicited.

A relatively inexpensive clinical instrument for the measurement of pitch-related parameters is the piano or electric keyboard. Isolated vowels or connected speech can be produced by the patient and pitch-matched on the keyboard by the clinician. With a piano or keyboard (or pitch pipe, for that matter), it is possible to estimate SFF because the tones produced by the human voice can be matched to the musical notes of these instruments. For example, in hertz, the typical adult male voice is near C3 (131 Hz), an adult female voice is near A3 (220 Hz), and a child's voice is between C4 and D4 (262 to 294 Hz). Each octave on a musical instrument is comprised of eight whole tones, with each tone represented by an alphabetical letter. Sharps and flats represent semitones. There are 12 semitones in an octave. Each C begins a new octave. Each octave represents a doubling of frequency of vocal fold vibration. Therefore, an increase from C3 to C4 represents a doubling of frequency (131 Hz + 131 Hz = 262 Hz). See Table 6.4 for a musical note–to–frequency chart.

Frequency Variability

This is the range of SFFs used in connected speech. Normal voices have some frequency variability, perceived by the listener as acceptable changes in prosody. In some dysphonic speakers, however, frequency can be either more or less variable than expected or tolerated by the listener. Increased frequency variability may be perceived as a child-like, sing-song prosody, while decreased frequency variability may be perceived as monotone. Abnormal frequency variability may have a functional, organic, or neurological basis.

Frequency variability is measured in terms of the standard deviation (SD) from the average F_0. It can be measured two ways: either the standard deviation of F_0 in Hz (F_0SD), or in semitones (pitch sigma). F_0SD in normal connected speech is around 25 to 30 Hz (Ferrand, 2007) but can be greater depending on the speaker's mood. For steady-state sustained vowels, F_0SD should be even lower (3 to 6 Hz); higher F_0SD values can indicate a patient's difficulty with control of frequency. Table 6.5 presents average pitch sigma data for adults and children (Siupsinskiene and Hugo Lycke, 2011).

TABLE 6.4 Musical Note–to–Frequency Chart

Note	Freq. (Hz)	Note	Freq. (Hz)	Note	Freq. (Hz)
A_1	55	A_3	220	A^5	880
B_1	62	B_3	245	B^5	988
C_2	65	C^4	262	C^6	1046
D_2	73	D^4	294	D^6	1175
E_2	82	E^4	330	E^6	1318
F_2	87	F^4	349	F^6	1397
G_2	98	G^4	392	G^6	1568
A_2	110	A^4	440	A^6	1760
B_2	123	B^4	494	B^6	1975
C_3	131	C^5	523	C^7	2093
D_3	147	D^5	587	D^7	2349
E_3	164	E^5	659	E^7	2637
F_3	175	F^5	698	F^7	7294
G_3	196	G^5	784	G^7	3136

Note: The notes are sequentially numbered, from left to right on the piano keyboard, starting with the first C-octave. All decimals are rounded off. The Visi-Pitch will only record between 0–1600 Hz.

TABLE 6.5 Average SFF Variability (Pitch Sigma) for Adults and Children

	Adult Males		Adult Females		Children	
	Mean	Range*	Mean	Range*	Mean	Range*
Average pitch sigma (ST)	14.5 (nonsingers)	7.5–21.0	10.7 (nonsingers)	5.2–16.1	8.9 (nonsingers)	4.0–20.7
	12.5 (singers)	3.7–21.0	9.9 (singers)	4.9–14.8	8.7 (singers)	3.0–13.0

*Plus or minus two (±2) standard deviations.

Maximum Phonational Frequency Range (MPFR)

MPFR is defined by Hollien and colleagues (1971) as "that range of vocal frequencies encompassing both the modal and falsetto registers; its extent is from the lowest tone sustainable in the modal register to the highest in falsetto register, inclusive." MPFR is one of the most frequently obtained voice measures (Hirano, 1989). It is reported commonly in semitones (ST). Table 6.6 presents MPFR data for adults and children (Siupsinskiene and Hugo Lycke, 2011). An MPFR of about two and a half to three octaves (30 to 36 semitones) is expected for healthy young adults, with a smaller MPFR expected in older adults (Kent, 1994) and those with dysphonia (Sataloff, 2005). The patient's MPFR should be determined as a prelude

TABLE 6.6 Maximum Phonational Frequency Range (MPFR) for Adults and Children

	Adult Males		Adult Females		Children	
	Mean	Range*	Mean	Range*	Mean	Range*
MPFR in semitones (ST)	34.2 (nonsingers)	27.0–41.0	29.5 (nonsingers)	22.2–36.7	22.4 (nonsingers)	16.0–29.0
	37.7 (singers)	29.0–47.0	34.4 (singers)	28.2–40.5	27.9 (singers)	19.0–34.0

*Plus or minus two (±2) standard deviations.

to identifying that person's best pitch level (the patient's easiest and most compatible voice pitch) at which to begin therapy probes.

Zraick and colleagues (2000) compared two methods for eliciting MPFR (stepping from lowest to highest note versus gliding from lowest to highest note) and reported that stair-step progression through the range resulted in a larger MPFR. Zraick and colleagues (2002) tried to determine whether the lowest or highest pitch should be obtained first and reported that obtaining the lowest pitch followed by the highest pitch resulted in a larger MPFR. Results of these studies (and others) indicate that MPFR should be interpreted in light of how it was elicited.

Average/Habitual Intensity

Vocal intensity corresponds with the acoustic power of the speaker. It is reported in dB SPL, and correlates with the auditory perception of loudness. Habitual loudness is the average loudness level used by the speaker for the majority of his or her vocalizations. For most speakers, habitual loudness should be loud enough to allow them to be heard over background noise but not so loud that it brings the listener discomfort or distraction (Awan, 2001). Normal conversational speech usually is in the range of 65 to 80 dB SPL, with an average for males and females (adults and children) of around 70 dB SPL (Baken, 1996). Older adults may exhibit a slightly less intense conversational voice.

Various methods have been proposed for eliciting habitual intensity. Key considerations when measuring intensity are the mouth-to-microphone distance, the level of ambient or background noise, speaking task, and SFF. Although no standard exists, a common mouth-to-microphone distance is 12 inches (or 30 cm). One should document the distance and use this consistently when comparing intensity values across sessions. Zraick and colleagues (2004) suggest that clinicians use more than one task to determine habitual loudness. For example, values elicited by having the patient count from 1 to 10, speak spontaneously, and read aloud could be averaged before a determination is made about whether therapy to address loudness is necessary. Table 6.7 presents average habitual speaking intensity data for adults and children (Siupsinskiene and Hugo Lycke, 2011).

A relatively inexpensive clinical instrument for the measurement of loudness-related parameters is the Level II sound level meter, purchased from a place such as RadioShack. Analog and digital versions are available. Most consumer sound level meters are sensitive from 40 to 130 dB SPL, with slow or fast response for checking peak and average signal levels. The sound level meter should have the ability

TABLE 6.7 Average Habitual Speaking Intensity for Adults and Children

	Adult Males		Adult Females		Children	
	Mean	Range*	Mean	Range*	Mean	Range*
Average intensity (dBA)	62.1 (nonsingers)	56.7–67.5	62.1 (nonsingers)	55.5–68.6	59.7 (nonsingers)	53.0–68.9
	61.2 (singers)	53.2–67.0	61.0 (singers)	52.1–69.9	61.5 (singers)	56.0–66.9

*Plus or minus two (±2) standard deviations.

to employ different weighting filters, with a C or Linear weighting being the most desirable for voice recordings. Typically, the sound level meter is held by the clinician at a distance of 30 to 50 cm from the speaker.

Intensity Variability

Intensity variability is the range of intensities used in connected speech. Normal voices have some intensity variability, perceived by the listener as acceptable changes in intonation. In some dysphonic speakers, however, intensity can be either more or less variable than expected or tolerated by the listener. In connected speech, decreased intensity variability may be perceived as monoloudness. Abnormal intensity variability may have either a physiological etiology (such as Parkinson's disease, vocal fold paralysis, or hearing loss) or may result from learned behavior. Intensity variability is measured in terms of the standard deviation (SD) from the average intensity. This SD reflects the range of intensities around the average intensity, measured in dB SPL. Intensity SD for a neutral, unemotional sentence is around 10 dB, but it can be higher depending on the speaker's mood.

Dynamic Range

Dynamic range is the physiologic range of intensities, from the softest nonwhisper to the loudest shout, which the patient can produce without undue physical strain. Speakers rarely speak at either end of their dynamic range (approximately 40 to 115 dB) for extended periods. Therefore, the clinician should focus attention on the dynamic range available to the patient around their habitual loudness. Table 6.8 presents average dynamic range data for adults and children (Siupsinskiene and Hugo Lycke, 2011). The dynamic range depends on the F_0 produced. It tends to be greatest for F_0 in the midrange and less for F_0 that is much lower or higher (Ferrand, 2007). The fact that F_0 and intensity co-vary leads some to propose the use of the voice range profile (VRP) to assess some patients.

The Voice Range Profile (Phonetogram)

Voice range profile (VRP) is the official term proposed by the Voice Committee of the International Association of Logopedics and Phoniatrics in 1992 to describe an individual's minimum and maximum intensity levels across his or her vocal range. Phonetograms are graphical representations of the VRP (see Figure 6.11). The patient is asked to phonate the vowel /i/ or /a/ at select frequencies across his or her frequency range (modeled by a tone-generator such as a piano or pitch pipe, or

TABLE 6.8 Average Dynamic Speaking Range for Adults and Children

	Adult Males		Adult Females		Children	
	Mean	Range*	Mean	Range*	Mean	Range*
Average dynamic speaking range (dBA)	30.2 (nonsingers)	21.9–38.5	28.1 (nonsingers)	19.0–37.0	26.1 (nonsingers)	15.6–35.5
	30.6 (singers)	17.4–44.0	29.9 (singers)	19.6–40.0	26.6 (singers)	16.8–36.0

*Plus or minus two (±2) standard deviations.

FIGURE 6.11 Voice Range Profile

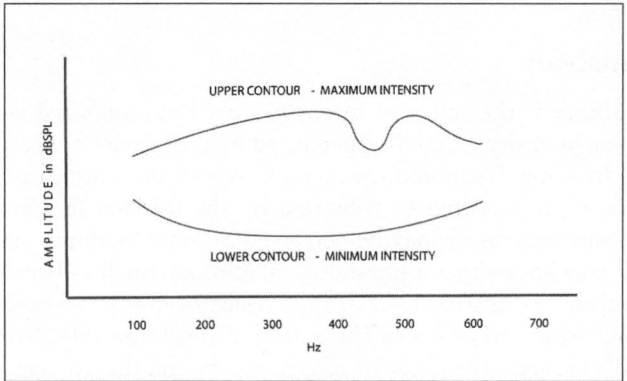

Note: The upper contour is the patient's maximum intensity at each frequency; the lower contour is the patient's minimum intensity at each frequency. A normal VRP should have an oblique-oval shape; at the physiologic extremes of vocal range, there is a minimal intensity difference between the soft and loud phonations. A compressed VRP indicates that the patient cannot achieve normal frequency and intensity ranges.

Source: Courtesy of KayPENTAX®.

presented by computer software), both as softly and loudly as possible. We typically obtain the lower VRP intensity contour before the upper intensity contour to avoid possible laryngeal fatigue, particularly in persons with dysphonia. The following VRP characteristics are usually reported: habitual frequency, total fundamental frequency range, lowest and highest fundamental frequencies, habitual intensity, total intensity range, lowest and highest intensity, and VRP shape and contour. The upper contour of the VRP represents the patient's maximum phonation threshold (maximum intensity at each frequency) and the lower contour represents their minimum phonation threshold (minimum intensity at each frequency). A normal VRP should have an oblique-oval shape; at the physiologic extremes of vocal range, there is a minimal intensity difference between the soft and loud phonations (LeBorgne, 2007). A constricted (compressed) VRP indicates that the patient has difficulty achieving normal frequency and intensity ranges. Obtaining a complete VRP for some patients can be challenging, leading some to propose various customized VRP protocols for clinical use (Awan, 1991; Holmberg and colleagues, 2007; Ma and colleagues, 2007; Schneider and colleagues, 2010; Wingate and Collins, 2005; Wingate and colleagues, 2007). Table 6.9 presents VRP data collected on children with normal and dysphonic voices (Heylen and colleagues, 1998). Table 6.10 presents VRP data collected on adults with normal and dysphonic voices (Ma and colleagues, 2007). VRP data is also available for male and female professional voice users (Heylen and colleagues, 2002) and trained versus untrained singers (Siupsinskiene and Lycke, 2011).

TABLE 6.9 Voice Range Profile Measures for Children with Dysphonic Voices Versus Children with Normal Voices, as Reported by Heylen and colleagues (1998)

Measures	Dysphonic[†] (n = 136)		Normal Voice* (n = 94)	
Frequency Measures:	Mean	SE[‡]	Mean	SE
Lowest frequency (Hz)	196.3	2.5	192.8	2.5
Highest frequency (Hz)	550.0	11.0	857.0	21.0
Total frequency range (Hz)	354.0	13.0	663.0	22.0
Number of semitones in modal register	13.8	0.3	18.0	0.3
Number of semitones in falsetto register	5.5	0.4	8.4	0.4
Total number of semitones	19.4	0.5	26.4	0.5
Intensity Measures:	Mean	SE	Mean	SE
Lowest intensity (in dB)	52.4	0.3	48.2	0.3
Highest intensity (in dB)	95.2	0.5	98.0	0.6
Total intensity range (in dB)	42.7	0.6	49.7	0.6

*Vocally healthy group composed of 53 boys and 41 girls.

[†] Dysphonic group composed of 87 boys and 49 girls.

[‡]SE = standard errors.

TABLE 6.10 Voice Range Profile Measures for Adult Females with Dysphonic Voices Versus Adult Females with Normal Voices, as Reported by Ma and colleagues (2007)

Measures	Dysphonic (n = 90)		Normal Voice (n = 35)	
Frequency Measures:	Mean	SD	Mean	SD
Lowest frequency (Hz)	127.65	20.99	115.01	12.00
Highest frequency (Hz)	854.98	251.25	1232.85	221.42
Total number of semitones	32.36	6.39	40.89	3.73
Intensity Measures:	Mean	SD	Mean	SD
Lowest intensity (in dB)	60.64	7.41	48.91	3.12
Highest intensity (in dB)	109.28	5.18	105.66	6.12
Total intensity range (in dB)	48.63	8.06	56.74	6.29

FIGURE 6.12 A Visi-Pitch™ IV in Clinical Use

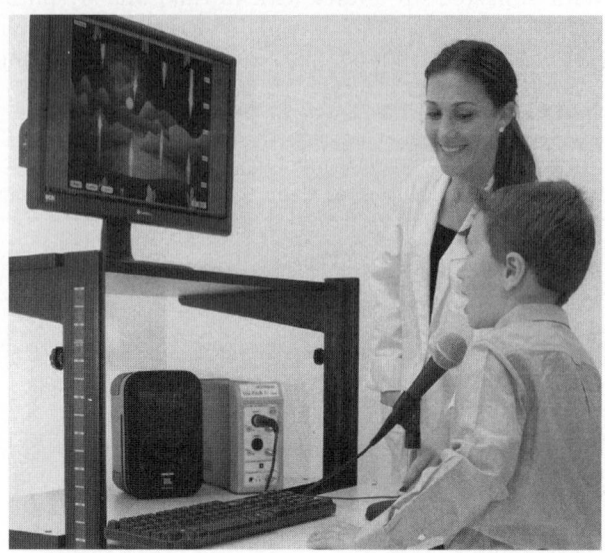

Source: Courtesy of KayPENTAX®.

The Visi-Pitch™ IV (Model 3950B; KayPENTAX Corp., Montvale, New Jersey) (Figure 6.12) is a widely used clinical instrument for measuring habitual pitch and loudness, frequency and intensity variability, and MPFR and dynamic range, among other things. The Visi-Pitch IV extracts acoustic parameters during speech production and presents these in real time, providing clients with clear, intuitive visual displays. Target vocalizations provided by a clinician can be compared to client attempts, both graphically and with auditory playback. Monitoring important speech/voice behaviors with concrete visual displays helps clients reach therapy goals more easily.

Vocal Perturbation Measures

Vocal perturbation is the cycle-to-cycle variability in the vocal signal. A small amount of cycle-to-cycle variability is expected in the normal voice. It results from aperiodic vibration of the vocal folds. Unlike the frequency/intensity variability previously discussed, vocal perturbation is aimed at identifying the short-term, cycle-to-cycle nonvolitional variability, not the longer-term, volitional word or utterance (prosodic) trends. Therefore, sustained vowels or steady-state portions of vowels extracted from connected speech are typically used to determine vocal perturbation. Software programs, such as the Analysis of Dysphonia in Speech and Voice™ (ADSV) (KayPENTAX Corp., Montvale, New Jersey), allow for analysis of vocal perturbation in connected speech and are now commercially available (Lowell and colleagues, 2011; Watts and Awan, 2010). Two vocal perturbation measures commonly obtained are jitter and shimmer.

Jitter is the short-term variability in fundamental frequency, while *shimmer* is the short-term variability in the amplitude. There are a variety of perturbation measures from which to choose, making valid selection and interpretation difficult (see Behrman [2007] and Ferrand [2007] for descriptions of the most common perturbation measures). Standardization is almost nonexistent when it comes to vocal perturbation measures, making them potentially less clinically useful, particularly when comparing research results across sites, clinicians, and equipment manufacturers (Brockmann-Bauser and Drinnan, 2011). It appears that there may be vowel, gender, vocal intensity, and fundamental frequency effects in a typical clinical task (Brockmann-Bauser and Drinnan, 2011). Further limiting the clinical utility of vocal perturbation measures is the fact that a direct correlation between jitter and shimmer and voice impairment does not exist (Kreiman and Gerratt, 2005). Also, because a coherent database of normative vocal perturbation values does not exist, vocal perturbation cannot be used to differentiate reliably between normal and abnormal voices (Behrman, 2007). Generally, jitter of less than 1.0% and shimmer of less than 0.5 dB are considered normal (Titze, 1994). Children demonstrate higher jitter and shimmer than adults, and older adults demonstrate higher jitter and shimmer than younger adults (Gorham-Rowan and Laures-Gore, 2006). Vocal perturbation measures should be interpreted in combination with other instrumental assessment data, auditory-perceptual data, and clinical impressions (Awan and colleagues, 2010).

Vocal Noise Measures

The human voice is not a pure tone. That is, it is made up of harmonic (periodic) and inharmonic (aperiodic) components. This is because vocal fold vibration is naturally aperiodic (irregular). In a voice with normal voice quality, the harmonic components should dominate, that is, have more energy (as measured in dB). In the dysphonic voice, the harmonic component is less dominant. In attempting to quantify the relationship between the harmonic and inharmonic components, researchers have proposed three ratios: (1) the harmonics-to-noise ratio (HNR), (2) the noise-to-harmonics ratio (NHR) and (3) the signal-to-noise ratio (SNR). The voice with normal quality is characterized by a high HNR or SNR and low NHR, whereas the dysphonic voice is characterized by a low HNR or SNR and a high NHR. Generally, an HNR of approximately 12 dB or greater is indicative of a voice with normal quality (Yumoto and colleagues, 1982), with higher normative HNRs commonly reported (Awan and Frankel, 1994; Horii and Fuller, 1990). Ferrand (2000, 2002) has reported that HNRs for children and older adults are lower than HNRs for young and middle-age adults. Many clinicians have rightfully questioned the usefulness of vocal perturbation and noise measures because they do not always correlate well with listener perception of dysphonia or patient perception voice handicap (Bhuta and colleagues, 2004; Eadie and Doyle, 2005; Wheeler and colleagues, 2006).

The Computerized Speech Lab™ (CSL) (Model 4500; KayPENTAX Corp., Montvale, New Jersey), shown in Figure 6.13, is a more comprehensive hardware system than the Visi-Pitch™, with optional software and database options. One of the more clinically useful CSL options for voice is the Multidimensional Voice Program™ (MDVP). This program analyzes and displays 33 different vocal parameters, including the more commonly reported vocal perturbation and vocal noise measures just described.

ELECTROGLOTTOGRAPHIC ANALYSIS AND INSTRUMENTATION

Electroglottography (EGG) is a noninvasive technique for obtaining an estimate of vocal fold contact patterns during phonation. A gold electrode is placed on each side of the thyroid cartilage at a level corresponding to the position of the vocal folds.

FIGURE 6.13 The Computerized Speech Lab™ in Clinical Use

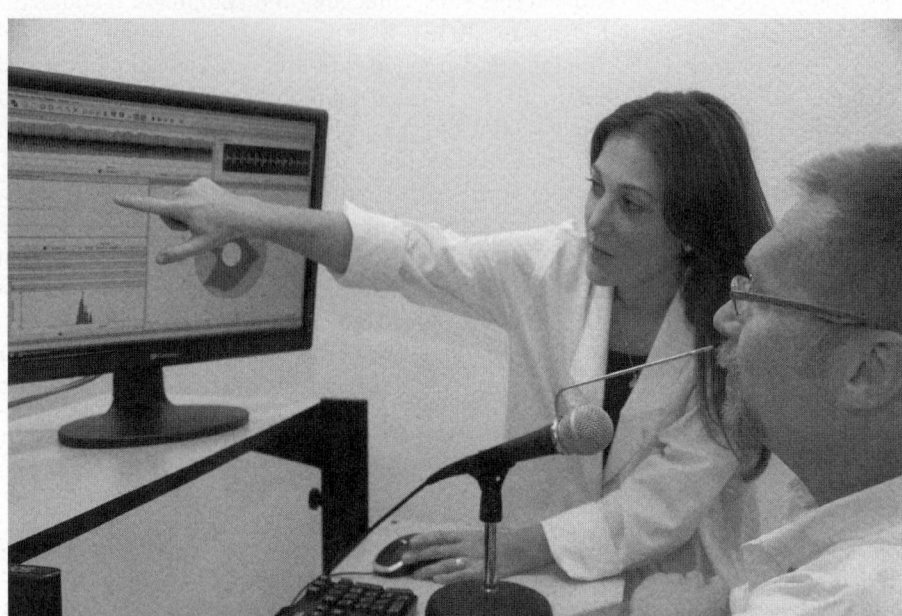

Source: Courtesy of KayPENTAX®.

A weak high-frequency electrical current is passed between the electrodes. As vocal fold contact area changes, there are changes in the electrical resistance between the electrodes. When the glottis is opening or open, resistance increases; when the glottis is closing or closed, resistance decreases. The resulting Lx waveform, called an electroglottogram or laryngogram, reveals summary information about vocal fold contact over time. The EGG can be used to visualize various types of voice quality. For example, Figure 6.14 shows electroglottograms for a prolonged /i/ vowel produced with a normal voice quality, a breathy voice quality, and a hoarse voice quality.

AERODYNAMIC MEASUREMENTS AND INSTRUMENTATION

Aerodynamic analysis of the voice is also becoming increasingly more possible and common in clinical practice. Aerodynamic measures reflect the patient's ability to use the larynx to regulate the flow of air for phonation. Prior to quantitatively assessing respiration, we suggest carefully observing the patient's breathing patterns. An inefficient breathing pattern or a lack of coordination between inspiratory and expiratory movements can contribute to dysphonia. For example, the patient may have to take more frequent breath groups, or may adopt increased musculoskeletal tension resulting in vocal hyperfunction. There are three basic types of breathing patterns: clavicular, thoracic, and diaphragmatic-abdominal, as described below:

- *Clavicular breathing.* This inefficient type of breathing is probably the easiest to identify. The patient elevates the shoulders on inspiration, using the neck

FIGURE 6.14 Electroglottograms

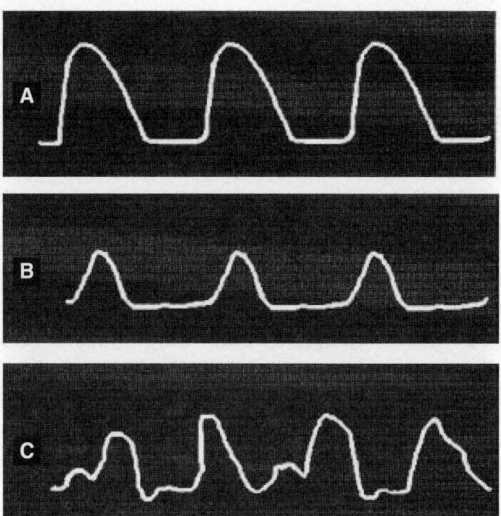

These three electroglottograms are productions of the /i/ vowel with (A) normal vocal quality, (B) breathy quality, and (C) hoarse vocal quality. The normal trace (A) demonstrates a sharp vertical rise, a narrow peak, an even return to baseline, and a substantial closed phase. Trace (B), the breathy voice quality, is represented in the sloping voice onset, rather than the vertical rise seen in the normal trace and the long open phase. Trace (C), the hoarse voice, is indicated by the lack of a uniform wave form from one cycle to the next.

accessory muscles as the primary muscles of inspiration. This upper chest breathing, characterized by noticeable elevation of the clavicles, is unsatisfactory for good voice for two reasons. First, the resulting weak and shallow inspiration does not provide adequate respiratory support for speech and voice. Second, overuse of many of the neck accessory muscles for respiration (particularly the sternocleidomastoids) may cause an increase in laryngeal tension (Prater and colleagues, 1999).

- *Thoracic breathing.* This type of breathing is characterized by expansion of the thorax and contraction of the abdomen during inspiration, reversed during expiration. It is the normal breathing pattern for most people. In some cases, however, thoracic breathing can be characterized by shallow breathing punctuated by breath holding or gasping.
- *Diaphragmatic-abdominal breathing.* This may well be the preferred method of respiration, especially if the patient has heavy vocal demands, as in singing or acting. This breathing pattern is characterized by abdominal and lower thoracic expansion on inspiration, with little noticeable upper chest movement, and a gradual decrease in abdominal and lower thoracic prominence on expiration.

Hixon and Hoit (1998, 1999, 2000) have written extensively about the clinical evaluation of speech breathing and have also published a comprehensive text on the evaluation and management of speech breathing disorders (Hixon and Hoit, 2005). In their writings, these authors emphasize the role of the speech breathing case history in the evaluation of patients. The speech breathing case history described by Hixon and Hoit (2005) includes the following sections: (1) alerting signs and symptoms; (2) airway risk factors; (3) medical evaluations, diagnoses, and treatments; (4) breathing and speaking experiences; and (5) client perceptions of speech breathing. Figure 6.15 lists some of the alerting signs and symptoms described (p. 196), and Figure 6.16 lists some of the abnormal client perceptions of speech breathing (pp. 200–201).

Aerodynamic measures obtained in the clinic include (1) lung volumes and capacities, (2) air pressure, (3) airflow, and (4) laryngeal resistance. In the sections that follow, we briefly describe each measure and the equipment needed.

Lung Volumes and Capacities

Part of evaluating respiratory adequacy is measuring the patient's lung volume. Lung volumes refer to the amount of air in the lungs at a given time and how much of that air is used for various purposes, including speech (Solomon and Charron, 1998). Only a small amount of the air in the lungs is exchanged during a single "quiet" respiratory cycle. The total volume of the lungs can be divided into *volumes* and *capacities* (see Table 2.1). Lung volumes, also known as respiratory volumes, refer to the amount of air in the lungs at a given time and how much of that air is

---

FIGURE 6.15 Alerting Speech Breathing Signs and Symptoms

Frequent coughing

Persistent hoarse voice

Coughing up mucus

Coughing up blood

Wheezing

Difficulty breathing

Chest pain

Numbness, weakness, coordination problems, or involuntary movements

Source: From Hixon and Hoit (2005).

FIGURE 6.16 Abnormal Client Perceptions of Speech Breathing

Frequent awareness of breathing

Hunger for air

Uncomfortable urge to breathe

Breathlessness

Shortness of breath

Hard work to breathe

High effort to breathe

Weak breathing muscles

Tired breathing muscles

Difficulty inhaling

Difficulty exhaling

Tightness in chest

Difficulty coordinating breathing movements

Need to think about breathing

Feelings of distress with breathing

Feelings of panic with breathing

Source: From Hixon and Hoit (2005).

used for various purposes, including speech (Solomon and Charron, 1998). Respiratory volumes include *tidal volume, inspiratory reserve volume, expiratory reserve volume* and *residual volume*. Lung capacities combine two or more of the respiratory volumes and include *inspiratory capacity, vital capacity, functional residual capacity,* and *total lung capacity*. These volumes and capacities are useful for diagnosing problems with pulmonary ventilation (Moini, 2012). Respiratory volumes and capacities vary depending on the patient's age, gender, level of physical exertion, and vocal training. Data reported by Hoit and Hixon (1987) and Hoit and colleagues (1989; 1990) indicate that, in general, lung volumes and capacities increase from infancy through puberty and then remain stable until advancing age, when they decrease slightly (see Table 6.11).

Air Pressure

Various air pressures are necessary for speech, including pressure inside the lungs, pressure below the vocal folds, and pressure inside the oral cavity. Air pressure is measured and expressed in units of cmH_2O. The total pressure that a person can generate may be as high as 50 cmH_2O or more, yet the pressure needed for conversational speech is only around 5 to 10 cmH_2O. Greater pressures than this may be required, however, depending on syllable stress and loudness demands (Stathopoulos and Sapienza, 1997). Pressure below the vocal folds is estimated indirectly by measuring oral pressure during production of the closed portion of a voiceless bilabial consonant such as /p/. When producing this consonant, the lips are closed, the velopharyngeal port is sealed, and the glottis is open; thus, pressures throughout the system are equal. Oral pressure is measured by a pressure transducer connected to a small tube placed just inside the mouth (Smitheran and Hixon, 1981).

TABLE 6.11 Group Means of Seven Age Groups of Subjects for Some Lung Volumes and Capacities (in Cubic Centimeters)

Subjects' Age Group	7	10	13	16	25	50	75
Males							
TLC	2120	3140	4330	6200	6740	7050	6630
VC	1670	2510	3550	5080	5350	5090	4470
FRC	980	1400	1970	2940	3120	3460	3440
ERV	530	770	1180	1810	1730	1500	1280
Females							
TLC	2070	2980	3740	4980	5030	5310	4860
VC	1580	2340	2999	3780	3930	3600	2940
FRC	970	1430	1690	2560	2420	2930	2590
ERV	480	780	940	1350	1320	1220	670

Source: Adapted from Hoit and Hixon (1987); Hoit, Hixon, Altman, and Morgan (1989); and Hoit, Hixon, Watson, and Morgan (1990).

Airflow

Laryngeal airflow is the volume of air passing through the glottis in a fixed period. It is measured in cubic centimeters (cc) or milliliters (mL) per second. For example, the /a/ vowel produced with a normal voice quality is characterized by an approximate laryngeal airflow of 100 cc/sec (Baken, 1996). That same vowel produced with a breathy voice quality (perhaps by a patient with large bilateral nodules) would be characterized by a laryngeal airflow of higher than 100 cc/sec due to excessively decreased glottal resistance to airflow. At the opposite end of the continuum, that same vowel produced with a strained-strangled voice quality (perhaps by a patient with adductor spasmodic dysphonia) would be characterized by a laryngeal airflow of less than 100 cc/sec due to excessively increased glottal resistance to airflow. Peak airflow (i.e., greatest flow) can be considerably higher than 100 cc/sec and depends on articulatory demands; for example, peak airflow during production of fricatives and stop consonants may exceed 500 cc/sec (Stathopoulos and Weismer, 1985). Children and older adults tend to demonstrate higher laryngeal airflows than younger adults (Stathopoulos and Sapienza, 1997).

Laryngeal Resistance

Laryngeal resistance is a measure derived from peak intraoral pressure and peak airflow during production of the /pi/ syllable repeated at a rate of approximately 1.5 syllables per second. Peak intraoral pressure is estimated from the /p/ portion of the syllable, and peak airflow is measured from the /i/ portion of the syllable. A breathy voice would suggest decreased laryngeal resistance, while a strain-strangled voice would suggest increased laryngeal resistance. When interpreting laryngeal resistance values, the clinician must examine the relative contribution of air pressure and airflow to that value.

The capacities and volumes we need to measure can be determined by using wet or dry spirometers. In the wet spirometer, a container floats in water placed in a larger container. As air is introduced into the smaller floating container, it floats higher in proportion to the volume of air introduced. The distance or rise of displacement is measured in terms of cubic centimeters or liters. Some spirometers are of the dry type. A flexible container enlarges on inspiratory tasks and decreases in volume on expiratory tasks, in both instances measuring the volume of displacement. Recent advances in technology have resulted in miniaturization and digitization of dry spirometers, allowing for ease of use and reduced cost compared to the wet spirometers.

Relatively inexpensive pressure measuring gauges and manometers are available for the measurement of airflow pressures. For example, Hixon and colleagues (1982) described a simple water manometer test that can be used to estimate the ability to generate respiratory driving pressure sufficient for voice and speech. The test requires a drinking glass that is 12 cm deep or deeper, filled with water, and calibrated in centimeters by a marker pen. A plastic straw is attached to the cup with a paper clip. The bottom tip of the straw is anchored at 10 cm below the rim. The patient is instructed to blow bubbles through the straw. If the patient maintains a stream of bubbles for 5 seconds with the straw at a depth of 10 cm (10 cm H_2O), the authors suggest that breath support is adequate for conversational speech.

The Phonatory Aerodynamic System (PAS) (KayPENTAX Corp., Montvale, New Jersey), shown in Figure 6.17, is the latest pneumotachograph-based system for

FIGURE 6.17 The Phonatory Aerodynamic System™

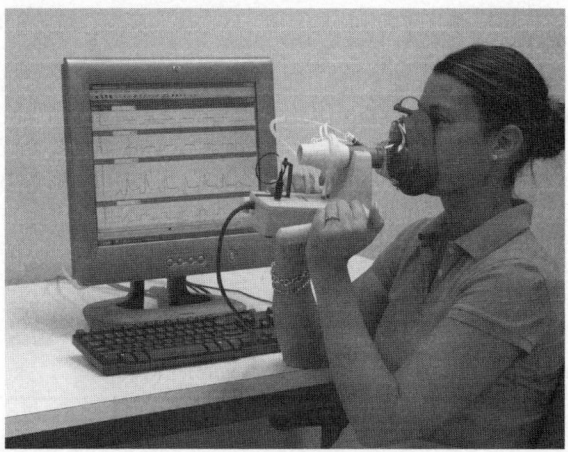

Source: Courtesy of KayPENTAX®.

aerodynamic analysis. The PAS allows the clinician to obtain measurements of average phonatory flow rate, sound pressure level, fundamental frequency, vital capacity, subglottal pressure (derived), glottal resistance, and vocal efficiency, among other parameters. Zraick and colleagues (2012) recently reported the first adult normative data for this system, obtained from 157 speakers over the age of 18 years.

PHONATORY-RESPIRATORY EFFICIENCY ANALYSES AND INSTRUMENTATION

As noted earlier in this chapter, the thoughtful clinician is able to generate a valid report based on noninstrumental means alone provided that clinician is well versed in normative measures of respiration, phonation, and resonance. This entails being familiar with a number of seminal research articles that report normative measures of speech and voice production, among them Kent and colleagues (1987), and Hixon and colleagues (1982).

Maximum Phonation Time (MPT)

MPT is the longest period during which a patient can sustain phonation of a vowel sound, typically /a/, at her or his most comfortable pitch and loudness. Maslan and colleagues (2010) describe current knowledge about the effect of age, gender, and number of trials on MPT values. They report that (1) children tend to have shorter MPTs, require more trials to learn how to maximally phonate, and show more variation than young adults; (2) young adults have less variability in MPT as a group and can phonate for a comparatively longer time than either children or older adults; (3) older adults have shorter MPTs; and (4) across all age groups, men can sustain a longer MPT on average than women. If laryngeal airflow is high, MPT is shorter than normal; if laryngeal airflow is low, MPT may be longer than normal.

As Kent and colleagues (1987, p. 368) note, however, MPT by itself cannot be used to distinguish a deficit in respiratory support (reduced phonation volume) from an inefficiency in vocal fold vibration (high airflow). Table 6.12 presents select normative MPT data for adults and children.

When eliciting MPT, the clinician should give standardized instructions regarding depth of inhalation, and he or she should provide a visual and auditory model and visual feedback about performance. There is some disagreement in the literature about how many trials should be elicited (one versus three to five), and whether one should take the longest utterance or an average of the utterances. Practically speaking, an average of three trials should result in a representative MPT for most patients. A timer and audio recorder are the only equipment needed to measure

TABLE 6.12 Select Maximum Phonation Time (MPT) for Normal Speakers Producing /a/

Source	Age Range (years)	Sex	Mean (sec)	Stand. Dev. or Stand. Error	Range (sec)
Finnegan (1984)	3–5	Male	9.3	2.4	4.5–14.1
		Female	8.5	2.1	4.5–12.6
	6–9	Male	15.5	4.1	7.5–23.6
		Female	14.8	3.6	7.7–21.9
	10–13	Male	21.1	5.6	10.2–23.1
		Female	16.3	4.1	10.4–24.3
	14–17	Male	18.5	5.9	11.6–34.8
		Female	15.6	5.1	10.5–30.9
Tavares and colleagues (2012)	4–6	Male	6.0	1.8	Not reported
	4–6	Female	6.2	2.0	
	7–9	Male	8.1	2.0	Not reported
	7–9	Female	7.9	2.0	
	10–12	Male	9.2	2.3	Not reported
	10–12	Female	9.1	2.0	
Ma and Yui (2006)	20–55	Combined	22.9	8.9	Not reported
Maslan and colleagues (2011)	61–70	Male	26.2	1.2	16.0–35.0
	61–70	Female	18.8	2.5	8.0–60.0
	71–80	Male	23.1	1.7	7.0–58.0
	71–80	Female	22.8	1.4	12.0–45.0
	81–90	Male	21.7	1.5	10.0–50.0
	81–90	Female	21.0	0.9	5.0–60.0

MPT. Speyer and colleagues (2010) have shown that an individual's MPT is highly consistent over a period of six weeks, and that clinician intra-rater reliability is high for repeated measurements of the same trial. Perhaps one of the most efficient uses of MPT is as a baseline against which future comparisons can be made during and at the conclusion of voice therapy.

s/z Ratio

The s/z ratio is also an indirect index of laryngeal airflow. To obtain the s/z ratio, the clinician asks the patient to first sustain the /s/ as long as possible, and then to sustain the /z/ as long as possible, each at normal pitch and loudness following a maximal inhalation. Verbal encouragement is usually given, and the longest /s/ and longest /z/ from one of three alternating /s, z/ trials is used to calculate the ratio. According to Boone (1971), who first proposed and developed this technique, persons with normal vocal folds could be expected to prolong the voiceless /s/ and the voiced /z/ phonemes for about the same length of time, resulting in an s/z ratio approximating 1. Eckel and Boone (1981) studied three groups of adult and pediatric speakers (those with vocal fold nodules or polyps, those with functional dysphonia, and those with normal larynges and voices) and reported s/z ratios > 1.40 in 95% of those speakers with nodules or polyps (p. 147). The s/z ratios for those speakers with functional dysphonia or normal voices were approximately 1.0 and did not significantly differ from each other. Across groups, however, there was a wide range of s/z ratios obtained: Some speakers with nodules or polyps or functional dysphonia exhibited s/z ratios less than 1.0, while some speakers with normal voices exhibited s/z ratios greater than 1.0. A number of subsequent studies of the s/z ratio with adults and children have been conducted, with most reporting quite variable results both within and across dysphonic and normal speakers (Fendler and Shearer, 1988; Gelfer and Pazerra, 2006; Hufnagle and Hufnagle, 1988; Larson and colleagues, 1990; Rastatter and Hyman, 1982; Soman, 1997; Sorenson and Parker, 1992; Tait and colleagues, 1980; Treole and Trudeau, 1997; Trudeau and Forrest, 1997; Van der Meer and colleagues, 2010). Procedurally, studies have differed in the type of instructions, number of trials, type and number of subjects, variables controlled (for example, loudness, pitch, motivation, training, respiratory effort), and age of the subjects (Gelfer and Palazar, 2006, p. 347). Elevated s/z ratios may be a red flag to check the glottal edge of the vocal folds for an additive lesion, or to suspect glottic insufficiency due to vocal fold paralysis (Miller, 2004), but this measure is by no means perfect. Table 6.13 presents select normative s/z duration data for adults and children.

VOICE DOSAGE ANALYSIS AND INSTRUMENTATION

Many voice disorders are chronic or recurring conditions that result from faulty and/or abusive vocal behaviors. Such behaviorally based disorders are difficult to assess and rehabilitate because patient self-reporting and self-monitoring are subjective and often unreliable. Instrumentation has recently become available that gives clinicians and researchers quantitative data on a patient's voice use throughout the day. The Ambulatory Phonation Monitor™ (APM) (KayPENTAX,

TABLE 6.13 Select s/z Ratios for Normal Speakers*

Source	Age (Years)	Gender	Maximum /s/ Duration			Maximum /z/ Duration			s/z Ratio		
			Mean	SD	Range	Mean	SD	Range	Mean	SD	Range
Tait and colleagues (1980)	5	Male	7.9	1.4	5.4–9.8	8.6	2.1	6.6–13.0	0.92	NR	0.82–1.08
	5	Female	8.3	4.0	4.8–18.3	10.0	3.3	5.2–16.0	0.83	NR	0.50–1.14
	7	Male	9.3	1.7	7.4–12.5	13.2	3.6	9.2–19.6	0.70	NR	0.52–0.97
	7	Female	10.2	2.6	7.3–16.0	13.1	4.0	9.1–20.0	0.78	NR	0.51–1.10
	9	Male	16.7	8.5	7.1–44.0	18.1	6.8	10.1–33.1	0.92	NR	0.66–1.50
	9	Female	14.4	3.1	9.3–20.9	15.8	5.2	8.5–24.2	0.91	NR	0.75–1.26
Tavares and colleagues (2012)	4–6	Male	5.77	1.94	NR	6.01	2.05	NR	0.96	NR	NR
	4–6	Female	5.91	1.88	NR	6.17	1.86	NR	0.96	NR	NR
	7–9	Male	7.47	1.92	NR	8.05	2.30	NR	0.93	NR	NR
	7–9	Female	7.74	1.92	NR	8.00	2.20	NR	0.97	NR	NR
	10–12	Male	9.22	2.23	NR	9.35	2.27	NR	0.99	NR	NR
	10–12	Female	9.10	1.96	NR	9.15	2.11	NR	0.99	NR	NR
Gelfer and Pazera (2006)	19–30	Male	25.04	10.10	9.18–43.77	27.33	8.07	15.43–41.23	0.91	0.25	0.46–1.36
	19–30	Female	16.92	5.46	9.13–29.07	17.47	3.86	11.67–26.17	0.97	0.25	0.55–1.57
Eckel and Boone (1981)	8–88	Both	17.73	7.65	5.0–38.0	18.60	6.97	5.0–37.0	0.99	0.36	0.41–2.67
Boominathan and colleagues (2012)	61–74	Male	NR	NR	NR	NR	NR	NR	1.21	0.08	NR
	60–65	Female	NR	NR	NR	NR	NR	NR	1.19	0.14	NR

NR = not reported.

Montvale, New Jersey), shown in Figure 6.18, is a portable device worn by clients to capture important parameters of vocal behavior over an entire day of normal activity (Cheyne and colleagues, 2003). The APM works via the use of an accelerometer that measures the vibration of the skin of the neck that occurs during phonation. The accelerometer signal is analyzed to provide percentage phonation time, fundamental frequency, sound pressure level, and vocal dosage. The APM may facilitate carryover of behaviors established in voice therapy by providing vibrotactile biofeedback to the user when voice usage parameters exceed limits set by the therapist. The Denver Center for the Performing Arts has also developed a vocal dosimeter that provides similar measures for research purposes (Popolo and colleagues, 2005). Griffin Laboratories has introduced the Vocalog™ Vocal Activity Monitor (Griffin Laboratories, Temecula, California). This instrument is a commercially available device that uses a neck-mounted contact microphone as the phonation sensor and provides simultaneous long-term monitoring and biofeedback for vocal SPL (Hillman and colleagues, 2011).

FIGURE 6.18 An Ambulatory Phonation Monitor™ in Use

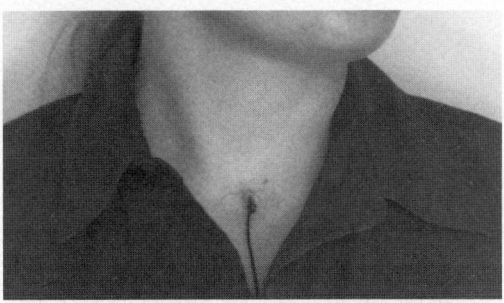

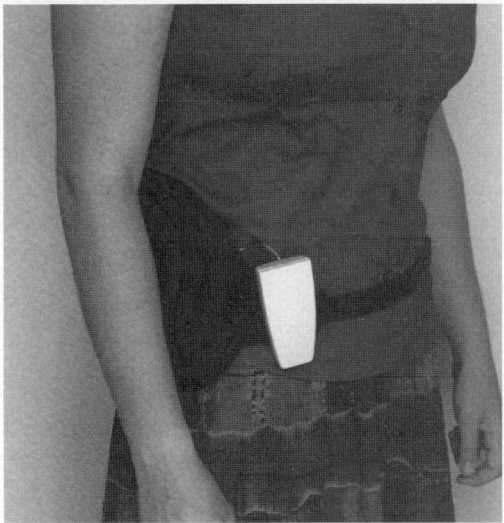

Source: Courtesy of KayPENTAX®.

CASE STUDIES

The following three case studies are new to this edition and are provided here to demonstrate the wide range of voice clients that we see at our clinics and the type of instrumental and noninstrumental approaches we perform. Just as important as the voice diagnosis is the clinician's ability to apply diagnostic probes to improve voice and to document those improvements in quantitative and qualitative language that is clear to the referring physician and the client and family. Each case study includes a summary and recommendations. Case 1 presents muscle tension dysphonia (see Chapter 3) in an elderly female with a complex medical history. Readers are asked to appreciate the effects of the client's hearing loss on her vocal behaviors. Case 2 involves a child client with vocal nodules (see Chapters 3 and 8). We report noninstrumental measures only because, in reality, many clinicians do not have access to digitized instrumentation. As noted at the beginning of this chapter, a valid voice evaluation can be performed noninstrumentally by a competent SLP. Individualized Education Plan (IEP) goals are included. Case 3 challenges the reader to engage in the practice of differential diagnosis, or the act of narrowing possibilities and reaching conclusions about the nature of the deficit (Duffy, 2005).

■ ■ ■ ■ ■ ■ ■ ■ ■

CASE STUDY 1

MTD IN AN ELDERLY FEMALE

HISTORY

Mrs. V is a 74-year-old female who was seen for a voice and laryngeal function study upon referral from her primary otolaryngologist. The history and physical summary noted that Mrs. V had experienced a change in swallowing and phonatory quality since anterior cervical discectomy and fusion (ACDF) surgery six months earlier. Mrs. V reported that she drinks about six to eight glasses of water per day, but throughout the 60-minute assessment, she drank only about two-thirds of a 6-ounce glass of water. Additional medical history includes asthma, osteoarthritis, GERD, diverticulitis, fibromyalgia, and sleep apnea, among others. She uses C-PAP PRN. She reports chronic back pain. Over the course of the assessment, it was also discovered that Mrs. V presents with reduced hearing acuity for which she is not aided. She responded positively to several signs and symptoms of laryngopharyngeal reflux (Belafsky and colleagues, 2002). She lives locally with her husband, who is retired. Mrs. V works as a paralegal assistant at an attorney's office.

■ ■ ■

ASSESSMENT

Perceptual and Noninstrumental Observations

Vocal quality today is strained and elevated in amplitude. Spoken phrases tend to grind to a vocal arrest toward phrase end, and the phrases themselves are monotone. As measured by the CAPE-V, during sustained phonation of /a/, the patient exhibits vocal strain (93 mm); moderate roughness (62 mm); and severe deficits in pitch (87 mm), characterized primarily by the inability to increase or lower pitch. Loudness is abnormally high (80 cm). Mrs. V speaks with very little anterior oral cavity movement; therefore, much of the voiced energy is reflected back into the oral cavity.

Voice Handicap Index (VHI). Mrs. V's total VHI score was 75, which is considered a severe self-perceived handicap.

Acoustic Observations. Acoustic recordings from the CAPE-V speech tasks were measured and demonstrated an average fundamental frequency (F^0) during sustained phonation of an /a/ of 127 Hz, which is well below normal limits for women. RAP, shimmer, and NHR were all above normal limits. Speaking fundamental frequency (SFF) ranged from 125 Hz to 135 Hz, which is well below the frequency range for women. Clinician models of pitch range changes did not elicit any immediate change in pitch. Mrs. V was observed to throat-clear on a number of occasions throughout the session.

Aerodynamic Observations. Phonation was brief at less than 5 seconds, with transglottal airflow greater than 200 ml/s.

Endoscopic Observations. The patient was seated in the exam chair in the clinic and positioned for a flexible endoscopic examination using a halogen light source. The KayPENTAX distal chip video laryngoscope was passed along the floor of the right nasal cavity. Nasoendoscopy revealed that, for a sustained vowel and speaking tasks, the patient revealed normal bilateral vocal fold abduction, but upon adduction, bilateral medial involvement of the ventricular folds were revealed during true vocal fold (TVF) vibration. This medial posturing of the ventricular folds served to dampen the vibration of the TVFs, which is a form of muscle tension dysphonia (MTD). This hyperfunctioning at the level of the supralarynx may have been secondary to irritation of the larynx—perhaps after extubation from the noted ACDF surgery. It is suspected that this maladaptive behavior had become habituated.

Probes. Before diagnostic probes were administered, Mrs. V was introduced to animated videos demonstrating vocal fold production and she was given a brief tutorial in the anatomy and physiology of voice production. She was then introduced to laryngeal function videos of past patients with MTD. She was asked to appreciate how the ventricular folds and anterior-posterior positioning of the arytenoids and epiglottis petiole restrict the movement of the TVF.

Diagnostic Probes. Mrs. V was introduced to the Voice Facilitating Approaches of focus, inhalation phonation, yawn-sigh, breathy voice, and confidential tone. She was encouraged to relax the jaw and neck and to reduce hyperextension of the head and neck. The tone-focus technique with nasals, liquids, and glides was administered with unremarkable results. The yawn-sigh; inhalation phonation; and confidential, breathy voice yielded brief periods of a higher pitch and normal vocal quality. SFF was re-probed and revealed a greater range of frequency, ranging from 155 Hz to 175 Hz. Mrs. V was able to engage in pitch shifts up for the penultimate or final word of the phrase. The ability to increase pulmonary pressure and TVF lengthening suggested a laryngeal and pharyngeal system that was experiencing greater mobility and flexibility. When this improvement was pointed out to Mrs. V, she said that, because of her hearing loss, *she had difficulty appreciating the results.* At this point, she also suggested that she might be engaging in a louder voice to increase sensory feedback, that is, to hear herself better.

This rapid increase in vocal quality was discussed with the patient and it was explained that improvement is typical when maladaptive behaviors are suppressed in a normal laryngeal system. It was suggested that Mrs. V return to this clinic for an additional session to video-record the facilitation approaches that were instrumental in reducing vocal hyperfunction and increasing normal vocal quality. Audio and video feedback have been shown to be powerful biofeedback tools to increase vocal quality and reduce maladaptive behaviors in a normal laryngeal system. Mrs. V said that she would appreciate such a DVD and would return for a final intervention session. Swallow strategies and signs and symptoms of LPR were also discussed, and Mrs. V said that she felt comfortable that many of the s/s of dysphagia were secondary to poor oral preparatory and transit behaviors, such as inadequate mastication of solid boluses. She was provided with dysphagia counseling. It was recommended that Mrs. V see a medical professional regarding s/s of reflux.

SUMMARY

Mrs. V is a 74-year-old female with complaints of strained and strangled phonation since ACDF surgery six months earlier. Fiberoptic endoscopy revealed a muscle tension dysphonia during phonation attempts, characterized by medial involvement of the false vocal folds. Perceptually, the voice was low in pitch and strained. Spoken phrases tended to grind to a vocal arrest toward phrase end, and the phrases themselves were monotone. The patient demonstrated little anterior mouth opening for speech. The Voice Facilitating Approaches of yawn-sigh, inhalation phonation, and breathy voice were successful in eliciting brief periods of improved vocal quality and pitch; however, Mrs. V reported that she had difficulty appreciating these improvements secondary to reduced hearing acuity.

RECOMMENDATIONS

Continue the vocal hygiene program and include increased hydration and reduction of throat clearing. Continue to discuss and practice the Voice Facilitating Approaches to reduce vocal hyperfunction: Those approaches that revealed the greatest improvement in vocal quality were inhalation phonation, breathy voice, and yawn-sigh. Open mouth approach will also be introduced. Discuss locating a local audiologist for a thorough hearing evaluation and acquisition of hearing aids. Discuss any signs and symptoms of reflux disease, secondary to patient reports of globus.

■ ■ ■ ■ ■ ■ ■ ■ ■

CASE STUDY 2

VOCAL NODULES IN A YOUNG MALE

HISTORY

Samir is a 7-year-old male who was seen for an evaluation of voice and laryngeal function per referral from his second-grade teacher. His teacher is concerned because Samir is reluctant to speak in class due to a hoarse and scratchy voice. The teacher has kept a diary of his vocal performance in class and has provided this to Samir's mother. Samir is being passed over by his peers to join in group reading projects because Samir's voice gives out on him completely at times. The school SLP has seen Samir for a few trial sessions of intervention involving mostly vocal hygiene counseling, and she accompanies Samir and his mother to today's voice assessment. Samir's mother brings with her a recent report from Samir's otolaryngologist. The otolaryngologist performed flexible nasoendoscopy the week prior and reports fullness on the medial margin of both vocal folds at the juncture of the anterior and medial third of the vocal folds. These space-occupying lesions are consistent with vocal nodules.

An initial interview reveals that Samir drinks a glass of orange juice at breakfast and a six-ounce carton of milk at school. He drinks a number of sweetened beverages during the day, but no established amount of plain water. Samir also presents with a history of allergies, for which he is therapeutically medicated. He has a history of middle ear infections; otherwise, birth and developmental history are unremarkable. Samir has a 5-year-old brother with no history of speech, resonance, or language disorders. His brother also attends the assessment. Interviewing revealed that Samir is very active in outside play, sports, choir, and martial arts. He tends to "give 110%" to everything he does, according to his mother.

■ ■ ■

ASSESSMENT

Perceptual and Noninstrumental Observations

Samir and his mother completed the pVHI, which revealed moderate perceived voice handicap. Questions regarding Samir's school and extracurricular activities are discussed. All present are seated at a round table an equal distance from a digital recorder with a multidirectional microphone. The discussion is later played back, and it is noted by Samir and his mother that they present with voices that are quite a bit louder than those of the two SLPs and Samir's brother.

Administration of the CAPE-V reveals Samir to exhibit moderate roughness (53 mm), moderately reduced pitch (64 mm), and loudness in the severe range (79 cm). Samir's spoken output is recorded and played back while the clinician matches several words on an electronic keyboard (see Table 6.4). Average SFF is B5 or 245 Hz, which is about 40 Hz below where it should be.

Samir is asked to talk about a typical day, and he is recorded via digital recorder. Playback reveals that he produces about three words before he runs out of breath, whereas eight words per breath are typical. MPT is 6 seconds, whereas the average MPT for same-age peers is about 12 seconds. In one minute of connected speech, he demonstrated 12 phonation breaks and six pitch breaks for 108 words, which represents 16% dysphonic events for the sample. He presents with a slightly hyperextended neck and head posture, and the strap muscles appear tense. He was observed to throat-clear extensively throughout the interview and clinical assessment.

VOICE FACILITATING APPROACHES

Samir and his mother were counseled about adequate water intake. It was explained that drinking too little water can result in a number of medical problems (Kent and Graubard, 2010), even beyond voice. Samir was provided with his own decorated water bottle and given a "doctor's prescription" to bring the water bottle to class. Silent cough (a quick exhalation of air up through an abducted glottis) and sniff-swallow (collecting mucus in the back of the nasopharynx and then swallowing) were demonstrated and recommended to reduce coughing and throat clearing.

Voice Facilitating Approaches of focus, yawn-sigh, and pitch shift up were introduced to bring the voiced energy from the larynx up into the facial mask and to increase the resonating chambers in the pharynx for good voice. Samir was provided with the concept of "just right voice," which is the pediatric equivalent of confidential tone (Chapter 7). By elevating the pitch from B5 (245 Hz) to C4 (262 Hz), vocal quality increased, and phonation and pitch breaks were reduced to less than 5% of the spoken output sample. Samir immediately noticed the improvements, remarking that it was much easier to voice and that he no longer had to "push the words out."

SUMMARY AND RECOMMENDATIONS

Samir is a 7-year-old male who presents with a gradual dysphonia that interferes with his education program at school. This dysphonia is limiting his classroom participation and places him at risk for reduced educational performance. Samir's mother and school SLP have been apprised of these findings and agree that an IEP is warranted. To summarize:

- *Breath support:* Samir presents with too little breath support for speech. He produces about three words per phrase. The average number of words per phrase is eight.
- *MPT:* Samir's MPT is six seconds. The average MPT for same-age peers is 12 seconds.
- *Pitch:* Samir presents with a pitch that is below normal limits for same-age peers. His speaking frequency is about a G3 (196 Hz), which is about 40 Hz below normal.
- *Quality:* Samir presents with a hoarse voice that sometimes stops completely. The CAPE-V reveals vocal parameters in the moderate to severe range.

EFFECTS OF DISABILITY ON PARTICIPATION IN GENERAL CURRICULUM

When Samir contributes in class, it is observed that his voice is hoarse at least 50% of the time, and aphonic (no voice) 30% of the time. His teacher states that he speaks in a "rough" and "low voice," and that during the week of March 14 to March 18, he lost his voice on three occasions. His vocal nodules have been verified by a medical doctor. Samir's hoarse voice interferes with his ability to participate in daily educational interactions.

Effects of Disability on Participation in General Curriculum

- *Priority educational needs:* To improve the quality of Samir's voice so that he can participate in all educational activities during the day.
- *Measurable annual goal:* During all oral school activities, Samir will use vocal hygiene and voice strategies to produce a clear, age-appropriate voice four out of five days a week for three school weeks.

SHORT-TERM OBJECTIVES

- Samir will identify and modify vocal abuse and overuse occasions with 90% accuracy by logging these events in his daily "just right voice" book (generated by the SLP).
- Samir will discriminate between "just right voice" samples of himself and two of his peers with 90% accuracy.
- Samir will demonstrate and teach vocal hygiene and voice strategies to family members and friends, as documented in his "just right voice" book.

- Samir will engage in "just right voice" when communicating orally in his classes as measured by his instructors, in eight out of ten opportunities.

EVALUATION PLAN

Samir's progress toward annual goals will be measured by:

- Teacher/clinician observations.
- Voice quality, pitch, and loudness data collected on a weekly basis.
- Review of Samir's "just right voice" book and related charts on a weekly basis.

- - - - - - - - - -

CASE STUDY 3

DIFFERENTIAL DIAGNOSIS OF DYSPHONIA IN AN ADOLESCENT WITH A COMPLEX MEDICAL HISTORY

This case emphasizes the importance of having a thorough understanding of the respiratory, phonatory, and resonance components of the voice mechanism and their intimate connections. This case also emphasizes the importance of conducting a full medical history interview and clinical examination because many voice disorders masquerade as other disorders.

HISTORY

Susan is a 13-year-old female who experienced pneumonia at three years of age. She developed pneumatoceles, air-filled cysts that develop within the lung parenchyma. She underwent tracheostomy and received mechanical ventilation for several weeks. According to her mother, who did not possess the medical records at the time of the current voice assessment, Susan was subsequently decannulated and underwent "tracheal reconstructive surgery." Pulmonary function studies show no evidence of lower airway compromise. She is on the standard medical regimen for asthma, although Susan says that those medications do not ease her breathing during exercise. A tracheobronchoscopy by a local pulmonologist suggests possible unilateral vocal fold paresis. Susan's current complaint is shortness of breath (SOB), which is mostly associated with exercise but can be exacerbated in instances of emotional distress. Susan and her mother are concerned because Susan cannot engage in many school activities, such as physical education. She is often late to class. At this time, she does not engage in any school field trips or extracurricular sports.

■ ■ ■

ASSESSMENT

Perceptual and Noninstrumental Observations

The voice is breathy and hoarse. Inhalatory stridor is observed during connected speech. As measured by the CAPE-V, during sustained phonation of /a/, the patient exhibits a consistently moderate amount of breathiness (53 mm); minimal strain (15 mm); moderately reduced loudness (67 mm); and severe deficits in pitch

(85mm), characterized by the inability to increase or lower pitch. Water monometer test (Hixon and colleagues, 1982) reveals that Susan is able to maintain a stream of bubbles for 5 seconds with a straw in water at a depth of 5 cm. This performance suggests sufficient breath support for most speech purposes. Maximum phonation time for a sustained /a/ is less than five seconds, which is well outside functional limits The s/z ratio is 1.0. Words per phrase for connected speech are reduced, at an average of four words per breath (average number of words per phrase group is eight, per Goldman-Eisler (1968). Diadochokinetic productions are normal at approximately six per second; however, Susan is not able to produce more than four seconds of sustained diadochokinetics. Reading for the Grandfather Passage reveals reading rate at approximately 120 words per minute, which is within functional limits, and Susan paused appropriately at the syntactic junctures.

Acoustic Observations. Acoustic recordings from the CAPE-V speech tasks were measured and demonstrated an average fundamental frequency (F^0) during sustained phonation of 283 Hz, which is elevated (mean F^0 for 13-year-old females is approximately 230 Hz.). Susan was not able to engage in normal pitch shifts; pitch range as measured on a keyboard and acoustically was limited to less than one octave, with basal at C4 (262 Hz) and highest production at B4 (494 Hz), as measured on an electronic keyboard and smartphone application (see Table 6.4). Young adults normally have a frequency range of 2.5 to 3 octaves, which indicates neuromotor control, adequate respiratory support, and ability to modify the shape and length of vocal folds (Bless, 1988). RAP was elevated at 1.46%, shimmer was elevated at 12.4%, and HNR was 9 dB.

Aerodynamic Observations. Phonation was brief at 3.5 seconds, with transglottal airflow greater than 200 ml/s.

Summary of Findings Thus Far. The patient is a 13-year-old female with a 10-year history of SOB following tracheostomy, mechanical ventilation, and reconstructive surgery. SOB grows worse with physical exertion. The patient reveals reduced MPT, elevated F^0 for sustained vowel and speaking tasks, and reduced pitch range. Voice is breathy and hoarse; s/z ratio is 1.0, suggesting same duration for exhalatory and vibratory phase. At the beginning of speaking and reading tasks, subject reveals sufficient respiratory support for linguistic demands, but this ability declines rapidly as the task proceeds.

Test Your Differential Diagnostic Abilities. Given the subject's complaints, medical history, and clinical assessments, suggest possible etiologies (mechanical or physiological or functional) that might underlie this dysphonia and shortness of breath.

Is it asthma? Asthma is an obstructive airway disease:

- Wheezing, coughing, difficulty exhaling due to obstruction in the airway.
- Triggered by allergies, viral infections, exercise, stress, cold air.

Symptoms/findings that *would* indicate a diagnosis of asthma:

- Patient has been on asthma medications since she was decannulated.
- Patient reported "trouble getting air out."
- SOB coincides with exercise and cold air.
- Asthma "fits" the medical history of tracheostomy secondary to pneumonia (Sataloff, 1997).

Symptoms/findings that would *not* indicate a diagnosis of asthma:

- Ten years of asthma mediation has failed to address SOB and wheezy respiration.
- No reported allergies.
- Pulmonary function studies by the pulmonologist revealed no lower airway expiratory obstruction.

Is it UVFP?

- Prior to voice assessment, Susan underwent tracheobronchoscopy. Although lower airway assessment was unremarkable, the otolaryngologist suspected left true vocal fold dysmotility or paresis.
- UVFP may occur after disease or trauma to the recurrent laryngeal branch of the Vagus.
- One vocal fold is normally "stuck" in a paramedian position off midline; phonation is breathy, rough, and short in duration. Dysphagia is not uncommon.

Symptoms/findings that *would* indicate a diagnosis of UVFP:

- "Fits" medical history of tracheostomy and reconstructive laryngeal surgery.
- Elevated airflow on phonatory function analysis.
- Breathy and hoarse vocal quality and reduced pitch range.

Symptoms/findings that would *not* indicate a diagnosis of UVFP:

- Although it is compromised, Susan has control of respiratory-phonatory valving for speech tasks.
- No diplophonia.
- No vocal improvement with facilitation techniques of half-swallow boom, head turn, and digital manipulation.

Is it paradoxical vocal fold movement?

- PVFM is an insidious laryngeal manifestation often mistaken for uncontrolled asthma.
- Vocal folds close when they should open and open when they should close.
- Tricky to diagnose because causes and presentation are so diverse.
- Susan's pulmonologist suspected PVFM because of the capricious nature of the SOB.

Symptoms/findings that *would* indicate a diagnosis of PVFM:

- SOB appeared to be associated with PVFM precipitators.
- Asthma had been ruled out.
- Previous medical testing revealed normal lower airway function.
- Susan reported some anxiety and depression.

Symptoms/findings that would *not* indicate a diagnosis of PVFM:

- Susan performed vocal and speech tasks while experiencing SOB. In our clinical experience, a person with PVFM is normally not able to perform those tasks.
- SOB resolves with rest.
- Too early to extrapolate limited observations of psychosocial disorders in PVFM to the larger population.

ENDOSCOPIC EVALUATION

The patient was seated in the exam chair in the clinic and positioned for a flexible endoscopic examination using halogen light source. The KayPentax distal chip video laryngoscope was passed along the floor of the left nasal cavity. Nasoendoscopy revealed a subgottal anterior laryngeal web, most likely a result of the reconstructive surgery performed 10 years earlier. The web was attached to the inferior and medial aspect of the anterior commissure bilaterally, ceasing about one-third of the distance from the anterior commissure, where the distance between the folds abducting becomes too great.

SUMMARY

The subglottal laryngeal web is consistent with the subject's medical history, symptoms, complaints, and clinical assessment. The web served to block incoming and outgoing air and to inhibit normal vocal fold vibration. The airway was estimated to be two-thirds to three-quarters occluded by the web. The web was associated with Susan's complaints of elevated pitch for speaking and sustained vowels, and reduced pitch range. It also contributed to the back pressure or buildup of subglottal air that might account for feelings of "spasms." The increased tissue at the glottis interfered with true vocal fold vibration and resulted in elevated measures of jitter and shimmer.

RECOMMENDATIONS

The patient and her mother were apprised of the findings, and Susan was referred to the local medical center for surgery to remove the web. She was encouraged to follow all recommendations by the surgical otolaryngologist. She was scheduled to return to this clinic after intervention for a brief reassessment followed by vocal hygiene counseling and any Voice Facilitating Approaches deemed necessary.

SUMMARY

The voice evaluation is the time when the clinician first meets the voice patient, providing opportunity for observation and testing. The evaluation begins when the patient is observed in the waiting room and continues as part of each therapy session, particularly as the clinician continually searches with the patient for new vocal behaviors. The clinician must continue to evaluate and observe the patient's respiratory, phonatory, and resonance functions. Whenever possible, these functions should be quantified with instrumentation. Auditory-perceptual judgments are also extremely valuable in describing the patient's voice disorder and the manner in which it is produced. The patient's perception of voice handicap is also important to assess. The patient's voice data are used for comparison purposes, to quantify vocal changes during the first visit, through subsequent therapy sessions, and in the final outcome session. Patient performance, both as observed and as measured, is offered to the patient as continuing feedback, which helps the patient become aware of voice performance. The evaluation enables the voice clinician to decide on which management steps to take for the patient, and to refer the patient to professionals in other disciplines when necessary. If voice therapy is indicated, the evaluation helps the clinician to develop a therapy plan and to predict the patient's prognosis.

GUIDED READING

Read the following article.

> Lee, L., Stemple, J. C., Glaze, L., & Kelchner, L. N. (2004). Quick screen for voice and supplementary documents for identifying pediatric voice disorders. *Language, Speech, and Hearing Services in Schools, 35*(4), 308–320.

Compile a list of the voice and resonance behaviors that are important to collect and assess in a child-related screening instrument. Create a miniversion of your own quick screen instrument.

Read the following reports.

> American Speech-Language-Hearing Association. (2004e). *Vocal tract visualization and imaging* [Position Statement]. Rockville, MD: Author. Available from www.asha.org/policy

> American Speech-Language-Hearing Association. (2004f). *Vocal tract visualization and imaging* [Technical Report]. Rockville, MD: Author. Available from www.asha.org/policy.

Describe the roles and responsibilities of the SLP with respect to vocal tract visualization.

PREPARING FOR THE PRAXIS™

Directions: Please read and answer the five questions that follow. (Please see page 319 for the answer key.)

1. In Case Study 1, the numeric value of 93 mm on the CAPE-V for vocal strain translates to:
   A. Mildly deviant
   B. Moderately deviant
   C. Severely deviant
   D. Within normal limits

2. In Case Study 1, the female client revealed a speaking fundamental frequency (SFF) ranging from 125 Hz to 135 Hz as measured instrumentally. If digitized instrumentation had not been available, SFF could easily be measured on an electronic

keyboard or smartphone application. In this case, the SFF would be approximately (hint: see Figure 6.4):

A. B2
B. F3
C. A3
D. C4

3. The throat clearing demonstrated by the child in Case Study 2 is most likely secondary to:
A. Behaviors he has adopted from his brother
B. Globus due to thickened mucus
C. Globus due to sensation of the vocal nodules
D. Reduced breath support
E. Both B and C

4. The maximum phonation time demonstrated by the child in Case Study 2 is:
A. Consistent with the mean MPT for normal speakers his age
B. Below the mean MPT for normal speakers his age
C. Within the range of MPT for normal speakers his age
D. Above the mean MPT for normal speakers his age

5. An IEP is warranted for the child in Case Study 2 because:
A. He speaks in a rough and low voice
B. He has been diagnosed with vocal nodules
C. His hoarse voice interferes with his ability to participate in daily educational interactions
D. He is in need of a "just right voice" book.

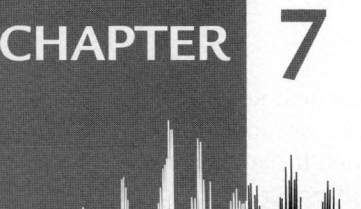

CHAPTER 7

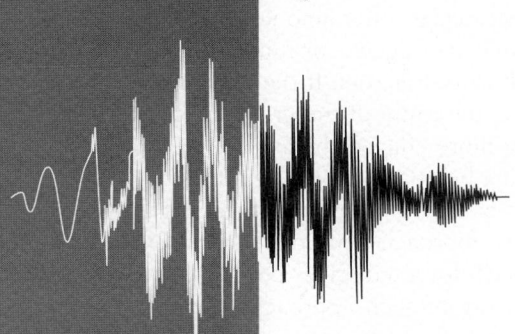

Voice Facilitating Approaches

▪ ▪ ▪ ▪ ─────────────── **LEARNING OBJECTIVES** ─────────────── ▪ ▪ ▪ ▪

After reading this chapter, one should be able to:

- Describe the reasoning for the suggestion that there is no one voice approach or program that is facilitative for all patients with the same voice problem.

- Define the concept of diagnostic probe and explain its importance in voice therapy.

- Identify the rationales and procedural approaches for the Voice Facilitating Approaches (VFAs).

- Identify at least one evidence-based practice article that supports the target VFA.

- Identify emerging technologies in voice intervention that appear to be promising tools when applied in conjunction with the guidance of the voice clinician.

Voice therapy is highly individualized, depending on the cause of the problem, its maintaining factors, the motivation of the patient, and the availability of appropriate management and treatment. Some voice problems may require only the management of professionals other than the profession of the speech-language pathologist (SLP), such as an otolaryngologist (ENT physician) who may successfully treat a papilloma or laryngeal cancer by laser surgery. On the other hand, using the case of unilateral vocal fold paralysis as an example, the patient is managed by both the SLP and the ENT physician, who will see the patient at different times during the recovery process. Many voice problems are managed by the SLP alone. For example, the SLP may help the patient with functional aphonia regain voice with voice therapy and then provide the follow-up that may be required to maintain normal voice.

What is offered for management and therapy (and by whom) is dictated by the presenting causal and maintaining factors that were identified at the time of the initial diagnostic evaluation. Even during voice therapy, there must be a continuous search for a possible change in the maintenance factors of the voice problem, which could then dictate a different management or therapy offering.

While many of the management strategies differ among voice patients according to whether their problems are organic, neurogenic, or functional, our VFAs may not be differentiated according to such causal factors. If the patient is exhibiting a problem in breath control, for example, the cause of the problem may get primary attention, but the techniques for using more efficient breath for voice are selected from a pool of approaches for improving breath control.

Perhaps the most commonly observed voice problems are related to vocal hyperfunction, for which many therapy approaches are designed to take the work out of speaking. A voice therapy approach for a particular person with vocal hyperfunction would be selected from an array of such approaches, with the selection again related to causal and maintaining factors. A young man who exhibits hard glottal attack might profit from learning to reduce his rate of speech, opening his mouth a bit more, learning more of a legato (smooth, easy flow) style of voicing, and practicing vocal chanting. His SLP would select the therapy approaches that help facilitate this easy, smooth style of voicing.

The authors were once approached by a computer scientist who suggested that the voice diagnostic–evaluation data could be fed into a software program, which would automatically tell the SLP what therapy methods to use with a recommended sequence of application. Such a cookbook approach to voice therapy is not possible. Rather, the SLP uses the presenting data and observations for decisions regarding management, selecting a particular approach for a trial beginning (known as a *diagnostic probe*). The patient's response to the probe and its effect on voice determine if that therapy approach will be used or eliminated in therapy, or if the approach can be combined with other approaches. Rarely is a particular voice therapy technique applied in isolation (Angadi & Stemple, 2012). For example, if a louder voice produces a clearer voice with less roughness, combining work on increasing respiratory volume, extending expiratory durations, improving patient posture, and increasing mouth opening could be combined with increasing loudness in a treatment session.

PATIENT COMPLIANCE AND EMERGING TECHNOLOGIES IN VOICE INTERVENTION

A number of voice researchers have performed retrospective studies over the years to try to find variables that determine why patients comply or do not comply with voice therapy. A study by Smith and colleagues (2009) looked at the attendance rates of 100 voice patients at a major academic urban medical center. Of the 100 patients scheduled for voice therapy, only 44 of those individuals complied. Suspected noncompliance factors ranged from clinician-related barriers, such as lack of empathy and lack of follow-up support, to clinic-related factors, such as inconvenient commutes and inflexible scheduling.

At our voice clinics, just as in many across the country and around the world, we encourage compliance by providing the voice patient with immediate success by applying what we call diagnostic probes or Voice Facilitating Approaches (VFAs) (described in this chapter). Once normal or near-normal phonation has been demonstrated, we capitalize on this success by making sure the client leaves with homework that includes an audio-video recording of the session. That is, if the aphonic patient has achieved vocal success by engaging in the VFA of focus and pitch shift down, we make a recording of these approaches and provide the recording to the patient at the end of the session or later, via the Internet.

Video-recordings of voice therapy have been shown to increase patient compliance (van Leer and Connor, 2012). In addition to video-recordings, other researchers advocate virtual reality approaches to voice intervention that simulate vocally challenging environments (Hapner and Johns, 2004). By placing him- or herself in a virtual, vocally challenging environment—such as a classroom—the voice patient is more likely to generalize the VFAs learned in clinic. Voice intervention via telepractice is also gaining momentum as a service delivery model (American Speech-Language-Hearing Association, 2001). Mashima and colleagues (2003) and Tindall and colleagues (2008) reported that voice intervention via videophone yielded voice outcomes similar to conventional voice therapy at a significant financial savings to the voice client.

VOICE THERAPY FACILITATING APPROACHES

In this text, we call our therapy approaches *Voice Facilitating Approaches* (VFAs). That is, the selected therapy technique facilitates a "target" or a more optimal vocal response by the patient. The VFAs are used with patients having various kinds of voice disorders: functional, organic, or neurogenic. Part of voice therapy is searching with patients to find the VFA that seems to help them produce the desired vocal response. Many patients with the same voice disorder, such as muscle tension dysphonia, may require different therapy approaches for the same problem. For example, in the same afternoon, we may see a patient who finds focus, or resonant voice therapy, effective in reducing vocal fold overvalving, while the next patient finds inhalation phonation and pitch shift up the keys to a less effortful voice. It is important to remember that, because a person's voice problem is often a combination of behavioral, emotional, physical, and structural issues, no one specific therapy approach is facilitative for all patients with the same voice problem. The experienced voice clinician has many voice therapy techniques to use for particular voice problems with certain patients. In addition to the current list of 25 approaches in this edition of *The Voice and Voice Therapy*, the SLP should be aware of the many other management and therapy approaches described in the literature: Titze (2006), Colton and colleagues (2006), Andrews and Summers (2002), Boone and Wiley (2000), Case (2002), Stemple (2000), Patel and colleagues (2011), and Denizoglu and Sihvo (2010). Smartphone and computer tablet software applications have made it even easier to use accessible and low-cost clinical tools with our voice patients. Angadi and Stemple (2012) list just a few of these apps, which includes virtual keyboards, pitch matchers, stopwatches, dB meters, voice recorders, and metronomes.

The VFAs in Table 7.1 are listed alphabetically. After each approach, a notation (×) indicates the voice parameters that the particular VFA has the potential to influence. For example, VFA #1, auditory feedback, can have an impact on both vocal loudness and quality, with less influence on voice pitch.

Accordingly, for the three columns in Table 7.1 (pitch, loudness, and quality) only the loudness and quality columns are marked with (×). Other techniques, such as yawn–sigh (VFA #25), influence all three parameters of pitch, loudness, and quality, and each column is marked with (×).

Experienced voice clinicians often combine therapy approaches in their search with the patient to find the target voice. Each of the 25 VFAs in Table 7.1 is presented from the following four perspectives: (1) kinds of problems for which the approach is useful, (2) procedural aspects of the approach, (3) typical case history showing utilization of the approach, and (4) evaluation of the approach.

TABLE 7.1 Twenty-Five Facilitating Approaches in Voice Therapy

Facilitating Approach	Parameter of Voice Affected		
	Pitch	Loudness	Quality
1. Auditory feedback		X	X
2. Change of loudness	X	X	X
3. Chant–talk		X	X
4. Chewing	X	X	X
5. Confidential voice		X	X
6. Counseling (explanation of problem)	X	X	
7. Digital manipulation	X		X
8. Elimination of abuses		X	X
9. Establishing a new pitch	X		X
10. Focus	X	X	X
11. Glottal fry	X	X	X
12. Head positioning	X		X
13. Hierarchy analysis	X	X	X
14. Inhalation phonation	X	X	
15. Laryngeal massage	X		X
16. Masking	X	X	
17. Nasal/glide stimulation			X
18. Open-mouth approach		X	X
19. Pitch inflections	X		
20. Redirected phonation	X	X	X
21. Relaxation	X	X	X
22. Respiration training		X	X
23. Tongue protrusion /i/	X		X
24. Visual feedback	X	X	X
25. Yawn–sigh	X	X	X

New to this ninth edition of *The Voice and Voice Therapy* is the addition of evidence-based practice (EBP) that supports each VFA. Evidence-based practice (EBF), for the purpose of this chapter, combines the information gleaned from all levels of evidence, ranging from the expert opinion of respected authorities to systematic reviews and randomized controlled clinical studies. Readers are encouraged to investigate these EBP resources further for at least a couple of reasons: (1) to gain an appreciation of the converging evidence for each of these approaches and (2) to use as rationales when generating goals and objectives for the VFAs.

1. Auditory Feedback

Kinds of Problems for Which the Approach Is Useful. The shift from analog to digital analysis in the late 1980s and 1990s revolutionized voice analysis and therapy. This certainly applies to immediate auditory feedback (and visual biofeedback later in this chapter) afforded by digitized instrumentation. Many voice patients profit from using some kind of auditory feedback in and out of voice therapy. Patients who displayed a window of voice improvement during the evaluation session (such as when masking was used as a diagnostic probe resulting in an immediate improvement in voice) often benefit from the use of auditory feedback during therapy sessions. Regardless of the causal factor of the disorder (organic, neurogenic, or functional), the patient's voice may improve with such feedback.

Auditory feedback is supported by motor planning and programming theory (Duffy, 2005; Callan and colleagues, 2000; Hodson, 1992). In a nutshell, this theory suggests that humans are able to alter and adapt motor-equivalent voice and speech production through integration of sensory information from peripheral mechano-receptors, one of those being acoustic feedback. Different kinds of auditory feedback may enhance patient response, such as using real-time amplification and letting patients hear themselves on headphones as they are speaking. The slight amplification is thought to bridge the gap between the disordered kinesthetic model and the correct one while using the auditory feedback loop. Voice improvement is best secured by listening in real time on amplification equipment that ensures a speech–voice range focus. Numerous smartphone apps and devices are available for these purposes.

Some patients with movement disorders might profit from the use of an auditory metronome that can pace either an increased or decreased rate of speaking for the patient. For example, a metronome set at about 60 words per minute can result in a marked slowing down of the Parkinson's patient's speech rate, which may improve voice quality, loudness and speech intelligibility. Others have been reported to benefit from delayed or frequency altered feedback, which serves to feed the voice back into the auditory system (McNeil, 2009; Yorkston, 2004). Some of those devices are manufactured by KayPENTAX Corp. (Montvale, New Jersey), Casa Futura Technologies (Boulder, Colorado), and Griffin Laboratories (Temecula, California).

Most voice patients profit from auditory modeling: hearing either his or her own voice on auditory playback or an external model (perhaps a speaking pitch note or the clinician's voice). Auditory modeling, to be effective, must be immediate. The clinician must stop recording, and play back for the patient the recording of the model and the patient response. The auditory playback is easy to achieve on most digital recorders or smartphones. It is important that the recording device have at least two ports for a speaker, or headphones, so that the client and clinician can hear the production immediately after generating it.

Procedural Aspects of the Approach. Let us separate the application approaches for three forms of auditory feedback: real-time amplification, metronome pacing, and loop playback.

1. Real-time amplification of speech and voice enables one to hear oneself more clearly than would be possible without such self-amplification and auditory focus.

Real-time amplification requires the clinician to use a device that features good quality amplification and playback.

a. The patient listens closely on the headphones to what he or she will be saying. Usually another voice is used, such as chanting or focus, which the patient will use while speaking. The patient then listens closely to the sound of the voice or speech while he or she is using the approach.

b. The patient evaluates the appropriateness of his or her response. If adjustments are needed, the patient listens with real-time amplification again.

2. The clicks or beats of a metronome may provide good auditory pacing for patients who need to decrease or increase their rate of speech.

a. The rate of clicks per minute is set on the instrument. All windup or electronic metronomes have a setting switch. The Auditory Feedback module by KayPENTAX Corp. (Montvale, New Jersey) offers variable rates, as do many smartphone apps.

b. The best pacing practice is achieved by the patient matching the clicks by shortening or prolonging the vowel duration of the practice material. Changing vowel duration is a preferred way to change rate rather than altering pause duration between words or phrases. Reducing the temporal length of the vowel is often suggested for individuals presenting with spastic or ataxic dysarthia (see Chapter 5).

3. Loop playback allows the patient to hear immediately what was just said. Early-generation instruments include the Phonic Mirror, the Language Master, and the Facilitator (1998). More current technology features digitized recorders that are stand-alone or embedded in smartphones as applications.

Typical Case History Showing Utilization of the Approach. Josie, a 49-year-old social worker, had a two-year history of functional dysphonia. At the time of the initial interview, it was found that elevating her pitch slightly at the end of a phrase or sentence seemed to eliminate all hoarseness. Immediate digitized auditory playback was very effective in helping her realize that raising pitch slightly in an upward inflection cleared the hoarseness from her voice. Working with her SLP using auditory playback, she practiced repeating sentences in two different ways: one, with the usual downward inflection (which caused hoarseness), and two, with an upward inflection. Using immediate auditory feedback in a few practice sessions appeared to be a primary approach in developing better functional voice outside the clinic, especially in her work as a social worker.

Evaluation of the Approach. Voice improvement is often enhanced by listening closely to one's voice. The use of auditory feedback is often an important step in therapy for articulation, language, fluency, and voice disorders. Real-time amplification, loop playback, and external metronomic pacing can be effective auditory aids in voice therapy. A holistic approach to correcting a voice disorder, such as listening to one's voice, is often preferred over fractionating various voice components (breathing, pitch, loudness, etc.) with separate practice for each component.

2. Change of Loudness

Kinds of Problems for Which the Approach Is Useful. Some patients have voices that have inappropriate loudness: a voice that is too loud or too soft. Many of the vocal pathologies experienced by children are related to excesses of loudness such as screaming and yelling.

Weak, soft voices may develop as a consequence of the prolonged hyperfunctional use of the vocal mechanism that results in the eventual breakdown of glottal approximation surfaces, for example, a patient with vocal nodules who loses much airflow around the nodules and is unable to produce an intense enough vocal fold vibration to achieve a sufficiently loud voice. Some speaking environments require a loud voice, and untrained speakers or singers may push for loudness at the level of the larynx rather than adjust their respiration. Inappropriate loudness of voice is most often not the primary causative factor of a voice problem, but rather a secondary, if annoying, symptom. Less common etiologies include motor speech disorders, including spastic and ataxic dysarthria (see Chapter 5). Reducing or increasing the loudness of the voice lends itself well to direct symptom modification through exercise and practice and, if other VFAs are being used, often does not even require the use of loudness techniques.

Procedural Aspects of the Approach

1. For a decrease in loudness:

   a. See that the patient has a thorough audiometric examination to determine adequacy of hearing before any attempt is made to reduce voice loudness. Once it has been established that the patient has normal hearing, the following steps may be taken.

   b. For young children, age three through 10, the change of loudness steps in *The Boone Voice Program for Children* (Boone, 1993) is useful. Ask the child to develop awareness of five different voices:
      • Voice 1 is presented as a whisper.
      • Voice 2 is presented as the voice to use when not wanting to awaken a sleeping person, a quiet voice.
      • Voice 3 is the normal voice to use to talk to family and friends.
      • Voice 4 is the voice to use to talk to someone across the room.
      • Voice 5 is the yelling voice to call someone outside.

   c. With patients over 10 years old, discuss with the patient the observation that he or she has an inappropriately loud voice. The patient may be unaware of the loud voice and should listen to digitized samples of his or her speech. The best demonstration for loudness variations include both the patient's voice and the clinician's, to provide contrasting levels of loudness. Then ask the patient, "Do you think your voice is louder than mine?"

   d. Focus on making the patient aware of the problem. Once the patient becomes aware that his or her voice is too loud, ask, "What does a loud voice in another person tell you about that person?" Loud voices are typically interpreted to mean that the speaker feels "overly confident" or "sure of himself"; or that the speaker is putting on a confident front when he or she is really scared; or that he or she is mad at the world, impressed with his or her own voice, trying to intimidate listeners, and so on. Some discussion of these negative interpretations is usually sufficient to motivate the average patient to learn to speak at normal loudness levels.

   e. Practice using a quiet voice (voice 2 in section b). The practice for the quiet voice can be facilitated by using digital recorders or other instruments that provide biofeedback for amplitude. Keeping the sound-level meter at a fixed distance, the patient can quickly learn to keep his or her voice at a lower intensity level to prevent the light (all or a few) from coming on.

2. For an increase in loudness:

   a. Determine first that the inappropriate softness of the voice is not related to hearing loss, general physical weakness (deconditioning), or a personality problem; for these cases, a symptomatic approach is not indicated. The steps that follow are for voice patients who are physically and emotionally capable of speaking in a louder voice.

   b. Discuss the soft voice with the patient. A digitized recording playback of the patient's and clinician's voices in conversation usually illustrates for the patient the inadequacy of the loudness. After the patient indicates some awareness of his or her soft voice, ask, "What does a soft, weak voice tell us about a person?" Inadequately loud voices are typically interpreted to mean that the speaker is afraid to speak louder, is timid and shy, is unduly considerate of others, is scared of people, has no self-confidence, and so on. Some discussion of these negative interpretations is usually helpful.

   c. By exploring pitch level and fundamental frequency, try to achieve a pitch level at which the patient can, with some ease, produce a louder voice. If the patient habitually speaks near the bottom of his or her pitch range, a slight elevation of pitch level will usually be accompanied by a slight increase in loudness. The Visi-Pitch IV, Sona-Speech, and even a musical keyboard or pitch-matching app have been useful in helping patients associate changes in pitch with relative changes in intensity. Certain frequencies produce greater intensities. When the patient finds the "best" pitch level, he or she should practice sustaining an /a/ at that level for five seconds, concentrating on good voice quality. He or she should then take a deep breath and repeat the same pitch at a maximum loudness level. After some practice at this "home base" pitch level, ask the patient to sing /a/, up the scale for one octave, at one vocal production per breath; then have him or her go back down the scale, one note per breath, until he or she reaches the starting pitch.

   d. Explore with the patient his or her best pitch, that is, the one that produces the best loudness and quality. Auditory feedback devices should be employed so that the patient can hear what he or she is doing. Some counseling may be needed about the practice pitch used because the patient may resist using a new voice amplitude and pitch level. Note that the practice amplitude level may well be only a temporary one and not necessarily the amplitude level the patient will use permanently. It is important that the work be pursued both in and outside therapy. A change in loudness cannot be achieved simply by talking about it. It requires practice.

   e. Sometimes respiration training (which we discuss later in the chapter) is necessary for a patient with a loudness problem. Remember, however, that even though loudness is directly related to the rate of airflow through the approximated vocal folds, little evidence indicates that any particular way of breathing is the best for optimum phonation. Any respiration exercise that produces increased subglottal air pressure may be helpful in increasing voice loudness.

   f. For patients who seem unable to increase voice loudness, we might employ the Lombard effect (Lau, 2008). The Lombard effect is observed when patients reflexively voice at louder levels when reading or speaking against increasing competing noise. For example, as the patient reads aloud, the clinician introduces about 75 dB of speech-range masking (see voice FA called Masking for application procedures).

3. Patients or people wanting to improve their voices sometimes demonstrate little or no loudness variation. Fluctuation in loudness can be helped by:

a. Make a digitized recording of the patient's voice. Ask the patient how he or she likes the voice on playback. People who become aware of the monotony of their voices and who are concerned about it can usually develop loudness variation (and pitch inflection) with practice.

b. Use an auditory playback system. Record speech or oral reading and then listen back immediately. Ask the patient about the relative appropriateness of loudness or loudness variation.

c. Most voice and diction books include practice materials for developing loudness variation in the voice.

Typical Case History Showing Utilization of the Approach. Curtis, a 31-year-old teacher, complained for more than a year of symptoms of vocal fatigue, that is, pain in the throat, loss of voice after teaching, and so on. Laryngoscopy revealed a normal larynx, and the voice evaluation found that the man spoke at "a monotonous pitch and low loudness level, with pronounced mandibular restriction, at times barely opening his mouth." Early efforts at therapy included the chewing approach, with special emphasis given to varying pitch level and increasing voice loudness using a sound-level meter. The patient was highly motivated to improve the efficiency of his phonation; he requested voice therapy three times a week and supplemented the therapy with long practice periods at home. After nine weeks of therapy, pre-therapy and post-therapy digitized recordings were compared, and the patient agreed with the clinician that he sounded "like a new man." Speaking in a louder voice for this patient seemed to have an immediate effect on his overall self-image, resulting in an almost immediate increase in his total communicative effectiveness. Not only did the patient achieve a better-sounding speaking voice, but he reported no further symptoms of vocal fatigue.

Evaluation of the Approach. Inappropriate loudness of voice penalizes the patient. Many of the VFAs described in this chapter have an effect on voice loudness, and inadequate loudness is also highly modifiable. This was demonstrated in a study by Schneider-Stickler and colleagues (2012). These researchers found that voice pitch ranges and amplitudes of call center agents were easily modified using biofeedback software. Results suggest that controlling amplitude can result in the treatment and prevention of abused and misused voices. Having immediate access to biofeedback allowed subjects to adjust for voicing made with appropriate amplitude, as well as pitch and speaking rate. The authors concluded that the use of a comfortable speaking voice, notably with respect to amplitude, is one of the most important factors in preventing vocal disorders.

3. Chant-Talk

Kinds of Problems for Which the Approach Is Useful. Voice problems related to hyperfunction are often helped by the chant approach. The chant in music is characterized by reciting many syllables on one continuous tone, creating, in effect, a singing monotone. We hear chanting in some churches and synagogues, performed by clergy and select groups. The words run continuously together without stress or a change in prosody for the individual word segments. In singing, the legato is very similar to the chant we use in voice therapy. A common dictionary definition of *legato* is "smooth and connected with no break between tones." The chant in therapy is characterized by an elevation of pitch, prolongation of vowels, lack of syllable stress, and an obvious softening of glottal attack. Once a patient can produce the chant in its extreme form (such as in a Gregorian chant), it can usually be modified to resemble conversational phonation. We have used chanting with other VFAs, such as chewing, open-mouth, and yawn-sigh.

Procedural Aspects of the Approach

1. The chant-talk approach is explained to the patient as a method that reduces the effort in talking. It is important to point out to the patient that the method will be used temporarily only, as practice, and will not become a permanent and different way of talking. Demonstrate chant-talk by playing a recording of a religious chant. Then imitate the recording by producing the same voicing style while reading any material aloud.

2. Urge the patient to imitate the same chant voicing pattern. Most patients are able to do this with some degree of initial success. For those who cannot chant in initial trials, present a chant recording again and then follow it with the patient's own chant production. Some lighthearted kidding is useful to tell the patient that the chant is a different way of talking and will be used only briefly as a voice training device. If the patient cannot chant after several attempts, use another VFA. For those patients who can chant, go on to step 3.

3. The patient should now read aloud, alternating the regular voice and the chant voice. Twenty seconds has been found to be a good time for each reading condition. Ask the patient to read aloud first in the normal voice, then in a chant, then back to normal voice, then in a chant, and so on.

4. Record the patient's oral reading. On playback, contrast the different sound of the normal voice with the chanted voice. Discuss the pitch differences, the phonatory prolongations, and the soft glottal onset.

5. Once patients are able to produce chant-talk with relative ease, they should try to reduce the chant quality, approximating normal voice production. Slight prolongation and soft glottal onset should be retained as the patient reads aloud in a voice with only slight chant quality remaining.

Typical Case History Showing Utilization of the Approach. Clara was a 28-year-old woman who worked at a call center selling telephone directory advertising. She began to experience increased dysphonia and "dryness of throat," particularly toward the end of a busy day of calling on customers. On endoscopic examination, she was found to have bilateral vocal nodules with unnecessary supraglottal participation during phonation. She spoke at an inappropriately low pitch, with mandibular restriction and noticeable hard glottal attack. Twice a week she received voice therapy designed to "take the work out of phonation." The chewing approach, coupled with the chant-talk approach, dramatically changed her overall voicing style. She was able early in therapy to incorporate the soft glottal attack of the chant into her everyday speaking voice. Other approaches, such as open mouth and yawn-sigh, were added with various self-practice materials she could use. The patient reported that she practiced throughout the day in her car, driving between appointments. In about twelve weeks, videoendoscopy revealed that the nodules had disappeared and that her supraglottal larynx stayed open during normal voicing. There was no evidence of hard glottal attack at the time of her clinic discharge.

Evaluation of the Approach. The chant-talk approach is easy for most patients to use. In addition to our experiences, McCabe and Titze (2002) also recommend the approach. These researchers introduced chant therapy and a placebo to public high school teachers who complained of vocal fatigue. Based on the changes of the subjects' responses to a fatigue task after the delivery of chant therapy, the researchers concluded that the principles learned by the subjects using chant-talk helped to reduce vocal fatigue. It is important to let the patient know that chanting is only a temporary behavior, designed to take the work out of phonation. We have found that the method works well with children, who seem to enjoy the "different" way of talking. For those patients who need to reduce hard glottal attack, the chanting approach seems to produce dramatic results for softening voicing onsets.

4. Chewing

Kinds of Problems for Which the Approach Is Useful. We see many people with vocal hyperfunction who appear to speak through clenched teeth with very little mandibular or labial movement. Such patients profit from using the chewing approach. We often kiddingly ask such patients, "Have you ever been a ventriloquist?" We then reply to their usual answer in the negative with "You certainly could be because you barely move your mouth when you speak." Many hyperfunctional voice patients, after being asked the ventriloquist question, develop immediate insight into their relative lack of mouth opening. Chewing is helpful for the patient who speaks with great tension and hard glottal attack. During simultaneous voicing and chewing, we often hear less strain in the voice, easier glottal attack, and an improvement in voice quality.

Procedural Aspects of the Approach

1. We first do what is necessary to help the patient become aware of the need for greater mouth opening while speaking. Following the ventriloquist question, we may ask the client to speak while in front of a mirror. Mirror intervention is a good method for instructing the patient specific to the relative amount of mouth opening he or she is using.

2. The clinician and patient look in a mirror as the clinician demonstrates exaggerated chewing. Care is given to have both good vertical and horizontal movements of the mouth. We pretend that we are chewing a stack of three crackers or a wad of French bread at one time with an open mouth. Ask the patient to imitate exaggerated chewing as has been demonstrated. Point out to the patient the amount of mouth opening by saying something like, "You see that we let our jaw drop down with our lips open wide. If we were actually chewing crackers, the crumbs would all drop out of our open mouth." Spend as much time as needed to develop good open-mouth chewing.

3. We now add light voice to the chewing. Here we have to be careful to avoid the same kind of monotonous sound, like "yam-yam-yam," that can come from chewing in the same pattern while voicing. To mix the sounds (and the mouth movements) a bit, we may have the patient say in a chantlike way nonsense words such as "ah-la-met-erah" or "wan-da-pan-da." Stay with such nonsense words until the patient masters the simultaneous chewing and speaking. It should be noted here that most children like to do chewing and take easily to the approach. Some adults may resist doing it or be unable to do it; if so, the approach should be abandoned and other approaches used, such as the open-mouth approach.

4. Once simultaneous chewing and speaking is established, ask the patient to count and chew. It will take several practice attempts before the patient can do it. Listen and watch the first attempts on video playback. Tell the patient at this point that the chewing is "a means to the end of producing a more relaxed voice." The patient should be counseled that the exaggerated chewing is used only temporarily and that we will soon cut down the movements to resemble more "the mouth movements of normal speakers."

5. Now use words and phrases for practice chewing. When the patient can do this, we then practice sentences. Avoid going too fast. Go back to earlier levels if the amount of chewing seems to be fading.

6. After the patient has mastered step 5, she or he should be taught how to diminish the exaggerated chewing to resemble more normal mouth movements. Practicing oral reading with chewing is a good final step. Video-recording the practice session allows the patient to study his or her success on video playback.

7. Ultimately, the patient just "thinks" the chewing method. By this time, the patient has developed an awareness of what oral openness and jaw movement feel like and has experienced the vocal relaxation that accompanies the feeling.

Typical Case History Showing Utilization of the Approach. Sara, a 44-year-old realtor, began to experience extreme vocal fatigue toward the end of her working day. At the voice evaluation, she reported, "Sometimes I lose my voice altogether at the end of the day, or after I talk a lot, it hurts right here" (she pointed to the general hyoid area). As she volunteered her history, little mouth opening was observed with her voice sounding at an inappropriate high pitch and the ends of sentences characterized by "squeezed phonation." On endoscopy, her vocal folds showed "posterior redness, suggestive of reflux with no middle or anterior pathology noted." A diagnosis of muscular tension dysphonia was made with a special notation made relative to speaking through clenched teeth. Early in voice therapy, the patient worked on developing better respiration skills for voicing and developing more natural oral movements (less mandibular restriction). There was some initial resistance by the patient to using the chewing approach, but after she began to experience increased oral relaxation as she practiced the chewing, she incorporated greater oral movements into her everyday speaking pattern. The patient experienced a very good voice result from both reduction of her reflux by a medical regimen and eliminating her dysphonia and vocal fatigue from voice therapy (with early emphasis given to using the chewing approach).

Evaluation of the Approach. The chewing approach is not a panacea for all voice problems, but its positive effectiveness in reducing muscular tension dysphonia or vocal hyperfunction is observed soon after it is applied. It appears that when oral structures are involved in the automatic function of chewing, according to Brodnitz and Froeschels (1954) who first introduced the technique, these oral structures (facial muscles, mandible, tongue) appear capable of "more synergic, relaxed movement."

It appears that relaxing the overall vocal tract while chewing also relaxes the phonatory function of the larynx and pharynx. By employing a commonly used action, such as chewing, the patient is able to achieve relaxation of the vocal tract from a holistic or gestalt point of view, without attempting to relax particular muscles. For the voice patient who appears to be talking between clenched teeth, the chewing approach is a good way to develop more open, natural oral movements. This approach may be contraindicated for the patient with temporomandibular joint (TMJ) syndrome. Chewing was listed as one of the VFAs studied by McCory (2001) in a retrospective audit of voice therapy outcomes in vocal nodules. Results revealed that this approach was consistent with best practice and that voice therapy is effective in the reduction, and in some cases elimination, of vocal nodules.

5. Confidential Voice

Kinds of Problems for Which the Approach Is Useful. Using a soft, confidential voice as an alternative to using a voice produced by much effort and hyperfunction was first described as the confidential voice by Colton and Casper (1996). Confidential voice has subsequently been studied by a number of researchers, who report that the approach is effective in reducing loudness, excessive vocal use, and abusive vocal patterns (Berhrman and colleagues, 2008). Confidential voice is similar to the soft voice recommended for children to use as the quiet voice, the second voice level of loudness that allows voicing at a quiet level "not loud enough to awaken someone sleeping nearby" (Boone, 1983). Both children and adults seem to be able to speak in the easy, confidential voice, which makes the approach useful in reducing overall vocal hyperfunction. The confidential voice, with its increased breathiness, not only reduces voice loudness, but also affects breath control; slows down speaking rate; and seems to create a more open, relaxed airway. The technique employs light voice (not whispering) and is used in a prescribed time period for reducing hyperfunction in functional dysphonia and in vocal hyperfunction resulting in vocal fold thickening and vocal nodules. The confidential voice is explained to both children and adults as a temporary way of talking, a means to an end for developing a better voice. In some populations, though, it is suggested as a long-term approach to be used with other technologies, such as portable amplification devices. Roy and colleagues (2002) found that teachers who employed portable amplification devices reported more clarity in their speaking and singing voice, greater ease of voice production, and greater compliance with the treatment program.

Procedural Aspects of the Approach. Much time can be saved in voice therapy by first seeing if the child or adult can imitate the SLP in producing the breathy, confidential voice. If this easy voice can be produced, the clinician explains how it will be used, as follows:

1. Repeat the confidential voice model and be sure the client understands how to produce it, a breathy voice with less loudness, as if one doesn't want to awaken a person sleeping nearby. We do not want a whisper, but a breathy, light voicing.

2. The breathy, light voice uses up more air. The slightly parted vocal folds and the open airway allow a greater volume of air to pass through than is normally experienced. Therefore, we explain that fewer words are said on one expiration when using the easy voice.

Clients with vocal hyperfunction may demonstrate a voice that is too loud. The prolonged use of inappropriate loudness levels may result in pathologies of the vocal folds, such as nodules or polyps. As explained by the clinician on the **video**, confidential voice is not a whisper; it is not elevating or lowering the pitch. It is simply a reduction of loudness in the voice. Grand Rounds: Describe how confidential voice might change the open-closed phases of vocal fold vibration.

3. Its temporary use is then explained. As often as one can find settings to use the breathy, confidential voice, the client should be encouraged to use it. There will be situations where such a light voice cannot be used, such as with a salesperson explaining a product to a customer. As soon as possible, however, the client should revert back to using the easy voice. It is important to let the client know about the temporary use of the confidential voice, perhaps by saying, "We will use this confidential voice only for a few weeks, or for as long as it seems to take to break up the effortful, hyperfunctional voice you have been using."

4. Specific instruction should be given for set time periods when the client does oral reading in the confidential voice.

It has been the authors' experience that both children and adults are able to produce the confidential voice with relative ease and soon enjoy voicing without all the work they previously used in voice production. For children and adults who cannot imitate the clinician easily in producing the confidential voice, we use the steps, listed here, for developing a soft voice from *The Boone Voice Program for Children* (Boone, 1993) or *The Boone Voice Program for Adults* (Boone and Wiley, 2000).

1. The patient is taught to be aware that voice loudness is divided into five levels: (1) whisper; (2) soft voice; (3) normal conversational voice; (4) louder, projected voice, and (5) yelling. Using the voice examples and cartoons from either the child- or adult-level programs, we select the second level, soft voice, as our target voice.

2. The clinician then reads aloud the voice examples at the second level of loudness, producing in effect the confidential voice. The client imitates the clinician, which may require some individualized coaching. Phrases and sentences are then practiced aloud at the soft voice level.

3. Once the client can produce the breathy, light voice with consistency, we follow the four steps described above in therapy.

Typical Case History Showing Utilization of the Approach. Dora was a 40-year-old teacher who taught computer science and computer applications. She experienced an increasing hoarseness that began to interfere with her teaching effectiveness. On endoscopy, she was found to have small bilateral vocal nodules. Following a 14-day period of voice rest, enforced by her laryngologist, she began voice therapy. The confidential voice was one of the first voice therapy techniques introduced, with which she had initial success. She found that she could use the easy, breathy voice in all situations, including in her computer classes when using a portable voice amplifier. Other voice therapy approaches were combined with confidential voice, including work on improving respiration, improving her head–neck posture, increasing greater mouth opening, increased hydration, and elimination of her tendency to clear her throat. After seven weeks, her voice therapy regimen (including the use of the confidential voice) was terminated, with her vocal nodules remarkably reduced and with the patient experiencing a normal voice in and outside the classroom.

Evaluation of the Approach. The use of the confidential voice replaces the hyperfunctional behaviors that the patient has been using in most voicing attempts. While using the confidential voice, nasoendoscopic viewing confirms that the vocal folds are slightly apart yet relaxed in their total anterior–posterior length, the laryngeal body remains lower, and the supralaryngeal mechanisms are relaxed and open.

The voice sounds free of squeezing or tightness. The easy, breathy voice was one of several techniques used to reduce vocal hyperfunction in 39 adults with functional dysphonia; 23 subjects (59%) experienced voice improvement (Boone, 1974). The results of using the confidential voice by five patients with vocal nodules was compared with five nodule patients in a control group not using confidential voice (Verdolini-Marston and colleagues, 1995). The confidential voice group improved in both voice quality and in reduction of the vocal nodules. Behrman and colleagues (2008) found that confidential voice is effective in reducing loudness, excessive vocal use, and abusive vocal patterns. Our clinical experience has found that the use of the confidential voice breaks up the hyperfunctional set the patient has been using for voicing, giving time for the elimination of undesirable vocal events and replacing them with more optimal vocal behaviors.

6. Counseling (Explanation of Problem)

Kinds of Problems for Which the Approach Is Useful. One cannot easily separate the person from his or her voice. Some voice problems may be among the visible symptoms of someone with serious personality problems, or sometimes the voice problem may be the cause of psychological maladaptive reactions. Counseling the voice patient, including direct explanations of the voice problem, may be more effective with the patient than applying various symptomatic voice therapy techniques. It is also important to be familiar with variables that may be more conducive to successful therapy.

Putting the voice problem in its proper perspective can often free the patient from overwhelming concern. Patients with hyperfunctional voice disorders, in particular, profit from hearing the clinician describe the voice problem in words they can understand. Clinical experience has taught us that if counseling can help individuals know why they have the voice problem, sometimes nothing more is needed to change a phonation style or to curb vocal abuse–misuse (Zraick, 2009). In the case of those dysphonias that are wholly related to functional causes (such as hyperfunction), it is important that clinicians not confront patients with the implication that they "could talk all right if they wanted to." Instead of saying, "You are not using your voice as well as you could," a clinician might say, "Your vocal folds are coming together too tightly." The latter statement absolves the patient of the guilt he or she might experience if the clinician indicated that the patient was doing things "wrong." Patients are more likely to be more receptive to a statement that puts the blame on the vocal folds. For patients with structural changes of the vocal folds, such as nodules or polyps, it may be necessary to explain that the organic pathology may well be the result of prolonged misuse, and that by eliminating the misuse, the patient will eventually experience a reduction of vocal fold pathology.

Procedural Aspects of the Approach. Counseling the patient is highly individualized. One of the most common counseling approaches in voice therapy is helping the patient to put his or her voice problem in its proper perspective. For some patients, the voice problem is the cause of all of their ills, such as poor job performance, social inadequacy, or general unhappiness. The clinician must have some sensitivity to the depth of the patient's overall attitude and self-image. We find that the Voice Handicap Index (Jacobson and colleagues, 1997) and the Voice Handicap Index–Partner (Zraick and colleagues, 2006) (see Chapter 6) are effective scales to begin to define and quantify patients' and family members' feelings about the dysphonia.

If the clinician senses psychological or social problems well beyond his or her counseling-psychological training to deal with such problems, referral should be made to professional counselors, psychologists, or psychiatrists. More often than not in voice therapy, a direct explanation of the patient's problem proves to be most effective.

In voice problems related to vocal hyperfunction, it is important to identify for the patient those behaviors that maintain the dysphonia. No exact procedure can be laid down, however; each case has its own rules. For problems related to abuse and misuse of the voice, identify the inappropriate behavior and demonstrate to the patient some ways in which it can be eliminated. In the vocal abuse reduction section of our voice program for children (Boone, 1993), we put much focus on having the child cognitively approach the problem of vocal abuse. By using comic pictures with an accompanying story text, we help the child understand the consequences of continued abuse and emphasize what can be expected (a better voice) if he or she reduces or eliminates such abuses. A voice program for adults (Boone and Wiley, 2000) provides descriptions of vocal hyperfunction and resulting voice problems of functional dysphonia and dysphonia related to vocal nodules or vocal polyps. Excellent animations of normal voice and maladaptive behaviors can be found at Blue Tree Publishing, either in educational modules or through software apps.

For truly organic problems, such as unilateral adductor paralysis, the same explanations must be made, but in terms of inadequate and adequate glottal closure. Most voice patients want to understand what their problems are and what they can do about them. Make use of medical and diagnostic information, but explain in language the patient can understand. Such imagery as "your vocal cords are coming together too tightly" or "you seem to place your voice back too far in your throat" may lack scientific validity but may help the patient understand the problem. Make explanations brief and to the point, but take care not to put the patient psychologically on the defensive during the first visit. If, after the evaluation, it appears that some psychological or psychiatric consultation is necessary, further diagnostic–therapy sessions may have to be held before the patient can agree to find out more about his or her feelings.

Typical Case History Showing Utilization of the Approach. Cora, a 62-year-old widow, came to the clinic with a voice problem that first resembled spasmodic dysphonia. As she volunteered her history, her voice sounded tight, strangled; it sounded as if she were crying. She differed from the typical patient with spasmodic dysphonia in the diagnostic session and early therapy periods by demonstrating normal voice repetition skills, and she could count or read aloud with normal phonation. Spontaneous narratives, however, about her former work as a department store buyer or details about her personal life were portrayed vocally with great struggle, sometimes accompanied by actual weeping. Early in voice therapy, her SLP was sensitive to the continuous observation that her voice symptoms were part of an overall picture of loneliness and general unhappiness about life. The woman was referred to a counseling psychologist, who, together with the SLP, has helped the patient make a happier life adjustment and consequently experience a better-sounding voice for most situations.

Evaluation of the Approach. With a little guidance by the clinician in helping the patient understand his or her voice problem, what causes it, and what can be done about it, the typical voice patient can often make progress in overcoming the voice problem. Both children and adults profit from an explanation of their voice problem and from understanding how particular behaviors, like yelling or clearing one's throat excessively, keep their voices in trouble. Sometimes an explanation of the problem is the primary treatment, with no other VFAs required. For patients who need much practice with various approaches, they seem to make better progress when they understand the rationale behind what they are practicing. Voice clinicians must remain sensitive to the psychological needs of voice patients and recognize that some of their patients have personal needs greater than improving their voices per se. Such patients should be referred appropriately to other counseling or psychological professionals.

7. Digital Manipulation

Kinds of Problems for Which the Approach Is Useful. Finger pressure on the thyroid cartilage can be applied by the clinician in different ways for different problems. For males who, for functional reasons, are using higher F_0 values than they should, light pressure anteriorly on the thyroid cartilage appears to nudge the thyroid cartilage back slightly, shortening the overall length of the vocal folds. This shortening thickens the folds, resulting in a lower F_0. This anterior pressure approach is particularly effective for postadolescent males whose pitch levels seem to remain at prepubescent levels (see Chapter 8).

Another form of digital manipulation is placing the fingers lightly on the thyroid cartilage to assess the vertical positioning of the larynx. During the swallow, in a fear–tension state, or when singing notes toward the upper end of one's singing range, the larynx appears to rise. Lowell and colleagues (2012) reported that radiographic findings revealed that the hyoid and laryngeal positions during phonation were more elevated in patients with primary muscle tension dysphonia than in those with no voice disorders.

Lowering of the larynx is achieved during the yawn-sigh (Boone and McFarlane, 1993) or singing at the lower end of one's range or during a very relaxed state. The digital monitoring of laryngeal height is a good technique for anyone who appears to have excessive laryngeal vertical movement or who is concerned about laryngeal posturing at high or low levels. Analysis of voice therapy effectiveness for patients with unilateral vocal fold paralysis (McFarlane and colleagues, 1991, 1998) is another form of digital manipulation found to be effective. McFarlane and colleagues found that finger pressure on the lateral thyroid cartilage wall can often produce better vocal fold approximation, resulting in stronger phonation.

Procedural Aspects of the Approach. The three digital procedures used in voice therapy are quite distinct from one another, both in the procedural steps used and the kind of voice problems for which they are helpful. We list the steps separately for each of the three procedures.

Digital Pressure for Lowering Pitch

1. With the exception of some men with falsetto voices, patients respond to digital pressure by producing a lower voice pitch. Ask the patient to prolong a vowel (/a/ or /i/). As the vowel is prolonged, apply slight finger pressure on the thyroid cartilage. The pitch level will drop immediately.

2. Ask the patient to maintain the lower pitch after the fingers are removed. If the patient can do this, he or she should continue practicing the lower pitch. If the high pitch quickly reverts back, repeat the digital pressure.

3. If the method is used to let the patient hear and feel a lower pitch, the patient should practice producing the lower pitch with and without digital pressure on the thyroid cartilage.

Monitoring the Vertical Movements of the Larynx

1. For a patient with excessive pitch variability and tension related to much vertical movement of the larynx, demonstrate how to place the fingers on the thyroid cartilage and monitor laryngeal vertical movement while phonating.

2. Ask the patient to produce a pitch level several full musical notes off the bottom of his or her lowest note. Keeping the fingers on the thyroid cartilage, ask the patient to lower pitch one note at a time to the lowest note in his or her pitch range. Usually, the larynx will lower its position in the neck at the low end of the pitch range. Then ask the patient to sing one note at a time up to the top of the singing range, exclusive of falsetto. Toward the top of the scale, the patient should feel (through the fingertips) a slight elevation of the larynx. Review both the lowering and rising of the larynx at the extremes of the pitch range.

3. Once the patient has experienced vertical movement in the preceding steps, point out that, in production of a speaking voice that is relatively free of strain, no vertical movement of the larynx should be felt during digital monitoring. Oral reading and speaking should be developed with little or no vertical laryngeal movements. Practice in oral reading with encouraged pitch variability can then be monitored by slight digital pressure of the thyroid cartilage, with the patient confirming (hopefully) no vertical movement.

Unilateral Digital Pressure for Patients with Unilateral Vocal Fold Paralysis

1. There appears to be a slight phonation improvement by pressing on the thyroid lamina on the side of the paralysis, but this is not always found. We begin, however, by having the patient posture the head straight forward (looking slightly down rather than upward). The patient phonates and extends a vowel. While the patient phonates, the clinician exerts medium finger pressure on the lateral thyroid wall on the side of the vocal fold paralysis. If a louder, firmer voice is produced with this pressure, continue various phonation tasks, coupled with finger pressure on the thyroid cartilage on the side of the involvement.

2. If a louder voice was not achieved in step 1, the patient continues to look forward while the clinician applies pressure to the opposite side of the thyroid cartilage (pressing the side opposite the vocal fold paralysis). Attempt various phonation tasks while exerting this lateral finger pressure.

3. If lateral pressure to either thyroid lamina while the patient looks ahead has not produced an improvement in voice, provide lamina pressure with the head turned to one side. If the head is turned to the left, first apply pressure to the left lamina; if unsuccessful, keep the head turned left with pressure then given to the right lamina. If this produces better voice, continue phonation tasks with the head turned to the left and finger pressure on the side that seems to produce the best voice.

4. The last posture is for the head turned to the right with each side pressed in an attempt to find the better, more functional voice.

5. It has been our experience that one cannot predict which head posture (straight ahead or turned laterally) and/or which side receiving finger pressure produces a better-sounding voice, whether or not the left or right vocal fold is paralyzed. More often than not, however, digital manipulation, following steps 1 to 4, often provides for the patient a better, more functional voice.

Typical Case History Showing Utilization of the Approach. Jeff was a 17-year-old male who had been raised exclusively by his mother until her sudden death about a year before. Since that time, he had lived with a maternal uncle who was concerned about the boy's effeminate mannerisms and high-pitched voice. Laryngeal examination revealed a normal adult male larynx. The boy was found to have a habitual pitch level of around 200 Hz, well within the adult female range, but below the level of falsetto. The most effective facilitating VFA for producing a normal voice pitch was to apply digital pressure on the external thyroid cartilage. The young man was able to prolong the lower pitch levels with good success, but any attempt at conversation would be characterized by an immediate return to the higher pitch. After three therapy sessions, he was able to read aloud using the lower pitch but was unable to use the lower voice in conversation except with his male clinician. Subsequent psychiatric evaluation and therapy were initiated for "identity confusion and schizoidal tendencies." Voice therapy was discontinued after two weeks, when it was clearly demonstrated that the patient could produce a good baritone voice (125 Hz) whenever he wanted. Unfortunately, follow-up telephone conversations several months after therapy revealed that he was using his high-pitched pretherapy voice exclusively.

Evaluation of the Approach. The effectiveness of any one of the three digital manipulation approaches can be determined immediately. Either the anterior digital pressure to the thyroid cartilage lowers voice pitch or it does not. If the speaking pitch is lowered with digital pressure, it affords an excellent "window" for the patient (such as a young man with puberphonia) to experience producing a lower-pitched voice. Tracking the vertical movements with light finger pressure can often help the patient appreciate the amount of unnecessary laryngeal movement he or she may be experiencing (Lowell and colleagues, 2012). In the search for a more functional voice after unilateral vocal fold paralysis, digital pressure on the thyroid lamina with or without head turning may uncover a functional voice. Developing such an uncovered voice in the patient with unilateral vocal fold paralysis may obviate the need for various surgical procedures in the quest for restoring a functional voice (McFarlane and colleagues, 1991, 1998).

8. Elimination of Abuses

Kinds of Problems for Which the Approach Is Useful. Many functional voice disorders are associated with behavior that can damage laryngeal structures and ultimately vocal performance. Learning to recognize and eliminate these behaviors helps maintain a functioning larynx and improve vocal performance (Stemple and Thomas, 2007). The voice can be abused or misused in many ways. Vocal abuse comprises various behaviors and events that have some kind of deleterious effect on the larynx and the voice, such as:

1. Yelling and screaming
2. Speaking against a background of loud noise
3. Coughing and excessive throat clearing

4. Smoking
5. Excessive talking or singing
6. Excessive talking or singing while having an allergy or upper respiratory infection
7. Excessive crying or laughing
8. Weight lifting with effortful grunts

Vocal misuse means improper use of voice, such as:

1. Speaking with hard glottal attack
2. Singing excessively at the lower or upper end of one's range
3. Increasing vocal loudness by squeezing out the voice at the larynx
4. Speaking at excessive intensity levels
5. Cheerleading (Case, 2002)
6. Speaking over time at an inappropriate pitch level
7. Speaking or singing (such as a prolonged show rehearsal) for excessively long periods of time

We could add other abuses and misuses to such lists. Identification and reduction of vocal abuse–misuse are primary goals in voice therapy for hyperfunctional disorders such as functional dysphonia with or without physical changes such as vocal nodules, polyps, or contact ulcers. Therapy cannot be successful until contributory vocal abuse–misuse can be drastically reduced. Figure 7.1 shows a vocal abuse graph that plots the number of abuses a young patient had recorded over a period of two weeks. Keeping such a chart may help the patient become more aware of his or her vocal behavior. Optimum usage of the voice, such as the vocal hygiene program outlined in Chapter 8, also requires identifying possible abusive voice situations and making deliberate efforts to minimize their occurrence.

FIGURE 7.1 A Vocal Abuse Graph

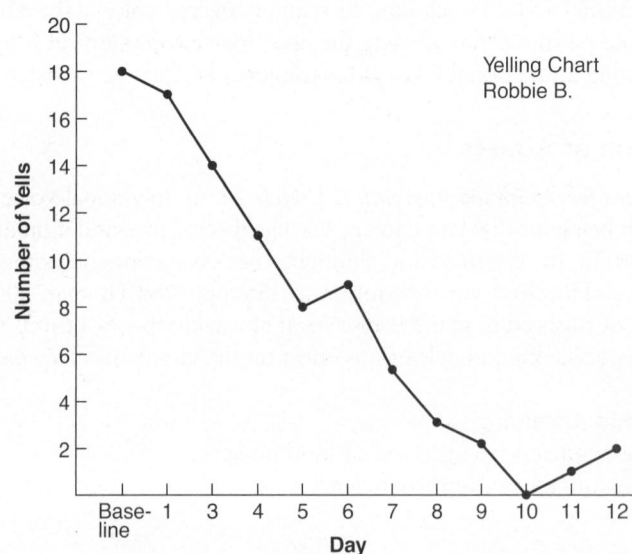

Procedural Aspects of the Approach

1. Time must be given early in voice therapy to identifying possible vocal abuse. Once a particular vocal abuse is identified, the patient and clinician should develop a baseline of occurrence. This will often require that the clinician hear and observe the patient in and outside the clinic environment, such as on the playground, at the pulpit, or in a nightclub. The number of times the particular event occurred must be tallied.

2. Children with vocal abuse must become aware of the impact of such abuses on their voices. With children, we use the "Vocal Abuse Reduction Program" (Boone, 1993), which recommends the following: an explanation of how additive lesions occur, using the story "A Voice Lost and Found"; a review of the child's abuses; and a systematic reduction of the child's abuses, using the voice tally card, the voice counting chart, and the hot-air balloon race (p. 7). The focus of the reducing abuse program is to make the child aware of the relationship of vocal abuse–misuse to increasing symptoms of voice. The story in the program is pictorially illustrated with various vocal behaviors related to changes of "the little bumps on the vocal cords."

3. Discuss identified vocal abuses with the patient, emphasizing the need to reduce her or his daily frequency. Assign to the patient the task of counting the number of times each day he or she engages in a particular abuse. Perhaps a peer or sibling could be brought in, told about the situation, and asked to join in on the daily count. Depending on the age of the patient, a parent, teacher, spouse, or business associate might be asked to keep track of the number of abuses that occur in his or her presence. At the end of the day, the abuses should be tallied for that day.

4. Ask the patient to plot his or her daily vocal abuses on a graph. Along the vertical axis, the ordinate, the patient should plot the number of times the particular abuse occurred; along the base of the graph, the abscissa, the individual days are plotted, beginning with the baseline count of the first day. Instruct the patient to bring these graphs to voice therapy sessions. Keeping a graph usually increases the patient's awareness of what he or she has been doing and results in a gradual decrease in the abusive behavior. The typical vocal abuse has a sloping decremental curve, indicating its gradual disappearance. Greet any decrease in the plots of the people observing the patient, but particularly in those compiled by the patient, with obvious approval.

Typical Case History Showing Utilization of the Approach. Joyce was a 27-year-old secretary who complained of a voice that was often hoarse and that tired easily every day. Subsequent indirect laryngoscopy confirmed a slight bilateral thickening at the anterior–middle third junction. A detailed history and observation of the patient found that she constantly cleared her throat. The throat clearing had become a habit. She rarely felt that she was able "to bring up any mucus" but just cleared her throat in an attempt to make her voice clearer. A high-speed motion picture depicting throat clearing was shown to the patient. She was counseled to try to reduce its occurrence. The patient subsequently began to tally her throat clearing and coughing as they occurred, plotting them on a graph at the end of the day. Within two weeks, she was able to change her throat-clearing habit. Her vocal quality improved immediately and she never needed formal, long-term voice therapy.

Evaluation of the Approach. Identifying vocal abuses and attempting to eliminate them by plotting their daily frequency on a graph are effective in helping young children with voice problems. Adolescents are equally guilty of vocal abuses and profit from keeping track of what they are doing. Typical adult abuses, such as throat clearing, are often eliminated after a week or two of graph plotting by motivated patients. The effectiveness of this approach, in fact, is highly related to the skill of the clinician in motivating the patient to eliminate the abusive behavior. The value of the plotting is more in developing awareness of the frequency of the problem than in the actual count per se. Reduction of vocal abuse has become a primary part of most voice therapy programs for children (Lee and Son, 2005; Andrews and Summers, 2000; Boone, 1993; Stemple and colleagues, 1994) and for adults (Boone and Wiley, 2000; Case, 2002; Stemple and Thomas, 2007).

9. Establishing a New Pitch

Kinds of Problems for Which the Approach Is Useful. Although it is well established that there is no absolute optimum pitch at which a particular person should speak, some people with voice problems may profit from speaking at a different pitch level. A change of pitch often has positive effects on voice, such as improving vocal quality and loudness. Speaking at the very bottom of one's pitch range requires too much force and effort. Similarly, speaking habitually toward the top of one's range can be vocally fatiguing. Because a number of instruments available today can portray fundamental frequency in real time (while one is phonating), awareness and feedback of one's ongoing pitch level play prominent roles in establishing new pitches through therapy (Watts and colleagues, 2003).

Procedural Aspects of the Approach

1. If pitch needs to be raised or lowered, describe where the patient is and where the target pitch is. The methods for determining habitual pitch and pitch range described in Chapter 6 can be applied here. Make a digital recording of the patient producing various pitches, including feedback about the old pitch and the projected target pitch. The playback should always be followed by some discussion comparing the sound and the feeling of the two pitches.

2. Most voice patients can imitate their own pitch models once they have been produced by the appropriate VFA. Occasionally patients cannot initiate a pitch to match a model, as Filter and Urioste (1981) found in testing college women with normal voices. A useful model can be produced by having the patient extend an /i/ at the target pitch level for about five seconds and recording the phonation. The patient will immediately hear the target production. The playback provides the patient with a continuous playback of his or her own voice model of the target pitch. Using the patients' own voices as their voice models has many advantages because they already have voicing experience producing the sounds they are now trying to match. Remain with the model /i/ for considerable practice before introducing a new stimulus.

3. Several excellent instruments available today can provide real-time display of fundamental frequency, both with a digital readout and on a monitor's display screen. Usually, these instruments permit the clinician to display patient voice values specific to frequency and intensity. The Visi-Pitch™ (KayPENTAX Corp., Montvale, New Jersey) offers split-screen capabilities, whereby a voice model can be put on an upper screen and the patient's production displayed on a lower screen, permitting comparisons between model and trial productions. Any instrument that can display fundamental frequency information can provide valuable feedback to a patient attempting to establish a new voice pitch.

4. Using any of the instruments described in step 3, the patient can receive exact feedback relative to the frequency he or she is using. Any deviation below or above the target F_0 can be given in immediate feedback. Of great benefit for the patient is developing the immediate awareness when he or she is producing the target F_0.

5. Establishing a new pitch is facilitated by working first on single words, preferably words that begin with vowels. Each word is repeated in a pitch monotone (using the target pitch). Occasionally a patient has more difficulty using the new pitch with certain words. Any such trouble words should be avoided as practice material because what is needed at this stage of therapy is practice in rapidly phonating a series of individual words at the new pitch level.

6. Once the patient does well at the single-word level, introduce phrases and short sentences. It is usually more productive at this stage to avoid practice in actual conversation because the patient is better able to use the new phonation in neutral situations such as reading single words, phrases, and sentences. When success is achieved at the sentence level, assign the patient reading passages from various voice and diction books. Success in using the new pitch level can be verified by using the instruments described earlier in step 3.

7. After reading well in a monotone, the patient may try using the new pitch in some real-life conversational situations. In the beginning, he or she may have more success talking to strangers, such as store clerks; patients often find it difficult to use the new pitch level with friends and family because their previous behavioral mindset may prevent them from utilizing their new vocal behavior. Whatever conversational situation works best for the individual should be the one used initially.

8. It is helpful in therapy to record the patient's voice as he or she searches to establish a new and different pitch level. When the patient is able to produce a good voice at the proper pitch level, his or her own "best" voice can then become the therapy model.

Typical Case History Showing Utilization of the Approach. John, a 10-year-old boy, was referred by his public school speech-language clinician for a laryngeal examination because of a six-month history of hoarseness. The findings included a normal larynx and a "low-pitched dysphonic voice." John could readily demonstrate a higher phonation, which was characterized by an immediate clearing of quality. In the discussion that followed the audio-recorded playback of his "good" and "bad" voice, John stated that he thought he had been trying to speak like his older brother. The clinician pointed out to him that his better voice was more like that of other boys his age, and that the low-pitched voice he had been using was difficult for others to listen to. In subsequent voice therapy with his school clinician, John focused on elevating his voice pitch to a more natural level. His success was rapid, and therapy was terminated after six weeks.

Evaluation of the Approach. The pitch of the voice changes constantly, according to the speaker's situation. In some patients, however, the pitch level appears to be too high or too low for the overall capability of the laryngeal mechanism. In other people, an aberrant pitch level is just one manifestation of the total personality. Patients with additive masses to the folds (nodules, papilloma, polyps, etc.) may have lower pitch levels than normal because the thicker vocal folds vibrate more slowly, emitting a lower fundamental frequency. As the lesion is reduced or eliminated, the frequency of the voice becomes higher, perhaps approaching normal limits. For patients with additive laryngeal lesions due to vocal hyperfunction, it is often best to work slowly toward increasing pitch level to approximate levels of the patient's age and sex peers. Some patients use aberrant pitch levels because of personality factors. Counseling such patients and helping them want to change pitch levels might well have to precede actual symptomatic therapy to alter pitch. Typically, however, voice patients who may need to change pitch levels can do so rather quickly, after experiencing marked improvement in overall voice quality because of pitch change (Schneider-Stickler and colleagues, 2012).

10. Focus

Kinds of Problems for Which the Approach Is Useful. Good focus of the voice is characterized by the voice coming "from the middle of the mouth, just above the surface of the tongue" (Boone, 1997, p. 71). Problems in "horizontal" voice focus occur when the tongue is too far forward or too far backward within the mouth. The "thin" or baby-sounding voice is produced by carrying the tongue high and forward. The back-focused voice is produced by carrying the tongue elevated in the back of the mouth.

The most common focus problem we see in patients with voice disorders is the voice sounding as if it were deep in the throat. Many patients focus on their throats as the anatomical site of their problem. Such patients profit from resonant therapy or the front-focus approach because it shifts their mental imagery from the throat to the upper vocal tract, that is, the face, cheeks, and the bridge of the nose (Boone, 1997; Verdolini, 2000).

Numerous intervention approaches employ focus or resonance as the primary or secondary treatment variable (Verdolini, 2000; Titze, 2006; Chen and colleagues, 2007). Common to them all is what Perkins (1983) wrote: a "voice that feels focused high in the head" is a more efficient voice, and it can survive extensive vocalization.

The clinician helps the patient focus on the area of his or her face under the cheeks and across the bridge of the nose. Most patients with chronic dysphonia experience both difficulty finding their voices and continued expectancy of vocal failure. They clear their throats continually, make phonation rehearsals, and worry about the poor vocal quality they are likely to have the next time they attempt to speak. For these patients, successful voice clinicians often employ two techniques—respiration training and placing the voice in the facial mask—for two reasons: (1) to improve respiratory control and resonance, and (2) to transfer the patient's mental focus away from the larynx and place it with the activator (respiration) and the resonator (supraglottal vocal tract).

Readers should note that focus is a successful approach for voice disorders beyond muscle tension dysphonia. Individuals with dyphonias secondary to unilateral vocal fold paralysis, or spastic dysarthria and ataxic dysarthria, have employed this approach successfully to balance oral–pharyngeal resonance for conversational speech (see Chapter 5).

Procedural Aspects of the Approach

1. An explanation of focus is facilitated by having the patient review Figure 7.2 with the clinician. Determination is first made about what kind of remedial focus is needed: Is the voice too far forward, too far back, or sounding deep in the throat? (Although mentioned in the line drawing in Figure 7.2, a nasal focus is not presented in this chapter as a focus problem.)

Patients with vocal hyperfunction tend to place undue attention on the larynx while attempting to produce voice. They mistakenly believe that if they push more forcefully at the vocal folds the voice will emerge stronger. The goal of Focus in the **video** is to transfer the patient's focus on the energy of the voice from the larynx to the nose, cheeks and lips. Nasal or facial focus eliminates overvalving at the glottis and supraglottis, thus opening the aditus for enhanced vocal resonance.

FIGURE 7.2 Voice Focus Sites

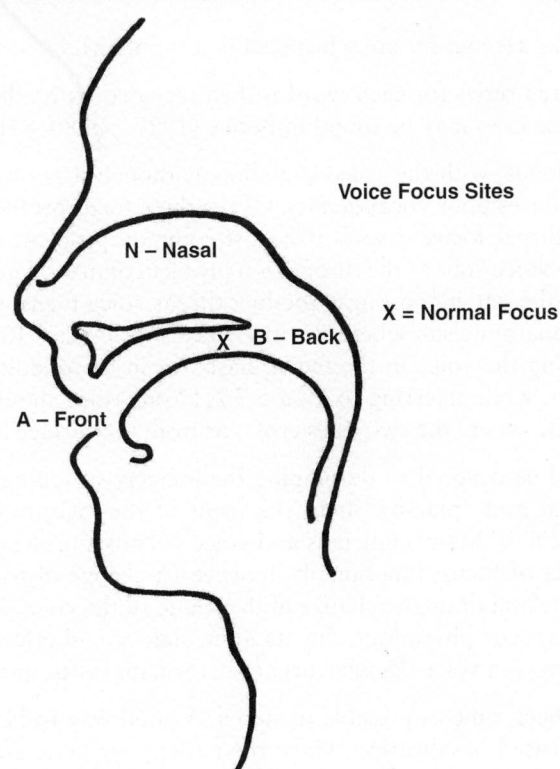

Voice Focus Sites

N – Nasal

X = Normal Focus

X B – Back

A – Front

2. For anterior focus, the clinician points to the left side, labeled "A = front" in Figure 7.2, saying to the client, "It appears that your voice sounds too far forward in your mouth. This seems to be caused by carrying your tongue high and forward in your mouth. This makes the voice sound babyish or thin." If possible, the clinician should imitate a thin, front-sounding voice, commenting afterward, "I made the thin voice with my tongue carried forward."

    a. Front-of-the-mouth focus can often be corrected by producing back-of-the-mouth sounds in rapid succession. We ask the patient to repeat "kuh-kuh-kuh-kuh" in a rapid series, stressing the back consonant /k/ and other low back vowel sounds like "kah," "guh," and "gah."

    b. Compare the old thin voice with the back voice, using some kind of immediate audio feedback.

3. For posterior-focused voice, the clinician points to the right side, labeled "B = back" in Figure 7.2. We say to the patient, "Your voice sounds back in your mouth, which seems to come from your tongue placed too far back. We can bring your tongue forward by practicing some front-of-the-mouth sounds."

    a. We seem to get posterior-to-anterior shift of focus quicker when only whisper is used on the first practice words. The patient is instructed to repeat front-of-the-mouth words like *peep, pipe*. Each word is said rapidly four or five times, like "peep-peep-peep-peep-peep."

b. Voiceless or *th* words like *this* or *that* are whispered in rapid succession, four or five times.

c. /s/ words like *see* and *sat* are whispered in a rapid series.

d. The whispered series for each word is then repeated with a light voice. Posterior focus exercises may be found in Boone (1997, pp. 80–81).

4. Poor vertical focus, with the voice sounding as though it is focused down deep in the throat, produces poor vocal quality. Of the three focus problems (front, back, and throat), the throat focus voice is the most common problem seen in the voice clinic. Getting the voice "out of the throat" is a problem of mental imagery. Although the clinician and the patient can hear the low-throat voice focus, it is not possible to find an exact anatomic site where the low voice is produced. Rather, we use the imagery of "placing the voice in the facial mask" or in the middle of the face. Or we tell the patient, while referring to Figure 7.2, "Your voice should sound like it's coming from the X, where the two lines cross, or from the surface of your tongue."

a. Time should be devoted to developing the imagery of taking the voice "out" of the throat and "placing" it in the front of the face, or the facial mask (Verdolini, 2000). Many clinicians and voice scientists profess skepticism over the construct of focus; functionally, however, a change of focus can produce an immediate and dramatic change in the sound of the voice. While we cannot demonstrate focus physiologically, its immediate sound effects produce measurable changes in voice (less perturbation, formant shifts, quality differences).

b. Devote as much time as possible to step a. A good way to begin higher focus is with increased nasalization. Have the patient say "one-a-one-a-one" with exaggerated nasality. Place the fingers along the bridge and sides of the nose to feel the sound vibrations in the nose. Use other monosyllabic nasal words like *mom, me,* and *many,* and exaggerate their nasality.

c. If the patient confirms feeling the vibrations of the nasal consonants and the nasalized vowels, practice reading short nasal sentences with exaggerated nasal resonance, such as "many men want some money." Practice reading /m-n-ng/ phrases and sentences. Contrast the feeling of the higher-focused nasal voice with the lower throat voice. The two voices should sound and feel different.

d. If the nasal consonants have facilitated a higher focus from the throat focus, introduce some high front vowels and words like *baby, beach,* and *take,* emphasizing the resonance in the facial mask.

e. This is a good time to listen critically to the higher-focused resonance. Use the audio playback or listen to the voice and look at the tracings on the Visi-Pitch. Contrast the old lower focus with the higher mouth focus, contrasting the sound and the "feel" of the two voices. Oral reading and conversation in the voice clinic should emphasize the feeling of higher focus and the "set" the patient assumes to achieve it.

Typical Case History Showing Utilization of the Approach. Lilly was a 49-year-old financial planner who decided that her voice was "too small for the kind of work I do." A subsequent voice evaluation found her to have a habitual voice pitch around 260 Hz (near middle C) with a thin, front-of-the-mouth resonance. An endoscopic examination found her to have a normal larynx. When she listened to her voice on audio playback, she commented, "That's the kind of baby voice I always seem to have." Our subsequent voice therapy emphasized developing a more posterior focus to her voice. In a few therapy sessions, she developed a voice that sounded like it came from "further back," with a noticeable improvement in overall voice resonance. She was also able to lower her voice pitch two full notes to 195 Hz (near an A3). After eight therapy sessions, she consistently showed a more mature voice with normal resonance. On a two-year follow-up interview, she continued to demonstrate a normal voice.

Typical Case History Showing Utilization of the Approach. J.J. was a high school teacher who had "lost her voice" after a serious bout of coughing and throat clearing during a particularly virulent upper respiratory infection (URI). When the infection cleared, she found she had no voice. A full endoscopic evaluation at the University of California at San Francisco found a normal laryngeal anatomy, but when J.J. tried to phonate, the true focal folds were unable to vibrate because the false vocal folds came together at the midline. It was explained to J.J. that the supraglottic structures in the larynx were assuming a protective posture secondary to the irritation that had accompanied the URI. J.J. was instructed to place her fingers lightly up to the bridge of the nose and lips and to produce nasals, such as "maninthemoon." Almost immediately she achieved easy phonation. She was instructed to attend to the "focus" of the energy, which she reported had transferred from the larynx to the lips. Nasals were transitioned into liquids and glides and finally to normal speech. A digitized recording was transferred to a DVD so that she could follow these steps at home in case she reverted to the protective laryngeal habit.

Evaluation of the Approach. For the patient with a thin, front voice; a back voice; or a low-in-the-throat voice, changing one's voice focus appears to be an easy goal to attain. Contrasting the sound of the voice from front, back, or low with a voice that sounds like it is coming from the middle of the mouth or higher in the facial mask is a vital step in using focus in therapy. If the patient can change the sound focus of his or her voice after clinician instruction and modeling, the impact on improving voice is almost immediate. Successful use of focus can be coupled with other VFAs, such as auditory feedback, establishing a new pitch, nasal-glide stimulation, and the open-mouth approach.

11. Glottal Fry

Kinds of Problems for Which the Approach Is Useful. As we learned in Chapter 2, the larynx vibrates in different ways to adjust airflow. This normally creates three types of vocal registers: falsetto or loft for the highest vocal frequencies, modal, and glottal fry. Blomgren (1998) writes that the fundamental frequency in the modal register is approximately 86 to 170 Hz for males and 175 to 276 Hz for females. This differs from the F_0 in the glottal fry register, which ranges from 24 to 72 Hz for both males and females, with the average fry at 48 Hz. We can actually hear each cycle of vocal fold vibration during glottal fry.

True glottal fry is produced in a relaxed manner with very little airflow and very little subglottic air pressure (Blomgren and colleagues, 1998; Zemlin, 1998). Glottal fry shortens the thyroarytenoid muscles and the vocal ligaments, which reduces the rate of vocal fold vibration. Glottal fry, considered a normal voice register, is valuable for patients with vocal nodules as well as for patients with other hyperfunctional problems such as polyps, cord thickening, functional dysphonia, and even spasmodic dysphonia and ventricular phonation. Although glottal fry can be an extremely powerful facilitating technique to improve voice in the dysphonic patient and is a useful diagnostic vocal probe, it has a second use, as well: It can be an index of vocal fold relaxation. To produce a glottal fry of 65 to 75 Hz, which is desirable, the vocal folds must be relaxed. A patient may not always be able to achieve this fry in the first session, but the accomplishment of a "good fry" of about 70 or 75 Hz is an indication that the larynx has been relaxed. The glottal fry can be produced on either inhalation or exhalation. After producing glottal fry phonation for 5 to 10 seconds and then being asked to say a phrase such as "easy does it," a patient with nodules often experiences normal or near-normal vocal quality for the first time in months.

Boone (1988) stated that the glottal fry is a successful VFA for treating puberphonia. It teaches the client to produce a lower pitch by relaxing and lowering the larynx, thus changing the features of the vocal folds. Fawcus (1986) suggested that the glottal fry might also be used to treat ventricular phonation, which occurs when the false vocal folds "ride" on the true vocal folds. The glottal fry discourages the tight and raised larynx phonations in vocal hyperfunction, thus encouraging the larynx to sit lower in the neck.

Procedural Aspects of the Approach

1. A common pencil eraser or a very dry, hard raisin can represent a vocal nodule. When placed between the pages of a hardcover book, the eraser keeps the pages apart with a gap on either side of the eraser; likewise, nodules produce a gap between the vocal cords. If the eraser is placed between two marshmallows instead of between the pages of a book, the marshmallows "wrap around" the mass of the eraser. In glottal fry, the compliant vocal cords can "wrap around" the nodules and improve approximation. A clinician can see this with stroboscopic videoendoscopy and demonstrate it to the patient.

2. Ask the patient to let out half of his or her breath and then say /i/ softly, holding it until it fades away slowly. Encourage the patient to stretch the /i/ as long as possible.

3. Once the patient has a well-sustained /i/ in the glottal fry mode, have him or her open the mouth medium wide and protrude the tongue. Then have the patient make the tone "larger" by "opening the throat." The desired tone is a deep, resonant, slow series of individual pops, which we describe as sounding "like dragging a stick along a picket fence."

4. Have the patient attempt to produce the same tone on inhalation as on exhalation. Some people are better able to produce the glottal fry on inhalation. Also have the patient alternately reverse the tone—first on exhalation, then on inhalation. Next, have the patient say words such as *on* and *off* and *in* and *out* in the glottal fry mode. Suggest that the patient slightly prolong these words and say them on both inhalation (*on, in*) and exhalation (*off, out*), alternately back and forth between ingressive and egressive airflow. Record the glottal fry so the patient has a model or target.

5. When the patient is able to produce these words well and can produce the sustained /i/ or /a/ in glottal fry, ask him or her to say, "easy does it," "squeeze the peach," or "see the eagle" in a normal voice. These are almost always produced with greatly improved or normal vocal quality. The patient will generally be able to say only a few words with the improved quality and will then need to go back to the glottal fry mode. Record these phrases and contrast them with the patient's typical voice. Also, ask the patient to judge the two ways of speaking.

6. When the correct glottal fry is learned, instruct the patient to practice for a few minutes several (10 or more) times each day. To assist the patient in practice, suggest that he or she tie practice to the environment—for example, by producing the fry each time he or she sees a bus or a red car, or during the last two minutes of each hour. The patient must be producing the fry appropriately before you allow practice.

Typical Case History Showing Utilization of the Approach. Mark, a 10-year-old boy, and Brian, an 11-year-old boy, were referred for voice evaluation by an otolaryngologist who had diagnosed bilateral vocal nodules. Both boys had low-pitched, hoarse voices with frequent phonation breaks during connected speech. They had had these voices for nearly one year. After teaching glottal fry as just described, we had contests to see who could fry the longest and at the slowest rate. We had the boys say words in the fry mode back and forth to each other. We saw each boy twice a week, once together and once individually, for 45-minute sessions. In three months, their voices were normal, and the nodules were completely gone. We should note that with one boy, we reduced vocal abuses during his soccer activity as well.

Evaluation of the Approach. The approach appears to work because very little subglottic pressure and very little airflow are required to produce the glottal fry. Therefore, there is little stress on the folds. The compliant folds seem to reduce the amount of friction as they meet during phonation, which allows the nodules to be reduced or reabsorbed even though the patient continues to talk. The new talking is produced with far less vocal fold tension.

12. Head Positioning

Kinds of Problems for Which the Approach Is Useful. Basic to good vocal performance (acting, lecturing, singing) includes good posture and head positioning. Also, changing head position may facilitate a better voice in patients with various kinds of voice problems (Aronson, 1990). In their study on interventions to reduce moderate to severe vocal hyperfunction, Van Lierde and colleagues (2004) included correction of head position prior to introducing subsequent intervention approaches. These researchers provided a table of various muscles and muscle groups that were influenced by head positioning changes.

Patients with unilateral vocal fold paralysis sometimes demonstrate a stronger voice by lateralizing head position, with or without digital pressure on the lateral lamina of the thyroid cartilage (see VFA #7, digital manipulation). Finding optimum head positioning has been found to be helpful in chewing and swallowing with patients with various neurological disorders (McFarlane and colleagues, 1998). The symptoms of dysarthria involving both speech and voice may be minimized in a particular patient by a specific head position. We find that a patient with symptoms of vocal hyperfunction can often experience a better, more relaxed voice by placing the head in a different position. Several distinct head positions can be tried in therapy in an attempt to find one that facilitates better voice:

1. Normal, straight ahead
2. Neck extended forward with head tilted down, face looking up
3. Neck flexed downward with head tilted down, face looking down

4. Neck flexed unilaterally with head tilted to either the left or right, with tilted face looking forward

5. Head upright and rotated toward the left or right, face looking in that direction

Any one head position may change pharyngeal–oral resonating structures so that a change in vocal quality (either better or worse) may occur.

Procedural Aspects of the Approach

1. Introduce the approach by demonstrating various head positions, either by photograph, video, or live demonstration. A simple explanation of the technique should accompany the demonstration: "Sometimes changing the positions of our heads can improve the sound of our voices. The head can be tilted either down or back, or to the left or right. Sometimes we can improve the sound of our voices simply by turning our heads to one side or the other. No one head position seems to help everyone. Let us try a few and listen to any changes in voice we hear."

2. The best voicing task to use to search for head position influence is the prolongation of vowels, such as /i/, /ɪ/, /æ/, /o/, or /u/. Once a helpful position is discovered, any kind of voice practice material can be used.

3. Many gradations in positioning are possible between the normal head position and one of the extreme head positions described previously. For example, when flexing the neck and bringing the head down in a gradual movement, perhaps at the beginning of the movement, a voice change can be noted. As soon as a change (if it occurs) can be noted, the head should be kept at that position without going to the full range of the movement.

4. Neurologically impaired patients may experience some oral–pharyngeal asymmetry from their disease; that is, one side of the neck or oral cavity may function better than the other side. A particular lateral movement of the head may make a sudden and noticeable improvement in voice in such patients. If so, ask the patient to practice voice material with the head in the lateral position. Head positioning, particularly to one side, is often effectively combined with lateral digital pressure (VFA # 7) on the thyroid lamina. Search with the patient to find the position that seems to increase subglottal pressure, resulting in a louder, more functional phonation (McFarlane and colleagues, 1998).

5. Patients with vocal hyperfunction, that is, patients who use too much effort to talk, often profit most from neck flexion with the chin tucked down toward the chest. Such downward carriage of the head seems to promote greater vocal tract relaxation. If an easy, target voice is achieved with neck flexion, this head-down position should be held during voice practice attempts.

Typical Case History Showing Utilization of the Approach. Mary was a 55-year-old wife and mother who had had vocal difficulties for the past five years. A subsequent voice evaluation found that she had a moderately severe functional dysphonia accompanied by neck tension with severe mandibular restriction, hard glottal attack, and an inappropriately high voice pitch. Voice therapy was scheduled twice weekly, with therapy focus on increasing her mouth opening and developing an easy glottal attack with "a legato phonatory style." The chewing and open-mouth approaches were unsuccessful until changing head position was added to the therapy.

Mary was instructed to "tuck in her chin," flexing the anterior neck muscles with her face looking downward. Keeping her chin down, she was able to reduce neck tension; she experienced immediate improvement in vocal quality. In subsequent therapy sessions, she developed an awareness that much of her past vocal strain was related to her tendency to hyperextend her neck; by using the opposite head position with anterior neck flexion, she was able to produce voice with relatively little strain. This change of head position, coupled with other therapy techniques designed to promote greater oral openness and ease of vocal production, helped Mary reestablish a normal voice.

Evaluation of the Approach. Changing to another head position by flexing or extending the neck can have an immediate positive effect on voice quality (Van Lierde and colleagues, 2004). Such an approach is seldom used in isolation; rather, it is usually combined with other voice therapy approaches, such as using the open-mouth approach or digital manipulation. Patients such as Mary with severe functional tension often profit from anterior neck flexion; however, voice problems caused by some neurogenic diseases are often minimized by using some of the other head positions described earlier in this section. Lateralization of the head by looking to one side or the other can often produce a stronger voice in patients with unilateral vocal fold paralysis. Changing head positions to facilitate better voice requires much trial and error. If a particular head position works, it should be used; if not, other head positions should be tried.

13. Hierarchy Analysis

Kinds of Problems for Which the Approach Is Useful. In hierarchy analysis, the patient lists various situations in his or her life that ordinarily produce some anxiety and arranges those situations in a sequential order from the least to the most anxiety provoking. Individual patients may instead prepare a hierarchy of situations, ranging from those in which they find their voices best to those in which they find them worst. This technique is borrowed from Wolpe's (1987) method of reciprocal inhibition, which teaches the patient relaxed responses to anxiety-evoking situations. After identifying a hierarchy of anxiety-evoking situations, the patient begins by employing the relaxed responses in the least anxious of them and, in therapy, works his or her way up the hierarchy, thereby eventually deconditioning his or her previously established anxious responses. The identification of hierarchical situations (less anxiety–more anxiety; worst voice–best voice) is a useful therapeutic device for most patients with hyperfunctional voice problems, which by definition imply excessive overreacting. Patients with functional dysphonia, or with dysphonias accompanied by nodules, polyps, and vocal fold thickening, frequently report that their degrees of dysphonia vary with the situation. Such patients may profit from hierarchy analysis. Case (2002) reports effective use of hierarchy analysis for particular aspects of voice, such as pitch or loudness.

Procedural Aspects of the Approach

1. Begin by developing in the patient a general awareness of the hierarchical behavior to be studied. If, for example, the patient is asked to identify situations in which he or she feels most uncomfortable, discuss with the patient the symptoms of being uncomfortable. Or if the patient is going to develop a hierarchy of situations in which he or she experiences variation of voice, discuss and give examples of a good voice or a bad voice. Explain that the patient must develop a relative ordering of situations, sequencing them from "good" to "bad." Some patients are initially resistant to this sort of ordering, perhaps because they never realized that there are relative gradations to their feelings of anxiety or relative changes in their quality of voice. They may not be aware that the degree of their anxiety or hoarseness is not constant.

2. Although the majority of voice patients are soon able to arrange situations into a hierarchy, a few require practice sequencing some neutral stimuli. On one occasion, a woman was taught the idea of sequential order by arranging five shades of red tiles from left to right, in the order of the lightest pink to the darkest red. Having done this, she was then able to sequence her voice situations, proceeding gradually from those in which her voice was normal to those in which it was extremely dysphonic.

3. As a home assignment, have the patient develop several hierarchies with regard to his or her voice. One hierarchy might center on how the patient's voice holds up with the family, another on how it is related to work situations, and a third on what happens to it in varying situations with friends. After these hierarchies have been developed by the patient at home, review them in therapy.

4. In therapy, use the "good" end of the hierarchical sequence first. That is, begin by asking the patient to recapture, if possible, the good situation. The goal of therapy is to duplicate the feeling of well-being or the good voice that the patient experienced in the situation rated as best. Efforts should be made in therapy to recall the good factors surrounding the more optimum phonation. If the patient is successful in re-creating the optimum situation, his or her phonation will sound relaxed and appropriate. The re-created optimum situation thus serves as an excellent facilitator for producing good voice. After some success in re-creating the first situation on the hierarchy, capturing completely his or her optimum response (whether this is relaxation, phonation, or both), the patient will then be able to continue with the second situation. Again the goal is to maintain optimum response. The rate of movement up the hierarchy depends entirely on how successfully the patient can re-create the situations and maintain optimum response. By using the relaxed response in increasingly more tense situations, the patient is conditioning him- or herself to a more favorable, optimum behavior.

5. Although some patients can re-create situations outside the clinic with relative ease, some cannot. As soon as possible, have the patient practice the optimum response outside the clinic under good conditions so that he or she will eventually be able to use it in the real world in more adverse situations. The patient must not lose sight of the goal of maintaining the good response in varying situations outside the clinic.

6. Not all patients can go all the way up the hierarchy, maintaining good voice at each level. Such patients should be counseled that most people experience anxiety or poorer voice in some situations, such as at the highest level of the hierarchy. Some practice might be given at one step lower in the hierarchy where good performance is still maintained.

Typical Case History Showing Utilization of the Approach. Jamie was a 28-year-old transsexual who was in counseling for gender transference from male to female. As part of her overall gender-change program, it was recommended that she "receive speech–voice therapy to develop a more feminine speaking style." In voice therapy, Jamie reported that her out-of-clinic voicing was continually changing, "very dependent on what kind of situation I find myself in." Jamie was employed full-time as a secretary-receptionist in an area agency for aging. Her SLP worked with her to develop this nine-step hierarchy, in which she found she had the best female voice all the way down to the level where it seemed hardest to convey her femininity:

Best Voice

1. I always have my best new voice with my mother.
2. The director of our agency. She is always a great listener to everyone.
3. I answer the phone at work with a very good voice.
4. The doctor at the clinic doesn't listen as well as he should. He wants me to try harder to be a woman.
5. Some salespeople are hard to talk to, especially car mechanics.
6. I think some people at the church are bigots.
7. I still date my old girlfriend who doesn't understand me anymore.
8. Meeting new men tends to make me nervous and my speech breaks down.
9. Talking with my dad is hardest. He won't accept me and still calls me Jim.

Worst Voice

Evaluation of the Approach. Most voice patients report great variability in voice quality, depending on how much they have been using the voice, the time of day, and the psychodynamics of the speaking situations. Hierarchy analysis is often helpful for dealing with vocal inconsistencies experienced while talking with different people in various situations (Hapner and Johns, 2004). By analyzing the hierarchical situations in which voice deteriorates or improves, the patient develops an awareness of the situational cues that are causing voice changes. Perhaps for the first time, the patient realizes that voice quality is not a constant and that vocal quality fluctuations are somewhat dependent on how relaxed one feels or how comfortable one is with his or her listeners. Therapy then focuses on using the best voice found low on the hierarchy. The patient attempts to use that optimum voice in situations in which he or she has previously experienced difficulty. Hierarchy analysis is consistently useful in voice therapy.

14. Inhalation Phonation

Kinds of Problems for Which the Approach Is Useful. Patients who have functional aphonia and functional dysphonia often profit from inhalation phonation. This can be a helpful technique for the patient who perseverates using ventricular phonation and often demonstrates difficulty "getting out of it." Likewise, it can be helpful for the patient with functional dysphonia who has developed some maladaptive voice that seems to resist change. On videoendoscopy, when the voice patient is asked to produce an inhalation voice, we see the true folds in a stretched position (lengthened in their respiratory length) suddenly adducted and set in vibration. It is the relative thinness of the folds on inspiration that seems to produce the high-pitched voice. The ease with which most patients can produce the technique (inhaling with voice and exhaling with a near-matched voice) makes the approach readily useful in establishing or reestablishing true vocal fold vibration. Inhalation phonation as a therapy technique for hyperfunctional phonation has been explored by Kelly and Fisher (1999), Orlikoff and colleagues (1997), and Lehman (1965). Robb and

colleagues (2001) suggested that vowel articulation associated with reverse phonation did not differ from expiratory phonation for the production of the /i/, although
it was affected for the production of the high and low back vowels. Therefore, it is
suggested that training be performed with the /i/. See the VFA *tongue protrusion /i/*
for additional benefits of the high-front tongue position in voice therapy.

Procedural Aspects of the Approach

1. This particular approach, which is similar to masking, is perhaps better demonstrated than explained. Demonstrate inhalation phonation by phonating a high-
pitched sound with your palms upturned. It is important to time the initiations of the
inhalation with palms upturned. Turn them up so you can mark for the patient the
contrast between inhalation (palms upturned) and exhalation (palms turned down).

2. After demonstrating several separate inhalations with phonation, say, "Now, I'll
match the high-pitched inhalation voice with an expiration voice." Inhale and then
exhale in a high pitch several times.

3. Ask the patient to make an inhalation phonation. He or she should repeat the
inhalation phonation several times. Now again repeat the inhalation–exhalation
matched phonation, taking care to make the associated palms-up and palms-down
movements.

4. After the patient has produced the matching hum, say, "Now, let us extend the
expiration like this." Demonstrate a continuation of the high pitch, sweeping down
from your falsetto register to your regular chest register on one long, continuous
expiration. Repeat this several times. Then say to the patient, "Once I've brought my
vocal cords together at the high pitch, I then sweep down, keeping them together, to
the pitch level of my regular speaking voice."

5. If the patient is unable to produce this shift from high to low, repeat the first four
steps. If the patient can make the shift down to the regular speaking register, say,
"Now you're getting your vocal cords together for a good-sounding voice." Take
care at this point not to rush the patient into using the "new" voice functionally.
Rather, have the patient practice some similar hum phonations. After some practice
just phonating the hum, give the patient a word list containing simple monosyllabic
words for "true" voice practice.

6. Once the patient is able to produce inspiration–expiration without difficulty, he
or she should be instructed to stop using the pronounced palms-up and palms-down
movements.

7. Stay at the single-word practice level until normal voicing is established. We often
spend several therapy periods practicing the new phonation as a motor practice drill
without attempting to make the voice conversationally functional. You might say,
"Now we're getting the vocal folds together the way we want them." This places
the previous aphonia or ventricular phonation "blame" on the mechanism rather
than on the patient. Counseling with the patient at this time is important. The motor practice gives the patient time to adjust to the more optimum way of phonating.

Typical Case History Showing Utilization of the Approach. Derek, a five-year-old boy,
was found to have small bilateral vocal nodules. His speech clinician placed him on
complete voice rest, which unfortunately was enforced for five continuous months.

At the end of five months, the nodules had disappeared, and Derek was instructed by both the physician and the speech pathologist to resume normal phonation. Despite all his efforts, Derek could only whisper. He became completely aphonic but whispered easily to all people with much animation and relative comfort. This functional aphonia remained for two months, after which he was instructed, "Go back and talk the normal way." Derek gestured that he wanted to use his voice but could not "find it." Therapy efforts for restoring phonation were begun about seven months after Derek's phonations had ceased. Inhalation phonation was initiated, and at the first therapy session Derek was able to produce a high-pitched inhalation sound and to follow his clinician well by matching the inhalation with an expiration sound. He was able to use an expiration phonation, appropriate in both quality and pitch, by the end of the first therapy session. He was scheduled for two other appointments within a 24-hour period, during which he practiced producing his regained normal voice. He was counseled that his "voice is working now and you'll never have to lose it again." The boy has had normal phonation since his voice was restored using the inhalation phonation technique. Counseling to curb yelling and other vocal abuses appeared to be successful because Derek has experienced no return of the bilateral vocal nodules.

Evaluation of the Approach. Some patients who experience either aphonia, dysphonia, or ventricular phonation for any length of time lose their ability to initiate normal true fold phonation. The longer the aphonia or dysphonia persists, the harder it might be to use normal voice. Inhalation phonation is a simple way to produce true cord approximation and voicing. The high-pitched voice on inhalation probably results from the folds being longer in their inhalation posture, and even though they may adduct on command, they remain in their longer configuration. This elongated posture thins them, resulting in the higher-pitched phonation (Robb and colleagues, 2001). The important part of the approach, however, is matching the inhalation voicing with exhalation voicing. Once the patient can produce the exhalation voice without the inhalation prompt, the inhalation practice is no longer needed.

15. Laryngeal Massage

Kinds of Problems for Which the Approach Is Useful. This particular approach follows the procedures, modified slightly, for manual circumlaryngeal therapy, as first presented by Aronson (1990), and further organized by Roy (2008) and Van Lierde and colleagues (2004), among others. Laryngeal massage involves the gentle manipulation and massage of the larynx. The approach is recommended for use with patients with functional voice disorders in which structural or neurogenic causal factors cannot be identified. While the most commonly used professional term for such voice disorders is functional dysphonia, a few authors have recommended that these functional disorders be classified as psychogenic dysphonia (Aronson, 1990) or muscle tension dysphonia (Morrison and Rammage, 1994). As introduced in Chapter 3, we use the term functional dysphonia generically to include hoarseness without identified structural or organic cause, ventricular dysphonia, puberphonia, falsetto, and voicing with discomfort (pain, scratchy throat, etc.). Stress, psychological conflict, and overall systemic tension often appear to worsen the symptoms of functional dysphonia. Manual circumlaryngeal therapy offers gentle laryngeal manipulation and massage, resulting in lower laryngeal carriage and greater intrinsic–extrinsic laryngeal muscle relaxation.

   A number of studies in the literature report reductions of hyperfunctional voice symptoms and normal vocal quality after a single therapy session using this laryngeal manipulation–massage therapy. Although the present authors can report good results with this technique, we have also achieved lower laryngeal posturing with greater muscle relaxation using the yawn-sigh technique (Boone and McFarlane, 1993). Therefore, in our clinical practice, we employ the yawn-sigh first for the patient with a high larynx and laryngeal tension. If the patient is not successful employing the yawn-sigh followed by focus, our next approach is the use of manual circumlaryngeal massage (VFA15).

Procedural Aspects of the Approach

1. The first step is a screen for a high larynx and likely excessive laryngeal–neck muscle tension. If neither of these are present, other VFAs are used. If either one or both are present, we continue.

2. The Yawn-sigh (see VFA 25) is attempted first. If a lower larynx and greater muscle relaxation are achieved by using the yawn-sigh, we do not apply laryngeal manipulation and massage.

3. We follow Aronson's (1990) procedures for reducing "musculoskeletal tension associated with vocal hyperfunction":

   a. Encircle the hyoid bone with the thumb and middle finger. Work back posteriorly until the major horns are felt.

   b. Apply light pressure with the fingers in a circular motion over the tips of the hyoid bone.

   c. Repeat this procedure with the fingers from the thyroid notch, working posteriorly.

   d. Find the posterior borders of the thyroid cartilage (medial to the sternocleidomastoid muscles) and repeat the procedure.

   e. With the fingers over the superior borders of the thyroid cartilage, begin to work the larynx gently downward and laterally at times.

   f. Ask the patient to prolong vowels during these procedures and note changes in quality or pitch. Clearer voice quality and lower pitch indicate relief of tension. Because of possible fatigue, rest periods should be provided.

   g. Improvement in voice is immediately reinforced. Practice should be given in producing voice in vowels, words, phrases, and sentences.

   h. Discuss with the patient how voice tension has been reduced. Repeat the procedures. Can the patient maneuver his or her own larynx to a lower position?

4. We find out whether the patient can experience the same lowering of the larynx with muscle relaxation by producing the yawn-sigh (VFA25). We discuss how both can be used when excessive laryngeal tension is experienced.

Typical Case History Showing Utilization of the Approach.

Carl was a 23-year-old graduate student in speech and hearing sciences who complained to his clinical supervisor that in certain situations he experienced "such tightness in my throat, I can hardly get my voice out." A subsequent voice evaluation found him to have unnecessarily high carriage of his larynx accompanied by some evidence of functional dysphonia.

He was asked to read Aronson's description of therapy for "musculoskeletal tension (vocal hyperfunction)" (Aronson, 1990, p. 339). Subsequently, the supervisor conducted a full one-hour manual circumlaryngeal therapy session with Carl that had an immediate result of lowering his laryngeal posture and relaxing his voice, resulting in "a voice that was always there with greater intensity and less perturbation." Carl was followed over an 18-month period (while in graduate school) and was able to maintain a normal voice following the one session of laryngeal manipulation and massage.

Evaluation of the Approach. One only has to see a demonstration of this manipulation–massage technique to be impressed with its sudden effectiveness in reducing muscular tension and producing a more relaxed, lower-pitched, resonant voice. We have been impressed with the results of laryngeal massage. Aronson has described his approach as "maneuvering the patient's laryngeal and hyoid anatomy," which fits the term *massage*, described as "the act of rubbing, kneading, or stroking the superficial parts of the body with the hand" (Blakiston, 1985, p. 913). Later studies by Van Lierde and colleagues (2004) and Roy and Leeper (2003) continue to support the role of manual circumlaryngeal techniques in the assessment and management of musculoskeletal tension in hyperfunctional voice disorders.

16. Masking

Kinds of Problems for Which the Approach Is Useful. Patients with functional aphonia are often able to produce normal phonation under conditions of auditory masking. Using masking with patients who have functional dysphonia often reveals a "window" of improved phonation. It appears that many such patients produce faulty voices because of poor real-time auditory monitoring. The use of masking in both diagnostic testing and therapy often reveals changed phonation states that can then be recorded and used as voice models in subsequent therapy. The masking VFA uses a voicing–reflex test, which audiologists administer as the Lombard test (Newby, 1972). The Lombard effect is believed to be an unconscious reflex that occurs when a speaker is trying to make him- or herself more intelligible by becoming (unconsciously) louder to listeners in a speaking situation with a loud background, such as a noisy restaurant (Lau, 2008). The normal hearing patient increases voice loudness reflexively when hearing a masking noise. In fact, the Lombard test was first introduced as a method of finding voice in patients with functional aphonia. When asked to phonate in a loud-noise background, patients with functional aphonia sometimes used light voice. In the voice–reflex situation, the patient wears earphones and is asked to read a passage aloud. As the patient is reading, a masking noise is fed into the earphones. The louder the masking, the louder the patient's voice. At loud masking levels, the patient cannot monitor well either the loudness or the clearness of his or her voice. Some patients with functional dysphonias actually experience clearer voices when they cannot monitor their productions because of loud masking. Some care should be given to the amount of masking intensity that is used, particularly when using white or pink noise masking (American Speech-Language-Hearing Association, 1991). The use of speech-range masking permits effective masking at relatively low intensity levels. Masking devices include the sine wave masking option on the Casa Futura, and the Computerized Speech Lab™ (CSL) by KayPENTAX Corp.

Procedural Aspects of the Approach. The masking approach is best used without any prior explanation. The increased voicing experienced under masking conditions is produced on a reflexive, nonvolitional basis.

1. Masking should be presented with the patient wearing headphones and not presented in an open-air field. The patient is seated by a masking source, such as the white noise of an audiometer or the speech-range masking of the Facilitator. The patient is asked to read aloud and to keep reading no matter what kind of interruption he or she may hear. We typically have the patient read (or very young children are asked to count) about 10 seconds, introduce masking for five seconds, go back to reading without masking, then reintroduce masking. We record the patient's oral reading, and on playback we can hear the changes in voice that are introduced when masking occurs.

2. A recording should be made as the patient reads aloud. An aphonic patient's whisper may change to voice under conditions of masking. It is important to have recorded the emergence of voice, which the patient can use in step 5. The dysphonic patient (functional, ventricular, or puberphonic) should also be recorded while using the masking approach. Marked differences in voice quality between the absence and presence of masking conditions will probably be evident.

3. Five- or ten-second exposures to masking are introduced to the patient bilaterally. The intensity levels should be in excess of 70 dB sound pressure level SPL, which is sufficiently loud to mask out the patient's own voicing attempts. Whenever an aphonic patient hears the loud masking, he or she may attempt some feeble vocalization. Under masking, a dysphonic patient will produce a louder voice and often a voice with more normal vocal quality as well.

4. Do not use the masking method beyond the trial stage with those few voice patients who do not demonstrate the voice–reflex effect. If it works well and produces voice improvement, the method may be used as part of every therapy period. One might then experiment by having the patient listen to recordings of him- or herself to see whether the patient can match volitionally his or her voice under masking conditions. Recordings can then be made contrasting the voice without masking (attempting to re-create the same voice as heard under masking) and the voice with masking. Try to have the voices sound alike.

5. A patient may profit from reading aloud under masking conditions, and then having the masking abruptly ended to see if he or she can maintain the better voice. Many other variations using the masking noise can be initiated by inventive clinicians.

Typical Case History Showing Utilization of the Approach. Lillian was a nine-year-old girl who had a history of vocal nodules that had been previously treated successfully with voice therapy. Several months after therapy had been terminated (because it was successful: no nodules, normal voice), Lillian developed a severe influenza that left her with no voice. She was completely aphonic and could communicate only by whispering and using good facial expressions and gestures. The aphonia continued for one month (over the December holiday break) before she returned to the voice clinic. The masking approach was used with Lillian after attempts at modeling and request for voice failed. Lillian was asked to read aloud under conditions of 70-dB masking. Her reading attempts were recorded on a digital recorder. As soon as masking was introduced, light phonation was heard and recorded. The masking and oral reading were stopped, and Lillian was asked to hear her good voice on the digital playback. The child clapped her hands in joy that she now had a returned voice. Further masking followed by ear training was used as her voice became stronger. After two follow-up therapy sessions, Lillian was discharged with a normal voice and provided with a DVD of her in-clinic intervention. She was encouraged to play this DVD should she again experience aphonia. Studies have suggested that target behaviors often improve with visual feedback when modeled by the patients themselves (Bandura, 1986, 1997).

Evaluation of the Approach. The masking approach is most helpful with aphonic patients. It is also helpful for patients with some form of functional dysphonia, young men with puberphonia, and clients presenting with dysarthria, notably of the hypokinetic type. If the masking noise is loud enough, in excess of 70 dB SPL, patients cannot hear their voices to monitor phonation. If required to continue speaking by reading aloud under conditions of masking, patients often produce relatively normal voices. Clinicians should use some care in confronting the patients on audio playback with their "good" voices. Improved voices under conditions of masking should be used as the patients' models for their own imitation phonations. Clinicians should use the masking approach with some degree of eclecticism—that is, if the approach works, use it; if it does not, quickly abandon it. Masking has been supported by EBP for decades. More recent findings that advocate masking come from Coutinho and colleagues (2009), who found that masking in the voice of individuals with Parkinson's disease (PD) revealed improvement in vocal quality and an increase in loudness.

17. Nasal-Glide Stimulation

Kinds of Problems for Which the Approach Is Useful. Clinicians frequently note that in voice therapy, certain stimulus sounds seem to facilitate an easier-produced, often better-sounding voice. If we harken back to our phonetics textbooks, we recall that nasals and glides are classified as sonorants. Sonorants entail little to no obstruction of voiced energy in the nasal and oral cavities; therefore, these sounds are very easy to produce. This is particularly true with children and adults having problems of vocal hyperfunction. Watterson and colleagues (1993) have found, in studying 15 adult voice patients with vocal hyperfunction and 15 matched control subjects, that nasal and glide consonants facilitated better voicing patterns and were judged by the hyperfunctional subjects as "easier" to produce. The concept of differences in vocal effort has been also investigated by Bickley and Stevens (1987) and Baken and Orlikoff (1988), generally finding that supraglottal resonance–articulatory postures have a direct relationship to laryngeal physiology and function. Using words that contain many nasal and glide consonants, usually coupled with other therapy techniques, often helps the patient produce desired "target" vocalizations. Using nasal-glide consonants as therapy stimuli is particularly useful for patients with functional dysphonia, spasmodic dysphonia, and dysphonias related to fold thickening, nodules, and polyps.

Procedural Aspects of the Approach. Most therapy techniques require the patient to say something. For example, in the open-mouth approach or in practicing focus, the patient is given a few stimulus words to say. Words that contain nasal or glide consonants often produce the best-sounding voice or the voice that appears made with the least amount of effort (as compared with words containing other consonants).

Nasals, glides, and liquids are phonemes that take little effort to produce, unlike fricatives, affricates, and stops. They are voiced and produced with a relatively open vocal tract and they are easy to sustain. Using words that contain many nasals and glides/liquids, usually coupled with other techniques, helps the clients in the **video** produce desired target vocalizations (e.g., my name means money). Grand Rounds: The m, n, ny, and w sounds also have a forward focus. How might these forward produced sounds help reduce muscle tension at the larynx?

1. The clinician can find a number of monosyllabic and polysyllabic words containing nasal consonants for the patient to practice saying as the response when using various VFAs. Here are a few examples: *man, moon, many, morning, many men, moon man, manual lawnmower, Miami millionaire, morning singing.*

2. A variation of the technique is to use nasal monosyllabic words and introduce an /a/ between each word. Ask the patient to say three words in a row with the neutral /a/ between each word. For example, "man a man a man" or "wing a wing a wing."

3. We use the same procedure for words containing glide consonants. It has been found, however, that nasal consonants combine very well with the /l/ and /r/ phonemes, and many of our glide words contain nasal consonants: *loll, lil, rare, rah, lilly, arrow, marrow, married, married women, one lonely memory, Laura ran around, remember many lawmen.*

4. Using monosyllabic /l/ and /r/ words with an /a/ between them, such as "lee a lee a lee" or "rah a rah a rah," seems to produce good voice.

Typical Case History Showing Utilization of the Approach. Louise was a 66-year-old housewife who was forced to divorce her husband of some 42 years. She experienced a number of somatic symptoms following the divorce, including a severe functional dysphonia. Endoscopic–stroboscopic examination revealed a high carriage of the larynx with moderate vocal fold compression. The yawn-sigh approach was found to be effective in lowering her larynx and encouraging a more optimal vocal fold approximation. Under the sigh condition, she was asked to say various words. It was found that words with many nasal and glide consonants facilitated the easiest to produce and best-sounding voice. Intensive self-practice and twice weekly voice therapy for nine weeks, supplemented by concurrent psychological counseling, resulted in a good functional return of normal voice.

Evaluation of the Approach. Clinicians are always looking for voicing tasks that facilitate good voice production. Recent research has validated that certain sounds, particularly nasal and glide consonants, facilitate easy voice production. Titze (2006) suggested that the semi-occluded vocal tract configuration of nasals and glides results in lower vibrational amplitudes at the glottis. This may be beneficial at reducing tension at the level of the glottis (Titze, 2006). Among patients with vocal hyperfunction, nasal-glide consonant words are perceived by patients as producing voice with less effort. Word stimuli containing many nasal-glide consonants appear to facilitate in voice therapy a voice that sounds better and is produced (according to patient self-evaluation) with less effort.

18. Open-Mouth Approach

Kinds of Problems for Which the Approach Is Useful. Some individuals may underestimate to what degree the mouth needs to be open for speech. Encouraging the patient to develop more oral openness often reduces generalized vocal hyperfunction. Increasing mouth opening can also reduce oral resistance and increase oral resonance (Kummer, 2001) The open-mouth approach promotes more natural size–mass adjustments and more optimum approximation of the vocal folds, and this helps correct problems of loudness, pitch, and quality. Opening the mouth more is also recommended to increase oral resonance and to improve overall voice quality.

The voice also sounds louder. Developing greater openness should be part of any voice therapy program wherein the patient is attempting to use the vocal mechanisms with less effort and strain. This approach is often combined in treatment with other VFAs.

Procedural Aspects of the Approach

1. Have the patient view him- or herself in a mirror (or on a video playback, if possible) to observe the presence and absence of open-mouth behavior. Identify any lip tightness, mandibular restriction, or excessive neck muscle movement for the patient.

2. Children seem to understand quickly the benefits of opening the mouth more to produce better-sounding voices. In our voice program for children (Boone, 1993), we use a brief story that illustrates two boys, one who talks with his mouth closed and one who speaks with his mouth open. We then introduce a hand puppet and ask the child if he or she has ever been a ventriloquist. The ventriloquist is described as someone who does not open the mouth, in contrast to the puppet, who makes exaggerated, wide-mouth openings.

3. The ventriloquist–puppet analogy also works well with adults. Let the patient observe the marked contrast between talking with a closed mouth and talking with an open one. Ask the patient to watch him- or herself speak the two different ways in a mirror. Instruct the patient that what he or she is attempting will at first feel foreign and inappropriate. The initial stages of letting the jaw relax are frequently anything but relaxed.

4. To establish further this oral openness, ask the patient to drop the head toward the chest and let the lips part and the jaw drop open. Once the patient can do this, have him or her practice some relaxed /a/ sounds. When the head is tilted down and the jaw is slightly open, a more relaxed phonation can often be achieved (Boone and Wiley, 2000).

5. For patients to develop a feeling of openness when listening, and as a preset to speaking, they must first develop a conscious awareness of how often they find themselves with tight, closed mouths. One way to develop this awareness is to have patients mark down, on cards they carry with them, each time they become aware that their mouths are closed unnecessarily. The marking task itself is often enough to increase a patient's awareness. Over a period of a week, the number of mouth closings should decrease notably. Another way of developing an awareness of greater orality is to have patients place in their living environments (on a dressing table, desk, or car dashboard) a little sign that says "OPEN" or perhaps has a double arrow or any other code that might serve as a reminder.

6. Greater oral openness requires a lot of self-practice to overcome the habit of talking through a restricted mandible. Steps 3 and 4 facilitate greater mouth opening and are good practice tasks. After some practice in using greater mouth opening, the patient should confirm what it looks like by viewing video playback in practice sessions. Practice materials for improving greater mouth opening may be found in practice kits for children (Blonigen, 1994; Boone, 1993) and in voice books such as Andrews (2006), Boone (1997), Brown (1996), Case (2002), Colton and colleagues (2011), and Stemple and colleagues (2010).

Typical Case History Showing Utilization of the Approach. Jennifer, a 17-year-old high school girl, was examined by an ENT physician about one year after an automobile accident in which she had suffered some injuries to the head and neck. Laryngoscopic examination found all visible laryngeal structures normal in appearance and function, despite the fact that, since the accident, the girl's voice had been only barely audible. The speech pathologist was impressed "with her relatively closed mouth while speaking, which seemed to result in extremely poor voice resonance." Voice therapy combined both the chewing and the open-mouth VFAs. It was discovered in therapy that, for three months after the automobile accident, the girl had worn an orthopedic collar that seemed to inhibit her head and jaw movements. It appeared that much of her closed-mouth, mandibularly restricted speech was related to the constraints imposed on her by the orthopedic collar. When using the open-mouth approach with her head tilted down toward her chest, she was immediately able to produce a louder, more resonant voice. The open-mouth approach was initiated before beginning chewing exercises, and both achieved excellent results. Therapy was terminated after six weeks, with much voice improvement in both loudness and quality.

Evaluation of the Approach. The end point of the vocal resonator is the open oral cavity, which contributes acoustically to the formation of the majority of phonemes (Sundberg, 1997). The voice, both normal and dysphonic, improves in quality with greater mouth opening. On opening the mouth a bit more, the voice usually improves immediately. Besides opening the mouth more while speaking, the approach also encourages slight mouth opening while listening. A gentle opening of less than one finger wide between the central incisors keeps the teeth apart and generally fosters a relaxed oral posture. The open-mouth approach has been particularly effective with performers who often open their mouths well during performance (acting, singing) but may forget the importance of opening their mouths during conversation.

19. Pitch Inflections

Kinds of Problems for Which the Approach Is Useful. The prosodic and stress patterns of the normal speaking voice are characterized by changes in pitch, loudness, and duration. In some individuals, the lack of pitch variation is noticeable because the resulting voice is monotonous and boring to listeners. Speaking on the same pitch level with little variation, which for the average speaker is impossible to maintain, requires the inhibition of natural inflection. It is usually observed in overcontrolled people who display very little overt affect. Fairbanks (1960), who describes pitch variation as a vital part of normal phonation, defines inflection and shift: "An inflection is a modulation of pitch during phonation. A shift is a change of pitch from the end of one phonation to the beginning of the next" (p. 132). Voice therapy for patients with monotonic pitch seeks not only to establish more optimum pitch levels, but also to increase the amount of pitch variability. Any voice patient with a dull, monotonous pitch level will profit from attempting to increase pitch inflections. Many patients with functional dysphonia related to vocal hyperfunction appear to speak with little pitch fluctuation, often part of a pattern of oral and mandibular tightness, with the lips and mandible in a fixed, nonmoving pattern. The SLP typically combines work on increasing loudness (intensity) with efforts to increase pitch variability; working on pitch alone is difficult without influencing loudness variations. Another population that may benefit from pitch inflection intervention is male-to-female transexuals who seek the experienced voice clinician to increase the naturalness of their prosody. Wolfe and colleagues (1990) found that female speakers had a higher percentage of upward intonation and downward shifts in conversational speech.

Procedural Aspects of the Approach

1. The patient must first become aware of his or her vocal monotony via digitized playback on a recorder or audiovisual instrument. Play samples that lack pitch variability and follow with samples of good pitch variability, as provided by the clinician. Follow the listening with evaluative comments.

2. Begin working on downward and upward inflectional shifts of the same word, exaggerating in the beginning the extent of pitch change. Helpful sources for increasing pitch variation may be found in Boone (1997), Boone and Wiley (2000), Brown (1996), McKinney (1994), Morrison and Rammage (1994), and Stemple and Holcomb (1988), among many others.

3. Using the same practice materials, have the patient practice introducing inflectional shifts within specific words, keeping loudness levels about the same.

4. Pitch inflections can be graphically displayed on many instruments, such as the Visi-Pitch IV or Sona-Speech (KayPENTAX Corp., Montvale, New Jersey). Set target inflections for the patient to see if the patient can make his or her pitch level reach the same excursions or movement as the target model on the monitor.

5. Record and play back for the patient various oral reading and conversational samples, critically analyzing the productions for degree of pitch variability.

Typical Case History Showing Utilization of the Approach. Tyrone, a 51-year-old economics professor, received severe course evaluations from his students, who complained of his "monotonous" voice. On a subsequent voice evaluation, during both conversation and oral reading, he used "the same fundamental frequency with only minimal excursion of frequency." His voice was indeed monotonous, not only in pitch but in loudness, too. He also used the same duration characteristics for most vowels. Tyrone was highly motivated to improve his speaking voice and manner of speaking. Subsequent therapy focus was on increasing pitch inflections and improving loudness variations. He was provided with digital recordings, which he practiced daily, matching the target model productions with his own voicing attempts. After six weeks of voice therapy and intensive self-practice, Tyrone demonstrated improvement in both his conversational and lecture voices. Unfortunately, his lack of overall animation and boring affect still resulted in poor course evaluations. However, his conversational voice with increasing pitch inflections appeared to make a much more favorable impression on those around him.

Evaluation of the Approach. Voice quality in functional dysphonias is often improved when overall effort in speaking is reduced. Speaking for an extended period of time in a monotone is tiring (to both the speaker and the listener). People who wish to improve the quality of their speaking voices can often profit from increasing pitch variability as they speak. Using auditory feedback, listening to one's voice on playback, and having naïve listeners judge the quality of inflection in a speaker's voice appears to be a good way of improving pitch variability in one's voice. At our clinics, we often record the patient's voice during speaking tasks, then randomize the recordings and present them to listeners who are not familiar with the patient. The listeners' judgments are powerful biofeedback to the patient. To judge the recordings, clinicians can use the GRBAS or the CAPE-V instruments (see Chapter 6).

20. Redirected Phonation

Kinds of Problems for Which the Approach Is Useful. Some children and adults with voice problems experience difficulty "finding" their voices. This is particularly more common among patients with functional aphonia or functional dysphonia in their attempts to find interactive phonation. In redirected phonation, the SLP searches with the patient to find some kind of vegetative phonation (coughing, gargling [Boone, 1983], laughing, throat clearing) or some kind of intentional voicing ("playing" the comb or kazoo, humming, singing, trilling [Colton and Casper, 1996], or saying "um-hmm" [Cooper, 1990]). If the patient has the capability of voicing one or more of these noncommunicative (other than "um-hmm") sounds, the sound(s) might be redirected into production of the speaking voice. After hearing the unintended phonation for speaking, the clinician counsels the patient, "Now your vocal folds sound like they are coming together well when you make that sound on the kazoo [or other voiced production]." This is usually followed by recording the phonation, such as the gargle or the "um-hmm," and then using it as the patient's beginning intentional voicing model.

Procedural Aspects of the Approach. The search for key phonations that can be redirected to the speaking voice for patients with functional aphonia or functional dysphonia is obviously highly individualized. While some patients will "uncover" phonation on nontalking tasks, many patients are never able to reveal any phonation, no matter what the task may be. Because there appears to be no preference for introduction of particular behaviors that may reveal phonation, we are listing alphabetically nine phonatory behaviors that have been reported as useful for redirecting phonation to the speaking voice:

1. ***Coughing.*** Asking the functional aphonic patient to cough has long been used to uncover a vegetative phonation that might be redirected to the "lost" speaking voice (Van Riper and Irwin, 1958). The patient produces a cough on command and is then instructed to prolong the cough with an extended vowel. See Chapter 3 for further description of ways to use the cough in searching for the voice in functional aphonia.

2. ***Gargling.*** The voice used in gargling can often be extended after the gargling ceases. During the gargle, the patient places the gargle solution in the mouth, tilts the head back, and agitates the solution in the back of the throat by making a prolonged expiratory phonation. The patient is asked to hold the gargle expiration for five seconds. Back vowels /k/ and /g/ are then introduced "on top" of the gargle. Keeping the same tilted upward head position, the patient is then asked to produce a "dry" prolonged gargle sound, using these back phonemes. The gargle voice is then redirected to communicative phonation practice materials.

3. ***Humming.*** An occasional dysphonic patient may develop a voice with less perturbation by humming a song. The clinician explains to the patient that "we are going to listen to a certain song you may know, and as we hear it, we'll hum together the tune we hear." If the patient can hum along, the humming should be recorded and

used as a possible target voice. In searching for the patient's best voice, we have on occasion found the voice during humming (and immediately afterward) as the best voice to build on in therapy.

4. *Laughing.* Humor and laughing can play an important part in voice therapy, particularly with the patient who displays excessive muscular tension while voicing. The typical patient does not realize that his or her laughter is a form of voicing. The laugh is recorded; presented on playback; and discussed from the points of view of pitch, loudness, and quality. Spontaneous laughter is usually relaxed and can provide for the patient a sharp contrast to a hyperfunctional voice, both in sound and overall body tension.

5. *Playing the comb or kazoo.* Occasionally, a patient with functional aphonia can produce voice while playing on a comb or blowing a tune through a kazoo. The aphonic patient may be unaware that his or her musical attempts when playing the comb or kazoo are producing vocal fold vibration, or voicing. The skilled SLP does not confront the patient with the discrepancy of a musical sound (voice) with no speaking voice. Instead, the patient is instructed to articulate a word (using nasal-glide words) "on top of" the tune being played. If this can be done, attempts are made to produce the same sounds without the tune of the comb or the kazoo.

6. *Singing.* Singing can sometimes be redirected as speaking voice phonation. Some patients with functional dysphonia present clearer voices with less perturbation while singing. If this can be demonstrated, an early therapy task is to combine singing and speaking by singing practice sentences. Similar to procedures used during chant-talk, the goal is to phase out the singing as a prelude to using the speaking voice. Efforts should be made, however, to continue using the improved breath control, ease of production, and better vocal quality that was used while singing.

7. *Throat clearing.* Many voice patients clear their throats continually in their search for clearer phonation. In fact, typical vocal hygiene programs eliminate habitual throat clearing as part of the program. For the functional aphonic patient, however, we may use throat clearing in our search for a speaking voice. If the aphonic patients can clear their throats, we ask them to do it with intention. Toward the end of the throat clearing, the patient is asked to continue the effort by prolonging a low back vowel. This vocalization is then used as a "starter sound" for production of monosyllabic words beginning with low back vowels. We have redirected a vegetative phonation into a speaking voice.

8. *Trilling.* For the typical person, producing a trill is a difficult task. If a voice patient can produce the trill, it can be a most helpful technique for developing a better voice. The trill is produced by the tongue tip on the alveolar ridge with the anterior tongue oscillating in the outgoing airstream. Colton and Casper (1996) have written, "The trill appears to 'jump start' the vibratory behavior of the vocal folds" (p. 289). For most voice patients, the trill seems to produce the best voice they are capable of making and is therefore useful in voice therapy for functional dysphonia and in improving the sound of the injured voice.

9. *Um-hmm.* We call um-hmm the voice of agreement. When person A is listening to person B in conversation, person A may agree with speaker B by saying "um-hmm" in an automatic, natural way. Much of Cooper's (1990) direct voice rehabilitation and training focuses on redirecting the patient's utterance of um-hmm into an easy and improved speaking voice. The voice produced by the um-hmm voice is reported by Cooper to be spoken at an appropriate pitch level with good facial mask resonance. We redirect this automatic phonation with dysphonic patients, using the um-hmm as a starter phonation, followed by other nasalized words, such as *um-hmm one, um-hmm man, um-hmm many,* on the same breath. Let the patient have an immediate auditory feedback of his or her um-hum productions by using a digitized playback system. Introduce phrases and sentences, monitoring the patient's productions to have the same pitch and quality heard on the single words.

Typical Case History Showing Utilization of the Approach. Sister Catherine was a 42-year-old nun who lost her voice while on a month-long renewal tour, during which she had to give daily lectures at a number of parochial schools. Subsequent laryngoscopy found her to have a normal larynx, and the speech-language pathologist found her to have "functional aphonia." Attempts at coughing and inhalation phonation were unsuccessful in early therapy attempts to help her "find" her voice. The gargle approach was introduced with immediate results. She was able to produce an expiratory phonation while gargling, with her head tilted back and her mouth wide open. The clinician rewarded her early gargle phonations with comments like "Now your cords are coming together." Catherine was reassured that her vocal folds could come together well and produce voice on expiration. After several repetitions with the gargle, voice was sustained without the need of gargling water. At the first therapy session, when gargle was successfully introduced, counseling and explanations about voice were all provided. Toward the end of the session, Catherine was able to produce good voice consistently by coupling her phonation attempts with chanting and the open-mouth approach. Within four therapy sessions, she reported having her normal voice back.

Evaluation of the Approach. In redirected phonation, the clinician searches with the patient to find some kind of voicing, such as coughing or playing a kazoo, then takes that phonation and redirects it into the speaking voice. For the patient with functional aphonia, the search for any kind of vocal fold vibration is often the first step in voice therapy. Any phonation uncovered is then applied to the speaking voice. The dysphonic patient has often adapted a number of poor voicing behaviors that might be better replaced by "um-hmm" or one of the other eight nonverbal phonations described here. Each behavior is made automatically by the patient, and once it has been redirected to the speaking voice, it is no longer needed. The search for nonverbal phonations is often part of the voice evaluation and is frequently used in the early phases of voice therapy. Once the patient resumes normal phonation, we find it very important to provide an audiovisual sample of the therapeutic intervention to the patient as soon as possible. We encourage the patient to use her smartphone to film the therapeutic session with the clinician. The patient performing the maneuvers him- or herself that is even more powerful (Bandura, 1986, 1997). If the patient does not have a smartphone, we film the session with a digital camera and provide a DVD of the session at the subsequent visit.

21. Relaxation

Kinds of Problems for Which the Approach Is Useful. It is not possible for most students, working adults, and retirees to have a world that is free of tension. As Eliot (1994) has written in describing the need for relaxation and a reduction in life's stresses, "When you can't change the world, you can learn to change your response to it" (p. 87).

Because encountering stress is part of the human condition, what becomes important is how we react to stress. Our patients with hyperfunctional voices often develop vocal symptoms as part of their stress reaction. Among the particular voice symptoms Boone (1997) related to stress are diplophonia, dry throat and mouth, harshness, elevated pitch, functional dysphonia, and shortness of breath. Accordingly, a frequent goal in voice therapy is to take the work out of phonation by using voice therapy techniques such as the open-mouth and yawn-sigh approaches along with symptomatic relaxation.

Symptomatic relaxation methods might well relax components of the vocal tract, but they may not lead to overall relaxation from stress reduction (Feldman, 1992). It is usually useless to imply to voice patients that if they would "just relax," their voice symptoms would lessen and their voices would improve. If our patients could relax, they would! The clinician must recognize that a certain amount of psychic tension and muscle tonus is normal and healthy; however, some individuals overreact to their environmental stresses and live with "a fast idle," expending far more energy and effort than a situation requires. When such psychic effort is causative or coupled with voice symptoms, some encouragement for increasing the patient's relaxation abilities is in order. By *relaxation*, we mean a realistic responsiveness to the environment with a minimum of needless energy expended.

Procedural Aspects of the Approach

1. For children, we develop an understanding of principles of relaxation, following some of the recommendations and materials offered by Wilson (1987) or Andrews and Summers (2002). For adults, it is helpful to have voice patients read the chapters on stress management and methods for reducing stage fright in Boone (1997) or read about posture and release in Brown (1996).

2. Introduce to the patient the concept of differential relaxation as outlined by Feldman (1992). The classical method of differential relaxation might be explained to the patient and applied. Under differential relaxation, the patient concentrates on a particular site of the body, deliberately relaxing and tensing certain muscles, discriminating between muscle contraction and relaxation. The typical procedure is to have the patient begin distally, away from the body, with the fingers or the toes. Once the patient feels the tightness of contraction and the heaviness of relaxation at the beginning site, he or she moves "up" the limb (on to the feet or hands, and thence to the legs or arms), repeating at each site the tightness–heaviness discrimination. Once the torso is reached, the voice patient should include the chest, neck, "voice box," throat, and the mouth and parts of the face. With some patients, we start the distal analysis with the head, beginning with the scalp and then going to the forehead, eyes, facial muscles, lips, jaw, tongue, palate, throat, larynx, neck, and so on. Some practice in this progressive relaxation technique can produce remarkably relaxed states in very tense patients.

3. Various biofeedback devices can help the patient develop a feeling of relaxation. Feedback such as galvanic skin response, pulse rate, blood pressure, and muscle responsiveness through electromyographic tracings all seem to correlate well with patients' feelings of anxiety and tension. By performing a particular relaxed behavior, such as yawning, a patient can confirm his or her particular arousal state by the biofeedback data. Using such biofeedback devices, the patient can soon learn what it feels like to be relaxed or free of tension.

4. Wolpe (1987) combines relaxation with hierarchy analysis. The patient responds to particular tension-producing cues with a relaxed response, such as feeling a heaviness or warmth at a particular body site, and maintains a relaxed response in the tension situation. The patient may instead develop a situational hierarchy specific to tension and voice by attempting to use a relaxed voice at increasingly tense levels of the hierarchy, as outlined in the adult voice program by Boone and Wiley (2000).

5. Head rotation might be introduced as a technique for relaxing components of the vocal tract. The patient sits in a backless chair, dropping the head forward to the chest. The patient then "flops" his or her head across to the right shoulder, then lifts it, then again flops it (the neck is here extended) along the back and across to the left shoulder. He or she then returns to the anterior head-down-on-chest position and repeats the cycle, rolling the head in a circular fashion. A few patients will not find head rotation relaxing, but most will feel the heaviness of the movement and experience definite relaxation in the neck. Once a patient in this latter group reports neck relaxation, he or she should be asked to phonate an "ah" as the head is rolled. The relaxed phonation might be recorded and then analyzed in terms of how it sounds in comparison to the patient's other phonations.

6. Open-throat relaxation can also be used. Have the patient lower the head slightly toward the chest and make an easy, open, prolonged yawn, concentrating on what the yawn feels like in the throat. The yawn should yield conscious sensations of an open throat during the prolonged inhalation. If the patient reports that he or she can feel this open-throat sensation, ask him or her to prolong an "ah," capturing and maintaining the same feeling experienced during the yawn. Any relaxed phonations produced under these conditions should be recorded and used as target voice models for the patient. Encourage the patient to comment on and think about the relaxed throat sensations experienced during the yawn.

7. Wilson (1987) includes an excellent presentation on various relaxation procedures for use with children, which seem to have equal applicability to adults. Most of the procedures described can immediately increase relaxation and reduce tension associated with speaking.

8. Ask the patient to think of a setting he or she has experienced, or perhaps imagined, as the ultimate in relaxation. Different patients use different kinds of imagery here. For example, one patient thought of lying in a hammock, but another person reacted to lying in a hammock with a set of anxious responses. Settings typically considered relaxing are lying on a rug at night in front of a blazing fire, floating on a lake, fishing while lying in a rowboat, lying down in bed, and so on. The setting the patient thinks of should be studied and analyzed; eventually, the patient should try to capture the relaxed feelings he or she imagines might result from, or may actually have been experienced in, such a setting. With some practice—and some tolerance for initial failure in recapturing the relaxed mood—the average patient can find a setting or two that he or she can re-create in his or her imagination to use in future tense situations.

Typical Case History Showing Utilization of the Approach. Mike, a 34-year-old missile engineer, developed transient periods of severe dysphonia when talking to certain people. At other times, particularly in his professional work, he experienced normal voice. Mirror laryngoscopy revealed a normal larynx. During the voice interview, the clinician noted the man's general nervousness and apparently poor self-concept. In exploring the area of interpersonal relationships, the patient confided that, in the past year, he had seen two psychiatrists periodically but had experienced no relief from his tension. Further exploration of the settings in which his voice was most dysphonic revealed that his biggest problem was talking to store clerks, garage mechanics, and persons who did physical labor; some of his more relaxed experiences included giving speeches and giving work instructions to his colleagues. Subsequent voice therapy included progressive relaxation. Once relaxed behavior was achieved, the patient developed a hierarchy of situations, beginning with those in which he felt most relaxed (giving instructions to colleagues) and proceeding to those in which he experienced the most tension (talking with car mechanics). After some practice, the patient was able to recognize various cues that signaled increasing tension. Once such a cue occurred, he employed a relaxation response, which more often than not enabled him to maintain normal phonation in situations that had previously induced dysphonia. As this consciously induced response continued to be successful, the patient reported greater confidence in approaching the previously tense situations, knowing he would experience little or no voice difficulty. Voice therapy was terminated after eleven weeks, when the patient reported only occasional difficulty phonating in isolated situations and increased self-confidence in all situations.

Evaluation of the Approach. The popularity of many relaxation and stress-reduction programs today is probably due in part to their offering people with excessive tensions some relief from their agonies. Symptomatic voice therapy focuses on faulty voices and sometimes the tensions associated with (if not the cause of) the vocal problems. A number of experienced voice clinicians (Glaze, 1996; Roy, 2008) have suggested that direct symptom modification, such as teaching relaxed responses to replace previously tense responses, breaks up the circular kind of response that often keeps maladaptive vocal behaviors "alive." In effect, we talk the same way today that we talked yesterday until we learn a better way to talk. Using the voice in a more relaxed manner with less competitive tension is a "better way to talk."

22. Respiration Training

Kinds of Problems for Which the Approach Is Useful. Singing teachers and vocal coaches often put more emphasis on respiration training for singers and actors than speech-language pathologists do for patients with voice disorders. While training in breath support is vital for the extremes of vocal performance produced by singers and actors, the typical patient with a functional voice disorder may need only some instruction for developing expiratory control (such as avoiding "squeezing" out final words of an utterance because of lack of adequate breath). Hoit (1995), in an excellent article summarizing studies of diaphragmatic–abdominal muscle physiology, makes a strong point for recognizing the difference in muscle function specific to whether the student or patient's body is supine or vertical. It would appear that increasing abdominal muscle participation while the patient is either sitting or standing has some relevance to the voice patient with vocal hyperfunction. Management of respiratory limitations related to neurogenic voice disorders and pulmonary disease are discussed in Chapters 5 and 8 of this text. The following procedures are useful with functional voice disorders when there is a demonstrated need to improve respiratory function for voice.

Procedural Aspects of the Approach

1. Provide the patient with a simple demonstration on how expiratory air can set up vibration. For example, place your lips gently together and blow through them, setting up a visual–aural demonstration. If the clinician has difficulty doing this, moistening the lips often facilitates the vibration and its audible sound. Continue with the explanation by discussing with the patient how outgoing air passes between the vocal folds, setting them into vibration, which we hear as voice.

2. After the patient is aware that the outgoing airstream sets the vocal folds in vibration to produce voice, a brief explanation of respiratory physiology is presented in words the patient can understand. For example, Case (2002) begins by saying in effect that as the chest gets bigger, the air comes into the lungs. As the chest becomes smaller, the air comes out, passing through the larynx. The steps for "getting bigger" and "getting smaller" are then described, often combined with demonstrations, with the patient practicing taking in a breath and letting the breath out slowly.

3. Demonstrate a slightly exaggerated breath, as used in sighing. The sigh begins with a slightly larger than usual inhalation (like a yawn) followed by a prolonged open-mouth exhalation, usually with light, breathy voice. Describe the type of breath used to produce the sigh as the "breath of well-being," the kind of easy breath one might take when comfortable or happy—the sigh of contentment. One of the authors (DRB) tells his patients to replicate "the kind of noise you make when you first see the Grand Canyon!"

4. Demonstrate the quick inhalation and prolonged exhalation needed for a normal speaking task. Take a normal breath and count slowly from one to five on one exhalation. See if the patient can do this; if he or she can, extend the count by one number at a time, at the rate of approximately one number per half-second. This activity can be continued until the patient is able to use the "best" phonation achieved during the number counts. Any sacrifice of voice quality should be avoided, and the number count should never extend beyond the point at which good quality can be maintained (Boone, 1997).

5. Various duration tasks, such as prolonging vowels, provide excellent practice in expiratory control. Prolonging an /s/, /z/, /a/, /å/, /æ/, or /i/ for as long as possible provides an expiratory measure that can be used for comparison. Take a baseline measurement in the beginning, such as number of seconds a particular phonation can be maintained, and see whether this can be extended with practice. Avoid asking the patient to "take in a big breath"; rather, ask him or her to take in a normal breath of well-being, initiating a lightly phonated sigh on exhalation. See if the patient can extend this for five seconds. If he or she can, progressively increase the extension to eight, 12, 15, and finally 20 seconds. The voice patient who can hold on to an extended phonation of a vowel for 20 seconds has certainly exhibited good breath control for purposes of voice. Such a patient would not have to work on breath control per se, but he or she might want to combine work on exhalation control with approaches such as hierarchy analysis (to see if he or she can maintain such good breath control under varying moments of stress) or breath-phrase coordination (that is, ensuring that the speaker takes in enough air to support a typical phrase without squeezing the glottis toward the end). It might help the patient to know that average spoken phrases are about eight words (Goldman-Eisler, 1968).

6. From various voice and articulation books, select reading materials designed to help develop breath control. Give special attention to the patient's beginning

phonation as soon after inhalation as possible to avoid wasting a lot of the outgoing airstream before phonating. Encourage the patient to practice quick inhalations between phrases and sentences, taking care not to take "a big breath."

7. With young children who need breathing work, begin with nonverbal exhalations. One way to work on breathing exhalation with little children is to use a pinwheel, which lends itself naturally to the game "How long can you keep the pinwheel spinning?" With practice, a child will be able to extend the length of his or her exhalations (the length of time the pinwheel spins). Another method of enhancing exhalation control is to place a piece of tissue paper against a wall, begin blowing on it to keep it in place when the fingers are removed, and keep blowing on it to see how long it can be kept in place. Both the pinwheel and tissue-paper exercises lend themselves to timing measurements. These measurements should be made and plotted graphically for the child; when a certain target length of time is reached, the activity can be stopped.

8. When working with a singer, actor, or lecturer who needs some formal respiration training, you might take the following steps:

   a. Avoid having the patient lie supine on his or her back for the purpose of observing abdominal protrusion on inhalation and abdominal retraction on expiration. As Hoit (1995) summarized, chest wall–abdominal muscle movements while supine are not the same as when sitting or standing in a vertical position. The only time we recommend watching supine abdominal movements is when the patient appears very tense; the tense patient may profit from watching the passive movements of the abdomen because the diaphragm's displacement moving toward the feet works to protrude the abdominal wall.

   b. Formal work on respiration requires good patient posture. Have the patient stand against a wall, with the buttocks and shoulders making some wall contact. Have the patient "stand tall," with the chin slightly tucked in as if the top of the head were suspended by a rope attached to the ceiling.

   c. Have the patient place one hand on the central abdomen and one hand laterally low on the rib cage (ninth through twelfth ribs). Instruct the patient to feel the abdomen and rib cage getting larger on inhalation. On exhalation, have them feel the abdomen tightening and the rib cage getting smaller. This exercise should be repeated as often as required to give the patient the awareness that the chest gets bigger on inhalation and it gets smaller on exhalation.

   d. The patient is encouraged to feel the abdomen tightening on expiration. Some practice should be given to following inhalation (accomplished primarily through chest wall expansion) by gradual tightening (contraction) of the abdominal muscles. As soon as the patient demonstrates some ability to contract the abdominal muscles on expiration, add phonation activities. The voice patient who has been speaking from the level of the throat, without adequate breath support, will feel the difference that a bigger breath makes when phonation is desired. The voice patient who needs respiration training in the first place must have respiration and phonation combined into practice activities as soon as possible.

   e. Ask the patient to prolong vowel sounds coupled with continuant-type consonants with and without abdominal muscle support. Provide immediate auditory feedback, such as by using a digital recorder, so that the patient can contrast the voice differences produced with and without abdominal support.

f. Develop with the patient the concept of increasing one's air volume by increasing chest expansion. Explain that with greater air volume available for expiration–phonation, it will be possible to say or sing more words per breath without squeezing or straining at the end of a phrase or sentence. It has been demonstrated (Plassman and Lansing, 1990) that subjects with perceptual cues (such as feeling chest wall expansion) can soon develop strategies to reproduce desired and greater lung volumes.

9. For serious problems in respiration, which are often related to diseases such as emphysema or bronchial asthma, the clinician should enlist the help of other specialists to help the patient improve efficiency. Physical therapists, respiratory therapists, and pulmonary medical specialists may have the expertise and pharmacologic means required to assist the patient. The voice clinician can often offer the patient ways of phrasing and using expiratory control to better match what the patient is trying to say and thus can supplement the intervention by these other specialists. For example, we have coordinated a breathing-for-speech program for quadriplegic patients, in which the speech pathologist and the physical therapist work closely with the patient to improve both general respiration and expiratory control for speech phrasing and better voice.

Typical Case History Showing Utilization of the Approach. Libby was a 45-year-old special education teacher who complained of vocal fatigue as a regular part of her teaching day. She felt that when she was not working, her voice was not a problem. Observation of Libby during her voice evaluation revealed that she often began to speak conversationally without an adequate inspiration. After five or six consecutive spoken words, her voice would become dysphonic and strained. Her voice problems seemed to occur when her air volumes were low and she was experiencing inadequate transglottal airflow. Subsequent voice therapy was designed to reduce the amount of work she was putting into vocalization and gave some priority to increasing her inspiratory volumes, reducing the number of words she attempted to speak on one breath, and teaching her to take catch-up breaths when she needed them. Loop recordings were used in therapy to monitor her breath support; she would read a 10-word sentence aloud and then immediately listen to a loop playback of the utterance, judging it for respiratory adequacy and lack of strain. After five weeks of twice-weekly voice therapy working on better respiratory control, Libby developed an easy phonatory style and a voice that served her well in her various life situations, including her teaching.

Evaluation of the Approach. A number of voice patients may profit from some kind of respiration training (Xu and colleagues, 1991; Silverman and colleagues, 2006; Van Lierde and colleagues, 2004). At the time of the initial voice evaluation, such patients may have done poorly on air-volume and pressure tests or exhibited poor expiratory control. Vocal attempts by such patients are often strained and involve too much effort; symptoms of vocal hyperfunction are common. A slight increase of inspiratory volume may produce an immediate effect of reducing vocal strain and improving overall vocal quality.

23. Tongue Protrusion /i/

Kinds of Problems for Which the Approach Is Useful. Many hyperfunctional voice problems are improved by the tongue-protrusion approach. This approach is especially helpful for patients with ventricular phonation (dysphonia plicae ventricularis) or "tightness" in the voice, such as when the laryngeal aditus (laryngeal collar) is held in a somewhat closed position. When the tongue is held in a posterior position or the pharyngeal constrictor muscles are contracted to constrict the pharynx, the voice sounds strained or "tight." A patient with such symptoms is asked to produce /i/ with the tongue extended outside the mouth (but not far enough to cause discomfort). This tongue-protrusion /i/ approach capitalizes on the physiology of the production of the /i/, whereby the tongue is shifted forward and raised toward the hard palate (Edwards, 2003). This works to offset the squeezing of the pharynx. The tongue must not protrude so far outside the mouth that it causes muscle strain in the area under the chin. The /i/ is produced in a high pitch either at the upper end of the patient's normal pitch range or at the lower end of the falsetto register. This approach can be used simultaneously with the glottal fry or the yawn-sigh.

Procedural Aspects of the Approach

1. Demonstrate to the patient what is expected by opening the mouth and protruding the tongue while producing a high-pitched, sustained /i/. Stress that the jaw is to drop open comfortably and that the tongue is to be extended comfortably. Many patients are reluctant, at first, to stick out the tongue in the presence of a stranger, so demonstrate and reassure them that this is just what you want. You may touch the patient's chin with the index finger to encourage a little wider jaw opening and say, "Roll the tongue out a little farther."

2. The patient should go up and down in pitch while sustaining the /i/ vowel, with the mouth open and the tongue out. Listen for improved vocal quality. When this is achieved, ask the patient to sustain the tone.

3. Have the patient chant "mimimimi" at this level with the tongue still out of the mouth. Then instruct the patient to slowly slip the tongue back into the mouth while continuing to produce the "mimimimi."

4. At this point, the pitch is usually still high. Demonstrating a sustained /i/ lowered by three steps from the pitch that the patient was producing often achieves a good quality on the first step or the first two steps, but a return to the poor voice may occur on the third step. Repeat the procedure, but only go down two steps. Sustain the second step. Repeat until the tone is established. You may need to return to the original open mouth and tongue protrusion if the target tone is lost.

5. When the new tone is established, gradually add words and phrases, for example, *be, pea, me, see the peach,* and *easy does it,* to the sustained /i/.

Typical Case History Showing Utilization of the Approach. Tammy, a 15-year-old girl, was referred with ventricular phonation of more than 18 months' duration. Her voice, which was consistently hoarse, rough, and low in pitch, was effortful to produce and made her sound like an older male speaker. Tammy had undergone a prolonged bout of flu prior to the onset of the ventricular voice, and she frequently coughed and cleared her throat violently. Strong glottal valving could be heard at times during connected speech. After seven sessions of individual voice therapy using the tongue-protrusion approach just described, Tammy's voice was normal in all situations at home, in school, and at work for the first time in more than 18 months.

Evaluation of the Approach. The tongue-protrusion /i/ approach appears to work because the tongue, when protruded, pulls its root out of the pharynx and opens the laryngeal aditus (Edwards, 2003). Also, the high pitch is made with a light, breathy approximation of only the true vocal cords. The production of voice with the tongue outside the mouth is sufficiently novel that it does not trigger the typical pattern of phonation that may have become habituated.

24. Visual Feedback

Kinds of Problems for Which the Approach Is Useful. With the advent of digitized audio-video feedback, there is great reliance on the device screen as a feedback device. For example, the patient can have a target F_0 line fixed on the screen, and the therapy task is to attempt to match the line with his or her same F_0 production. Converging of the lines is visual reinforcement of a "correct" production.

When we used various forms of auditory feedback as a VFA, we recognized that the auditory system may well depend on auditory feedback as a primary mode for modifying speech–language–voice behaviors. However, most voice patients also profit from receiving *visual feedback* relative to respiratory physiology, acoustic parameters of voice, and various digital feedback values (air volumes, pressure flow, F_0, percentage of nasal resonance, and so forth). For example, patients working on nasalance problems often profit from using the Nasometer™ (KayPENTAX Corp., Montvale, New Jersey), which provides real-time audiovisual feedback relative to the acoustic balance between oral and nasal resonance; the data generated by the Nasometer™ II can provide visual feedback specific to the success of increasing or decreasing one's nasal resonance. Visual feedback can provide the patient with data specific to his or her voice measurements, compared with the data found on the same vocal behaviors in the normal population. Visual feedback is valuable in voice therapy with any kind of patient who is working to improve or optimize vocalization.

Any of the evaluation instruments we use in our diagnostic voice evaluations that have visual screens, reference lines, or readouts can be used for visual feedback. In addition, with the client's permission, we regularly film the therapeutic part of the session using a digital camera or our laptops or smartphones, and send the session home with the client either via a DVD or a YouTube™ video. Audiovisual access to the intervention session provides good feedback for the patient or for the parents of a child with a voice problem who may see the child's voice progress as depicted visually. Providing visual feedback for the patient can play a prominent role in voice therapy.

Visual feedback has been studied scientifically by a number of researchers and is yielding promising results. Van Leer and Connor (2011) found increased client self-efficacy and compliance with intervention employing video augmentation.

Procedural Aspects of the Approach

1. Visual feedback instruments should be introduced to the patient. For respiration, any of the measuring devices for air volume and pressure flow described in Chapter 6 may be useful, particularly in comparing early performance with performance after therapy. Real-time measurements of respiration, such as how long one can prolong /s/, can be useful. Flexible videoendoscopy can provide the patient with visual confirmation of adequacy of velopharyngeal closure, pharyngeal and supraglottal participation during voicing, and/or detailed visualization of vocal fold movements. Stopping and restarting video playback provides visual feedback of actual oropharyngeal physiology.

2. The term *feedback* implies ongoing monitoring of some kind, giving back performance information to the patient as he or she is performing. Biofeedback (monitoring galvanic skin response, blood pressure, stress, etc.) is generally fed back to the patient visually, providing changing numeric values or changes in the pitch and amplitude traces on the screen. Some forms of biofeedback include tactual or proprioceptive monitoring, both of which have little relevance to voice feedback because both the pharynx and larynx are not particularly endowed with tactual or proprioceptive receptors. Acoustic and laryngeal physiology monitoring, when converted to visual images, can provide useful feedback, particularly when used jointly with another VFA. For example, look at Visi-Pitch tracings and perturbation numeric values when visually tracking voice production under deliberate changes in loudness (VFA number 2). Ask patients to match the visual feedback they may be seeing with the auditory feedback of what they have just said.

3. Real-time visual feedback of patient posture, head position, mouth opening, and other body positioning can be viewed in a mirror. Prior to the advent of computerized digitized feedback, much voice therapy was done with the clinician and the patient side by side in front of a mirror. Real-time posturing feedback can also be done with a video camera with a direct feed into a playback monitor, perhaps with a zoom close-up or a side view, which couldn't be accomplished by looking directly into a mirror. The best postural visual feedback is video playback. Particular posture positions, such as verticality of head or degree of mouth opening, are recorded and either played back immediately or deferred as feedback later in the therapy session.

4. Many computer-assisted clinical software programs have vital visual feedback available for patients of all ages. For example, the KayPENTAX Corp. (Montvale, New Jersey) software modules provide real-time portrayals (digital, line tracings, and animations) for voice parameters such as pitch or loudness. Among many other acoustic modules is the visual feedback available in the Computerized Speech Lab™ (CSL) software programs (KayPENTAX, Montvale, New Jersey), which permit looking at 22 parameters of a single vocalization and then comparing the data with built-in threshold results.

5. The SLP can find an endless number of software programs that provide visual feedback on some aspect of voice performance. However, try to use only those programs that provide some ongoing auditory feedback coupled with visual feedback.

Typical Case Showing Utilization of the Approach. Bill was a 21-year-old college student with vocal nodules and a severe dysphonia. At the time of his voice evaluation, it was found that he spoke at the very bottom of his pitch range. When he elevated pitch two or three notes, his voice became remarkably clearer. Using the Visi-Pitch, we were able to set pitch boundaries within which we wanted him to practice. If he dropped his voice too low, he could see his tracing go below our target lines. Jitter and shimmer values dropped considerably near B2 on the virtual keyboard app, which we used as a target pitch. Bill profited from his clinical practice on the Visi-Pitch, which provided him with immediate visual feedback relative to both his pitch usage and the perturbation values that shifted with the pitch of his voice. Audio-video feedback, as provided by a smartphone app, was also effective for Bill in practicing an easy glottal attack with a slightly higher voice pitch. At the end of eight weeks of twice-weekly voice therapy, endoscopic examination found Bill to have "a normal larynx, free of vocal nodules."

Evaluation of the Approach. As instrumentation is developed that can portray various aspects (respiration–phonation–resonance) of voice, it can play an important role in providing visual feedback to patients (see Ju and colleagues, 2011; Rizzo and Kim, 2005). Once a target behavior has been isolated for a patient, such instrumentation can provide ongoing feedback on the appropriateness of patient production. Feedback presents various visual portrayals (values of frequency, jitter, shimmer, and so forth) of what the patient is hearing. Various facilitating efforts in therapy often produce changes in the sound of voices that are confirmed by different feedback devices. Not to be forgotten for visual feedback is the mirror, especially for those who have adopted a limited mouth-opening manner of voicing and speaking. Once an optimal voicing pattern has been established, the use of feedback devices is no longer necessary.

25. Yawn-Sigh

Kinds of Problems for Which the Approach Is Useful. The yawn-sigh is one of the most effective therapy techniques for minimizing the tension effects of vocal hyperfunction. In vocal hyperfunction, we characteristically see the larynx rise, the tongue lifted high and forward, the vocal folds tightly compressed, and the pharynx constricted (Boone and McFarlane, 1993). The yawn-sigh provides a dramatic contrast: The larynx drops to a low position, the tongue is more forward, there is a slight opening between the vocal folds, and the pharynx is usually dilated. The yawn-sigh is frequently combined with other therapy approaches for problems such as functional dysphonia; spasmodic dysphonia; and dysphonias related to thickening, vocal fold nodules, and polyps. Any patient who might profit from a lower, more relaxed carriage of the larynx is a candidate to receive laryngeal massage as outlined in VFA15 or to use the yawn-sigh approach. The yawn-sigh approach also allows the patient to become more independent in reducing vocal hyperfunction because once the client has demonstrated independence with this approach, he or she does not require clinician intervention, as do a number of the laryngeal massage maneuvers described previously.

Procedural Aspects of the Approach

1. With children, explain this approach using the pictures and narrative from Boone (1993). Showing a child the appropriate pictures, we read:

> This girl usually has a tight mouth. She uses too much effort when she speaks. Her voice does not sound good. (Demonstrate) This girl is opening her mouth wide and yawning. She is very relaxed. When she sighs at the end of the yawn, it will be her best voice. (p. 141)

2. With teenagers and adults, explain generally the physiology of a yawn; that is, a yawn represents a prolonged inspiration with maximum widening of the supraglottal airways (characterized by a wide, stretching opening of the mouth). Then demonstrate a yawn and talk about what the yawn feels like.

3. After the patient yawns, following your example, ask the patient to yawn again and then to exhale gently with a light phonation. In doing this, many patients are able to feel an easy phonation, often for the first time.

4. Once the yawn–phonation is easily achieved, instruct the patient to say words beginning with /h/ or with open-mouthed vowels, one word per yawn in the beginning, eventually four or five words on one exhalation.

5. With teenage and adult clients, yawn-sigh exercises are available, with explanations that the patient can read in Boone (1997, pp. 121–126).

6. Demonstrate for the patient the sigh phase of the exercise, that is, the prolonged, easy, open-mouthed exhalation after the yawn. Then, omitting the yawn entirely, demonstrate a quick, normal, open-mouthed inhalation followed by the prolonged open-mouthed sigh.

7. As soon as the patient can produce a relaxed sigh, have him or her say the word *hah* after beginning the sigh. Follow this with a series of words beginning with the glottal /h/. Additional words for practice after the sigh should begin with middle and low vowels. Take care to blend in, toward the middle of the sigh, an easy, relaxed, relatively soft phonation. This blending of the phonation into the sigh is often difficult for the patient initially, but it is the most vital part of the approach for the elimination of hard glottal contacts.

8. Once the yawn-sigh approach is well developed, have the patient think of the relaxed oral feeling it provides. Eventually, he or she will be able to maintain a relaxed phonation simply by imagining the approach.

Typical Case History Showing Utilization of the Approach. Jerry, a 47-year-old manufacturer's representative, had a two-year history of vocal fatigue. He often lost his voice toward the end of the workday. After a two-week period of increasing dysphonia and slight pain on the left side of the neck, an ENT physician found that Jerry had "slight redness and edema on both vocal processes." The subsequent voice evaluation also found that he spoke with pronounced hard glottal attack in an attempt to "force out his voice over his dysphonia." Using the yawn-sigh approach, Jerry was able to demonstrate a clear phonation with relatively good resonance. His yawn-sigh phonations were recorded on loop and fed back to him as the voice model he should imitate. Because Jerry reported some stress in certain work situations, the hierarchy analysis approach was used to isolate those situations in which he felt relaxed and those in which he experienced tension. Thereafter, whenever he was aware of tense situational cues, he employed the yawn-sigh approach to maintain relaxed phonation. Combining yawn-sigh with hierarchy analysis proved to be an excellent symptomatic approach for this patient because his voice cleared markedly, and no recurrence of the periodic aphonia was evident. Twice-weekly therapy was terminated after 12 weeks, and the patient demonstrated a normal voice and a normal laryngeal mechanism.

Evaluation of the Approach. The yawn-sigh is a powerful voice therapy technique for patients with vocal hyperfunction (Blonigen, 1994; Brewer and McCall, 1974; Xu and colleagues, 1991; Boone and McFarlane, 1993). During the yawn-sigh, the pharynx is dilated and relaxed. When the patient is asked to sigh an /i/ or an /a/, the voice comes out with little effort and sounds relaxed. For some patients with continued vocal hyperfunction, the voice produced on the sigh will feel relaxed, in dramatic contrast to the patient's normally tense voice.

SUMMARY

We have included 25 Voice Facilitating Approaches (VFAs) that can be used in symptomatic voice therapy. We have provided extensive documentation of peer-reviewed evidence to support each approach. Most VFAs can be used individually; there is clinical advantage to combining certain approaches together with particular patients. For example, a typical voice therapy session might include counseling, use of the confidential voice, head positioning, visual feedback, and the yawn–sigh, combined or used sequentially. Voice therapy for most voice problems requires continuous assessment of what the patient is able to do vocally. The selection of which therapy approach to use is highly individualized for the particular patient, and no one approach is helpful for the same voice problem with every patient.

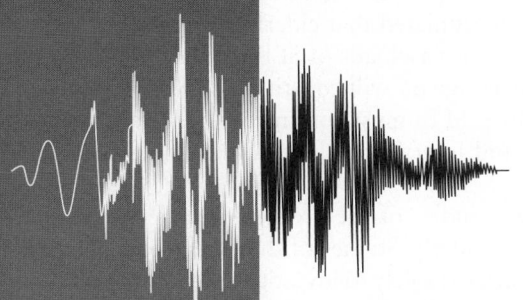

CHAPTER 8

Therapy for Special Patient Populations

After reading this chapter, one should be able to:

- Understand the laryngeal and voice characteristics of the aging voice and describe its management.

- Understand the laryngeal and voice characteristics of pediatric dysphonia, and describe its management.

- List the professional voice use populations who are at risk for dysphonia, and describe the management of dysphonia in these populations.

- Describe the speech and voice characteristics of the Deaf and Hard of Hearing populations and approaches to these behaviors.

- Discuss the speech and voice management approaches to the transgender populations.

- Describe respiratory-based voice problems and management.

- Describe paradoxical vocal fold movement and its management.

$\mathbf{W}$e have reviewed various voice disorders in Chapters 3 through 5: functional/behavioral, organic, and neurogenic. In this chapter, however, we consider special voice conditions and their treatment that do not necessarily fall under the headings provided in previous chapters. We will provide descriptions of the voice problems, with focus given to management strategies and the use of possible Voice Facilitating Approaches. Laryngeal cancer and its management by the speech-language pathologist (SLP) is presented in Chapter 9. Resonance disorders and their management are presented in Chapter 10.

VOICE THERAPY FOR PARTICULAR POPULATIONS

The Aging Voice

About one in every eight Americans is 65 years or older, and this number is increasing as the baby boom generation grows older (U.S. Bureau of the Census, 2010). This group represents the fastest growing segment of the U.S. population, with the over-85 group showing the largest percentage increase of any population segment (Barry and Eathorne, 1994). It has been estimated that elderly clients with communication impairments constitute 19% of the caseloads of SLPs (Slater, 1992). By the year 2050, it is expected that people over age 65 will constitute 39% of the speech-language impaired population. Therefore, SLPs must continually seek new methods of prevention, differential diagnosis, and intervention with older adults (Shadden and colleagues, 2011).

There are very few epidemiologic studies of the prevalence, risk factors, and psychosocial impact of dysphonia in the elderly. Studies of the epidemiology of dysphonia in this population have been restricted solely to investigations of those seeking treatment; thus, the true prevalence of voice disorders in the general elderly population remains largely unknown. Roy and colleagues (2007) interviewed 117 people over age 65 using a questionnaire that addressed three areas related to voice disorders: prevalence, potential risk factors, and psychosocial consequences/effects. They reported that the lifetime prevalence of a voice disorder in this population was 47%, with 29% of participants reporting a current voice disorder (Roy and colleagues, 2007, p. 628). The majority of respondents (60%) reported chronic voice problems persisting for at least four weeks. Seniors who had experienced esophageal reflux, severe neck/back injury, and chronic pain were at increased risk. Voice-related effort and discomfort, increased anxiety and frustration, and the need to repeat oneself were specific areas that adversely affected quality of life. In a similar epidemiologic study of persons under the age of 65, Roy and colleagues (2005, p. 1998) reported that the lifetime prevalence of a voice disorder was 30%, with 6% of participants reporting a current voice disorder (see also Cohen and Turley, 2009; Golub and colleagues, 2006). Cohen and colleagues (2012a) reported that adults over the age of 70 years were two and a half times more likely than those under the age of 70 years to be diagnosed with a voice disorder; in fact, adult males over the age of 70 years were the most likely persons to experience a voice disorder. The risk of an elderly person having a voice disorder is greater if the person also has a hearing loss, and having either disorder is more likely to lead to depression (Cohen and Turley, 2009).

The term *presbyphonia* refers to the clinical condition of elderly patients presenting to the otolaryngologist (ENT) with gradual weakening of the voice (Kendall, 2007, p. 137). Patients complain of an inability to project their voice over background noise and of a hoarse voice quality that deteriorates throughout the day. Visual examination of the larynx may reveal mild bowing of the vocal fold margins, a spindle-shaped glottis, prominent arytenoid cartilage vocal processes, and vocal fold edema (Bloch and Behrman, 2001; Pontes and colleagues, 2005). Laryngostroboscopy may reveal asymmetry of vocal fold vibration, and electroglottography may reveal predominance of the open phase (Winkler and Sendlmeier, 2006). High-speed digital imaging reveals more anteriorly placed glottal gaps (Ahmad and colleagues, 2012). Presbyphonia is correlated with poorer health-related quality of life and a tendency to avoid social situations (Costa and Matias, 2005; Golub and colleagues, 2006; Verdonck-de Leeuw and Mahieu, 2004; Plank and colleagues, 2011).

Presbyphonia is not the most common cause of dysphonia in the elderly. Possible other causes of dysphonia include: vocal fold atrophy (with or without vocal fold bowing), benign vocal fold lesions, laryngitis, malignant vocal fold lesions, muscle tension dysphonia, tremor, spasmodic dysphonia, and vocal fold immobility. A recent examination of 775 patients over the age of 65 years with dysphonia by Davids and colleagues (2012) indicated that vocal fold atrophy was the most common cause of dysphonia, comprising 25% of cases, followed closely by spasmodic dysphonia (23%) and vocal fold immobility (19%). A thorough evaluation is warranted in any elderly patient presenting with hoarseness. Poor general health correlates to negative objective vocal and laryngeal changes, showing that *physiologic* age may be a greater factor than *chronologic* age in some patients with dysphonia. Considering this information, one might well conclude that management and therapy should be more focused on *various disease processes* than on *aging per se*.

Because the acoustic features of voice are affected by respiratory, phonatory, and resonance events, each must be appreciated when developing an understanding of the presbyphonia voice (Baken, 2005; Ringel and Chodzko-Zajko, 1987). The first comprehensive studies reporting age-related changes in speech breathing were conducted in the late 1980s by Hoit and colleagues (1987; 1989). Across these two seminal studies the investigators examined speech breathing in 30 males and 30 females in three age groups (25, 50, 75 years). Speech breathing changes were assessed both from extemporaneous speech and reading. The major findings of Hoit and Hixon (1987) were that elderly males demonstrated larger rib cage volume initiations, larger lung volume excursions, and larger lung volume expenditures per syllable than younger men, particularly during extemporaneous speaking. The major findings of Hoit and colleagues (1989) were that, compared to younger women, elderly females demonstrated larger rib cage excursions during reading, increased frequency of inhalation during reading, increased air expenditure during unphonated intervals during reading, and larger lung volume initiations during extemporaneous speaking. The speech breathing changes reported by Hoit and her colleagues correspond with reports that changes in general pulmonary functioning with aging become measurable at around age 40 years (Rochet, 1991).

Much of what we know about the acoustic characteristics of the voice of older speakers comes from the work of Linville and her colleagues (see Linville, 2001) and Mueller and his colleagues (see Caruso and Mueller, 1997) (see Table 8.1). Many of their findings correlate well with what we know about the effects of aging on the

TABLE 8.1 Synopsis of Voice Changes with Advanced Age

Finding	Literature Source
Speaking fundamental frequency (SFF) raises in men and lowers in women.	Awan (2006); Brown, Morris, Hollien, and Howell (1991); Linville (1996); Xue and Deliyski (2001).
Maximum phonational frequency range (MPFR) is reduced in men and women.	Hollien, Dew, and Phillips (1971); Linville (1987); Ptacek and Sander (1966); Ramig and Ringel (1983).
SFF is less stable in men and women.	Linville, Skarin, and Fornatto (1989); Xue and Deliyski (2001).
Amplitude is less stable in men and women.	Linville (1996); Linville, Skarin, and Fornatto (1989); Xue and Deliyski (2001).
Standard deviations of SFF and amplitude increase in men and women.	Linville and Fisher (1985); Orlikoff (1990); Xue and Deliyski (2001).
Maximum intensity of vowel productions is reduced in men and women.	Morris and Brown (1994).
Perturbation increases (jitter, shimmer, spectral noise) in men and women.	Awan (2006); Decoster and Debruyne (1987); Ferrand (2002); Linville (2002); Linville, Skarin, and Fornatto (1989); Xue and Deliyski (2001)
Formant frequencies are lowered in men.	Benjamin (1997); Linville (2002); Linville and Fisher (1985); Linville and Rens (2001); Liss, Weismer, and Rosenbek (1990); Rastatter and Jacques (1990); Scukanec, Petrosino, and Squibb (1991).

larynx and supraglottal vocal tract. See Kahane and Beckford (1991) for extensive review of this topic.

In both men and women, speaking fundamental frequency (SFF) changes as an individual moves from young adulthood into old age. However, the pattern of change is quite different for the two genders: SFF in men lowers from young adulthood into middle age and then rises again into old age; in women, SFF remains fairly constant into middle age, then drops slightly and remains unchanged through old age. Maximum phonational frequency range (MPFR) also appears to be altered by the process of aging. Postmenopausal (presumably, middle-age) women are able to produce lower basal tones than their younger or older counterparts; however, this does not significantly expand total MPFR capabilities. At the other end of the MPFR, a reduction in the ceiling tone is a well-known finding in female speakers, even for those who have had professional voice training. In men, there does not appear to be an effect of aging on MPFR. Fundamental frequency and amplitude are reported to be less stable in older speakers; the standard deviations of these measures also tend to increase with age. Increased perturbation (that is, jitter, shimmer, spectral noise) in the voice of aging speakers has also been reported. Speech intensity has also been reported to change with aging. Vocal intensity during conversational speech has been reported to increase with aging in men, but not in women, and in both genders, reductions of maximum intensity of vowel productions has been reported.

Resonance characteristics of voice vary as a function of aging as well. Centralization of vowels is reported to be a common tendency of older speakers, and as a result, formant frequencies of vowels have been shown to differ in older versus younger speakers (Liss and colleagues, 1990). Lengthening of the vocal tract in older speakers is also thought to contribute to changes in formant frequencies (Kahane, 1981), chiefly a lowering of these frequencies across vowels (Linville and Rens, 2001). In addition to investigations into the effects of aging on formant frequencies, the effect of aging on nasal resonance has been investigated, though not as extensively. Hutchinson and colleagues (1978) reported that nasalance (see Chapter 10) in 50- to 80-year-old speakers is higher than the norms of younger speakers reported by Fletcher (1973). Scarsellone and colleagues (1999) reported slightly lower nasalance in elderly speakers when their maxillary dentures were removed versus when these dentures were in place, leading these investigators to conclude that existing normative data for nasalance could be applied to elderly speakers regardless of the status of their maxillary dentition.

Some general characteristics of the voices of elderly people lead to their identification as older speakers. A number of studies going back to the 1960s have demonstrated a relationship between older speakers' chronological age, sex, and vocal characteristics, and listener perceptions of their vocal age (Linville and Fisher, 1985; Ryan and Burk, 1974; Shipp and Hollien, 1969). From this clinical literature, a number of conclusions can be drawn. First, young adult listeners are capable of discriminating between younger and older adult voices with a high degree of accuracy (Huntley and colleagues, 1987; Ptacek and Sander, 1966), though listeners tend to slightly overestimate the age of younger speakers and underestimate the age of older speakers (Ryan and Capadano, 1978). Second, young adults are also quite good at distinguishing relatively minor differences in ages of older speakers, for example, distinguishing among 60-, 70-, and 80-year-olds (Hummert and colleagues, 1999). Third, young adults have a better than chance ability to estimate within five years a speaker's chronological age (Hollien, 1987). Fourth, listeners are able to reasonably estimate an older speaker's weight and height from their voice, and can do so almost as well as they can from viewing facial photos (Krauss and colleagues, 2002). Listeners perceive older speakers more negatively than younger speakers, particularly on competence dimensions (Hummert and colleagues, 1999).

Tremor, hoarseness, breathiness, voice breaks, decreased loudness, slower speaking rate, and a change in habitual pitch are specific acoustic characteristics that have been identified in perceptual studies of the elderly voice of both males and females (see Ramig and Ringel [1983] and Gorham-Rowan and Laures-Gore [2006] for reviews). The changes in habitual pitch, however, appear to be sex-dependent. In middle-age males, an increase in habitual pitch seems to signal advancing age, while in middle-age (postmenopausal) women, a decrease in habitual pitch signals advancing age. These acoustic cues are likely the product of age-related physiological changes to the vocal tract. Some of the physiological changes that have been identified include the lengthening of the vocal tract or oral cavity, reduction in pulmonary function, laryngeal cartilage ossification, increased stiffening of the vocal folds, and reduction in vocal fold closure (see Zraick and colleagues [2006] for a review).

Management of presbyphonia can involve three treatment approaches, either singly or in combination: (1) laryngoplasty, (2) thyroplasty, and (3) voice therapy (Johns and colleagues, 2011). Voice therapy is usually the first-line approach. Strengthening exercises for respiratory and phonatory control likely increase neuromuscular coordination. Stemple and Thomas (2007) have reported that vocal function exercises may improve a patient's laryngeal physiology, potentially improving voice. Counseling the patient about the need for good vocal hygiene may be helpful. Direct work on improving respiratory efficiency can help the older person develop better expiratory control, perhaps saying more words per breath. Direct work on increasing the speed of one's speech can have a "rejuvenating" effect on the sound of the older patient's voice. Among other VFAs we have found useful are auditory feedback, focus, glottal fry, masking, respiration training, and visual feedback (see Chapter 7). Berg and colleagues (2008) have reported that voice-related quality of life improves in patients with age-related dysphonia who participate in voice therapy. If a patient fails voice therapy, procedures to improve glottic closure may be employed. Such procedures are often used to manage vocal fold paralysis (see Chapter 5) and include laryngoplasty and medialization thyroplasty. Future treatments holding promise include the use of gel-based injectable materials for vocal fold regeneration (Bartlett and colleagues, 2012).

CHECK YOUR KNOWLEDGE

1. List three age-related anatomical/physiological changes that account for the sound of the aging voice.
2. Describe four auditory-perceptual features of the older person's voice.

Pediatric Voice Problems

As noted in Chapter 1, it is estimated that more than 7.5 million American children have some trouble using their voices (National Institute for Deafness and Other Communication Disorders, 2007). Dysphonia can be detrimental to children both psychosocially and academically. In the psychosocial realm, studies have revealed that childhood dysphonia has an adverse effect on the listener's perception of the child: Children are judged more negatively with regard to their physical appearance, their personality, and their cognitive skills by peers and adolescent and adult judges (Ruscello and colleagues, 1988), including teachers (Ma and Yu, 2009). It is possible

Elimination of abuses is critical not only to the vocal health of older individuals, but across the life span. This **video** introduces silent cough and sniff-swallow, two techniques that are designed to replace coughing and throat clearing. Grand Rounds: Describe the physiology of silent cough that reduces the collisionary forces of the vocal folds.

for children to express themselves about the impact of their voice disorder (Verduyckt and colleagues, 2011). Connor and colleagues (2008, p. 197) have shown that the attitudes of children and adolescents with dysphonia can be negative. In their interviews with children with dysphonia, these clinical researchers discovered that children and adolescents often felt that their dysphonic voice received undue attention; anger, sadness, and frustration were also expressed.

Academically, some adverse effects of dysphonia on a child's educational performance can include limited participation in speaking activities, fear of participating in oral reading activities, and limited participation in classroom discussion with peer groups. To address reduced academic performance as a function of dysphonia, Hoffman and colleagues (2004) describe eligibility decisions for students with dysphonia in school-based settings that fall within the framework of the Individuals with Disabilities Education Act (IDEA). These authors outline six school-based service delivery options for the voice-disordered child that are effective under IDEA guidelines (see also Chapter 6).

Children differ from adults in the way they produce their voice because pediatric laryngeal anatomy is distinct from adult laryngeal anatomy. As described in Chapter 2, among those differences are the size of the larynx; the proportion of membranous versus cartilaginous structure; and the position of the larynx, which in the child lies between the first and third cervical vertebrae, descending to between the sixth and seventh cervical vertebrae in the adult. The differences in anatomy are evident in the physiology of the voice. The child may find that his or her smaller lung capacity and resonating chambers in relation to an adult's render a voice that is softer and less versatile than the adult's (Sapienza and Stathopoulos, 1994). The child may try to compensate for this by placing excessive demands on the voice, thus beginning a cycle of muscle tension dysphonia, potentially leading to vocal nodules (Schalen and Rydell, 1995; Boyle, 2000).

Medical Factors Associated with Pediatric Voice Disorders. Most etiologies underlying dysphonia in children are benign and generally easy to treat (McMurray, 2003); however, children presenting with hoarse voices must have a thorough voice evaluation because some voice disorders are life-threatening (see Chapter 4 and Voice Therapy for Respiratory-Based Voice Problems later in this chapter). Dysphonia, such as that experienced from laryngeal papilloma, can present a significant and fatal airway obstruction. Cysts, while not life-threatening, can cause dysphonia by increasing the mass of the vocal fold. Chapter 6 features a medical history checklist to help the clinician zero in on the factor or factors that might underlie a dysphonia. For example, repeated otitis media and sinusitis might underlie allergies or laryngopharyngeal reflux. In fact, laryngopharyngeal reflux disease (LPRD) is increasingly recognized as a factor underlying pediatric dysphonia (Block and Brodsky, 2007). Laryngeal symptoms associated with pediatric LPRD include chronic cough, globus sensation, throat clearing, and laryngospasm (Karkos and colleagues, 2006). More atypical reflux symptoms reported in the literature are stridor (Heatley and Swift, 1996), paradoxical vocal fold motion (Wilson and colleagues, 2009), sinus infection (Phipps and colleagues, 2000), otitis media (Kotsis and colleagues, 2009), and subglottic stenosis. Even though accurate diagnosis of LPRD in children is challenging (Theis and Heatly, 2009), LPRD should be considered by ENTs, pulmonologists, gastroenterologists, and SLPs in the differential diagnosis and subsequent management of pediatric voice disorders (Ford, 2005).

The SLP should also ask about the amount of hydration the child is taking in because poor water intake in combination with caffeinated beverages may pull fluid from the body (Glaze, 1996). Any psychosocial and emotional aspects affecting the child at home, in school, or elsewhere also need to be addressed because there are links between psychological and musculoskeletal stress (Russell and colleagues, 2010). We once encountered a young teen who developed significant hypertension of the lips, cheeks, and neck muscles and larynx each time her mother changed her work schedule and left the teen in charge of her younger siblings. The Voice Facilitating Approaches in Chapter 7 were effective in rediscovering the voice within the first few minutes, but it was the underlying psychosocial demands on the teen that were the major issue. In this case, we referred the family to a child psychiatrist for counseling.

Functional Factors Associated with Pediatric Voice Disorders. Once a medical cause is ruled out, and the child has been diagnosed with a voice disorder of a functional nature, it is the realm of the SLP, the family, educators, and other individuals important to the child's life to identify the environments in which the abuse-misuse occurs and to develop strategies to reduce these instances of misuse (see Chapter 7). If the child is very young, say, younger than 5 years of age, parent counseling may be in order. Direct voice therapy with the child may be deferred until the preschooler is cognitively able to understand the importance of curbing particular hyperfunctional behaviors, such as yelling and making continuous "funny" noises. The primary voice management role in the preschool child is the identification and possible treatment of laryngeal disease rather than as a preliminary evaluative step for voice therapy.

> We often pair children in therapy because it encourages them to actively listen to and describe each other's vocal quality in terminology that is easy to understand and generalize outside of the clinic. Watch this **video** to see how these children engage in constructive feedback of each other's vocal quality. Grand Rounds: Describe one biofeedback activity that you might implement for a child dyad voice therapy session.

For older children, successful voice clinicians must build into their schedules actual visits to playgrounds, music rooms, churches, and other venues where the child spends his or her day. The overall thrust of voice therapy for vocal hyperfunction in school-age children is identifying their voice abuses and voice misuse (see VFA #8 in Chapter 7) and reducing the occurrence of such behaviors. More than once, we have discovered that the vocal misuse originates in the child's classroom itself. Much has been written about the occupational hazards of teaching; it comes as no surprise that vocal abuse and overuse might be identified in classrooms, which are notorious for poor acoustics and robust dynamics (McAllister and colleagues, 2009). When we encounter a classroom situation that appears to be contributing to a dysphonia, we contact the teacher and ask him or her to enlist as a partner in a vocal education and hygiene program. The teacher often views this program as an immediate benefit for all concerned, and we help the teacher adapt a list of behaviors and rationales that discourage vocal abuse and encourage just right voice, the child's equivalent of confidential tone. One classroom teacher even allowed our graduate students to enter the classroom and engage the children in a play depicting healthy and unhealthy voices. The play concluded with the following list of reminders to maintain a healthy voice in the future:

1. Build quiet times into one's day.
2. Walk over to a friend to talk.
3. Drink plenty of water.
4. Select a just right voice buddy to help maintain those good vocal habits.

In our voice clinics, we review the anatomy and physiology of the laryngeal mechanism using DVDs and Internet-based content, although still photographs are also powerful visual tools to aid the patient's comprehension. We use age-appropriate descriptive terminology to discuss the mechanics of normal voice and vocal abuse. Some examples we use are discussing the soreness and redness of palms after clapping hands forcefully and asking the child to describe what his or her vocal folds would feel like if they clapped all day. We attempt to video-record the child interacting with his family in free play or discussion. We review the video and discuss pitch, loudness, and vocal quality. This audio and video feedback indirectly draws everyone's attention to the distinctive qualities of voice, and the child and the family can begin to talk about voice using the same language.

A specific approach that we have found successful with children is making every attempt to pair child voice clients in therapy (Von Berg and McFarlane, 2002a). This arrangement has been found to be conducive to early and lasting success. At the beginning of the therapy session, unstimulated acoustic measures are collected from each child using the Visi-Pitch (KayPENTAX Corp., Montvale, New Jersey) or similar instrumentation. If the clinic does not have this type of instrument, a digital voice recorder or smartphone application is sufficient. The children listen to their voices and discuss any changes from the previous session. The children discuss vocal parameters using the same terminology developed during the audio- and video-recording of the family session discussed earlier. Each child is challenged to describe techniques that might move the voice closer to a just right voice. Voice Facilitating Approaches are introduced, and each is followed by a child production, using a novel phrase-generating task. The children analyze each other's productions, which is a powerful way to increase each child's understanding of her or his dysphonia and how to improve vocal quality. We often audio-record and immediately replay these sessions because the children are motivated to critique and repair their own dysphonia.

In Chapter 7, we identify the various biofeedback technologies currently available to support voice intervention in the general population; these technologies are also available for pediatric voice intervention. Readers are encouraged to investigate innovative approaches that employ virtual reality (Hapner and Johns, 2004; King and colleagues, 2011) and video self-modeling (Bandura, 1997).

CHECK YOUR KNOWLEDGE

1. List and describe three medical factors that can contribute to a child having a voice disorder.
2. List and describe three environmental factors that can contribute to a child having a voice disorder.

Professional Voice Users

In this **video**, we see that the act of chewing encourages an overall relaxation of the jaw, neck and laryngeal muscles for those patients with vocal hyperfunction. Many patients consider it a one-size-fits all tension reducer. Grand Rounds: Investigate Brodnitz' and Froeschel's reflexive chewing theory.

The professional user of voice exerts unusual demands on respiration, phonation, and resonance. We use the term *professional voice user* for the actor, singer, teacher, salesperson, minister, telemarketer, politician, broadcaster—people whose primary occupational competence (and probable success) is shaped by their voices. Their success in using their voices is always competing with demands of excessive phonation, background noise, and environmental pollution (Bovo and colleagues, 2007). The SLP may begin a vocal hygiene program designed for awareness of avoiding excessive phonation time and making attempts to reduce competing background noise. However, Holmberg and colleagues (2001) have found that a vocal hygiene program alone is not always associated with a good voice. It appears that a vocal hygiene program needs to be coupled with some vocal instruction provided by a vocal coach, singing teacher, or SLP to help the professional voice user maintain a functional professional voice (Hazlett and colleagues, 2011).

One of the obstacles we experience in working with the professional voice user is the relative "performance innocence" of the teacher or clinician. The professional uses his or her voice often beyond the normal limits we generally associate with heavy voice use. The SLP who has never performed beyond these supposed limitations may experience difficulty convincing the performer about what to do to correct a voice problem. Similar to the voice clinician who wants to communicate with the voice scientist or the scientist who likes to dabble clinically, the SLP's "performance naiveté" may be revealed to the professional performer once the SLP strays beyond his or her zone of training and competence.

Another obstacle to working successfully with the professional voice user is the lack of meaningful language between the performer and the SLP. For example, the actor or singer may have been taught a way of breathing for performance that is at variance with new voice science findings specific to respiration. Imagery abounds with performers, and the clinician cannot take away this imagery without replacing it with descriptions that will enhance performance and encourage using vocal mechanisms in a healthy manner. The skillful clinician can often use performers' imagery about what they are doing by not attacking it directly, but by modifying it by demonstration of less muscle effort producing similar vocal output. Excesses in muscle tension while performing have been categorized by Koufman and colleagues (1996), finding that much unnecessary supraglottic muscle tension occurs, particularly among "bluegrass/country and country/western and rock/gospel singers." When excessive muscle tension appears to cause laryngeal problems, voice therapy directed toward decreasing the excessive glottal and supraglottal muscle tension can be effective (Lowell, 2012). Excessive muscle tension can be reduced by using VFAs such as auditory feedback, change of loudness, chant talk, chewing, counseling, focus, changing glottal attack, laryngeal massage, open-mouth, relaxation, and yawn-sigh (see Chapter 7).

Most professional voice users have auditory recordings of their voices. At the first meeting between the performer and the SLP, an audio recording is made. It is sometimes useful to compare the client's previous recordings with the new one made at the time of evaluation. Part of the initial voice evaluation requires close listening to playback, possibly stopping and restarting to identify possible problem areas. Auditory feedback may play an important role in helping the performer identify what needs to be accomplished in future voice therapy situations. The SLP may use helpful auditory modeling in future therapy sessions (Boone, 1998), employing one or more applications available for playback listening and imitation. Perhaps the most effective auditory feedback is providing the client with real-time playback of what the client just said, and then comparing it with some kind of desired voice target. Fortunately, the myriad of handheld electronic devices, such as the iPad™ or iPod™, offer the performer many auditory feedback applications that may be recommended by the SLP (van Leer and Connor, 2012).

In many professional voice situations, the performer must speak above unreasonable background sound levels. Clinically, it has been found that hard rock concert performers and classroom teachers are the two performer groups who most frequently use their voices in excessive noise background settings. Among the many research studies looking at noise-level impact on vocal performance, Ferrand (2006) and Stathopoulos and Sapienza (1993) have found that excessive noise may compromise respiratory function, pitch changes, voice quality, and overall phonatory stability.

When actors, public speakers, politicians, ministers, and broadcasters consult with the SLP for problems with voice, the SLP should have them first complete questionnaires regarding their use of voice and their perceived voice-related quality of life (Portone and colleagues, 2007; Zraick and Risner, 2008) (see also Chapter 6).

Questionnaire and voice evaluation data should be reviewed to determine what type of voice therapy is indicated. The services of either the SLP or the vocal coach (VASTA, 2012) may then be provided. A blend of both specialties is often an ideal combination for the professional user of voice who is experiencing some vocal difficulties (Zeine and Walter, 2002; Hazlett and colleagues, 2011). Consideration is often given to providing vocal hygiene counseling and information along with voice therapy, although there is some research that finds equivocal value of vocal hygiene alone (Roy and colleagues, 2001); however, combining vocal hygiene and voice exercises for teachers with self-reported voice symptoms has been found to produce significant voice improvement (Gillivan-Murphy and colleagues, 2006). Following simple vocal hygiene guidelines often produces immediate benefit for the professional user of voice.

Singers often experience functional and/or organic problems of voice, and they are often referred to the SLP for consultation and possible voice therapy (Boone and Wiley, 2000). A special voice handicap scale for singers has been developed (Cohen and colleagues, 2007) that provides information relative to the constancy and impact of the problem on singing performance. For the SLP with a limited background in music performance and singing, consideration should be given to consultation with a singing teacher (NATS, 2012). The SLP often finds with professional singers that their vocal problems seem to originate from things they do when not singing, such as excessive throat clearing, smoking, lack of hydration, or talking too much before and after performance (Boone, 1997).

Of all professional performance groups, teachers appear to be the professional group experiencing the most vocal problems (Ferrand, 2012). Looking at voice disorders in a population of 550 primary school teachers, Munier and Kinsella (2008) found that "27% suffered from a voice problem, 53% reported an 'intermittent' voice problem, while only 20% had no voice problem." Summarizing multiple studies on voice problems in teachers, Grillo and Fugowki (2011, p. 149) reported that "between 15% and 32% of teachers reported experiencing a voice disorder in their teaching careers." Roy and colleagues (2004, 2005) have found an overwhelming prevalence of voice disorders in teachers compared with other adults in the same-age population. A large epidemiologic study in Brazil (Behlau and colleagues, 2012) of 1,651 teachers compared with 1,614 nonteachers found the prevalence of voice disorders among teachers was 11.6% versus 7.5% for nonteachers. Prolonged voicing times and talking against noisy backgrounds were identified as frequent causes of teacher voice problems. Among research studies looking at effectiveness of voice disorder prevention programs for teachers, Duffy and Hazlett (2004) and Bovo and colleagues (2007) report significant voice improvement for experimental subjects (versus control groups) in the programs.

The individual teacher, when consulting with the SLP, sometimes benefits from a classroom visit by the SLP to see and hear the teacher in action. The SLP may find the teacher in the classroom using much vocal hyperfunction while teaching, in sharp contrast to normal voicing efforts observed in the voice clinic. The SLP who hears high noise levels in the classroom may recommend that the teacher use a voice amplifier. Also, the teacher may profit from vocal training that uses both respiration support training and resonant voice therapy. In a study reviewing outcome effects of three treatments (using a voice amplifier, resonant therapy, or respiratory muscle training) for teachers with voice disorders, Roy and colleagues (2003) found that post-treatment results on the Voice Handicap Index (VHI) yielded positive support for teachers with voice problems using some kind of portable voice amplifier in the classroom. Teachers with clinical voice problems require a full medical and SLP diagnostic evaluation, followed by appropriate medical management and individualized voice therapy designed by the SLP for that particular teacher.

CHECK YOUR KNOWLEDGE

1. Which population of professional voice users is most at risk for developing a voice disorder? Explain.
2. What interventions might help a teacher with chronic job-related dysphonia?

Deaf and Hard of Hearing

Speech and voice characteristics in the absence of auditory feedback have been described in individuals with severe to profound hearing loss. Allegro and colleagues (2010), citing the work of others, describe the specific characteristics related to voice, including alterations in fundamental frequency, formant frequency transitions, phonation range, and vocal intensity. They also describe changes in speech, including difficulties with articulatory placement and precision, prolonged vowel durations, reduced speaking rate, and deviations in voice-onset timing. Nasality is more prominent in profoundly deaf children and adults. The earlier the onset of deafness or profound hearing loss, the more severe the aforementioned voice and speech symptoms are likely to be.

Voice production following cochlear implantation (CI) has been an area of emerging study in recent years, both in children and adults. In an early study of adult cochlear implant (CI) recipients, Svirsky and colleagues (1992) used an on-off study of auditory deprivation on voice. They found that when the CI was turned off for 24 hours, participants demonstrated elevated fundamental frequency (F0), increased intraoral pressures, and lowering of the second formant. With the restoration of auditory input via the CI, these voice parameters began to normalize. More recently, Ubrig and colleagues (2011) compared the vocal characteristics of postlingually deaf adults before and after CI. These clinical researchers reported a significant reduction in perceived overall voice severity, strain, loudness, and instability; a significant reduction in F_0 in male speakers; and F_0 variability in both genders.

In an early study of pediatric CI users, Seifert and colleagues (2002) found positive changes in voice pitch, elevated second formant, resonance, and rate of speech in older children who underwent CI. Campisi and colleagues (2005) identified unique voice characteristics in pediatric unilateral CI recipients related to the long-term control of vocal pitch and intensity. Their study cohort contained both pre- and postlingually deafened users of CIs. They reported that long-term control of amplitude variation improved to normal levels postimplantation, but long-term control of F_0 variation remained impaired. No significant differences were found between the results of the pre- and postlingually deafened CI users (see also Allegro and colleagues, 2010). Holler and colleagues (2010) reported a similar finding in their study of children with bilateral cochlear implants.

Although elevated voice pitch and excessive pitch variability are common findings in those with severe hearing loss, the anatomy and physiology of the larynx and vocal folds are the same as those of the normal hearing population. Children who are hard of hearing profit from developing an awareness of other voices, as well as an awareness of their own pitch levels, by using amplification feedback and instrumental tracings of pitch. Instrumental and software programs that provide good visual feedback of pitch and pitch variability may play primary roles in voice training. Such computer programs can also provide real-time feedback relative to excesses in voice loudness (too loud or not loud enough). The SLP provides display boundaries on the screen for pitch, pitch variability, and loudness; the child must keep his or her voice values within these boundaries.

A useful voice training method by the SLP is to provide "cue arrows" pointing in the desired direction of pitch change. For a typical Deaf child attempting to lower the voice, for example, cards should be printed with a down arrow. These cards should be placed wherever possible in the child's environment—in the backpack, on the bureau or desk, and so on. Also, the classroom teacher and voice clinician can give the child finger cues by pointing toward the floor. Another method for developing an altered pitch level is to place the fingers lightly on the larynx and feel the downward excursion of the larynx during lower pitch productions and the upward excursion during higher ones. The ideal or optimum pitch is produced by minimal vertical movement of the larynx. Any noticeable upward excursion of the larynx, except during swallowing, immediately signals that the voice may be at an inappropriately high pitch level. Once an appropriate pitch level has been established, the child may read aloud for a specified time period, placing the fingers lightly on the thyroid cartilage to monitor any unnecessary vertical laryngeal movement.

The typical voice of a Deaf child who has had no training in developing a good voice is characterized by alterations in nasal resonance, often accompanied by excessive pharyngeal resonance, which produce a cul-de-sac voice. The major contributing factor to these resonance alterations is the excessive posterior posturing of the tongue in the hypopharynx, which markedly lowers the second format (Wirz, 1986; Monsen, 1976). The tongue is drawn back into the hypopharynx and creates the peculiar resonance heard in Deaf speakers; this back resonance sounds similar to the resonance sometimes heard in speakers with athetoid cerebral palsy or oral verbal apraxia. The cul-de-sac voice has a back focus to it. In addition, the hearing-impaired child or adult may demonstrate marked variations in nasal resonance: too much nasal focus (hypernasality) or insufficient nasal resonance (hyponasality). Such nasal resonance variations may be due in part to the posterior carriage of the tongue, as well as to the inability to monitor acoustically the nasalization characteristics of the normal speaker.

Altering the tongue position to a more forward carriage and tongue protrusion (see Chapter 7) can contribute greatly to establishing more normal oral resonance in the voice. In addition to the procedures outlined in Chapter 7 for altering tongue position, more detailed procedures and therapy materials for both children and adults are available in *The Boone Voice Program for Children* (Boone, 1993) and *The Boone Voice Program for Adults* (Boone and Wiley, 2000). Once the tongue has been placed in a more neutral setting (Laver, 1980), the patient needs to practice making vocal contrasts between back-pharyngeal resonance and normal oral resonance. The patient needs to develop an awareness of what it feels like to use the lips, the tongue against the alveolar processes, the tongue on the hard palate, and other front-of-the-mouth postures. Such front focus seems to develop only after intensive practice doing tasks that encourage anterior tongue carriage.

For severely Hard of Hearing children and young adults who have had CIs or who wear hearing aids, computer programs and workbooks are designed for auditory processing and for developing listening skills These same materials are available for working on speech and voice (Erlmer, 2003; Mokhemar, 2002). Innovative software programs are also available for children and adults from CTS Informática (Parena, Brazil) and Griffin Laboratories (Temecula, California).

An innovative approach to improving the voice of CI users was explored by Holt and Dowell (2011). In their study of adolescent CI users, participants received vocal actor training. The workshop training focused on activities such as breath control, appropriate modulation of the voice, articulation of speech sounds, use of the soft palate, resonance, expressivity, and becoming aware of vocal habits that may impede speech. Voice and psychosocial variables were compared pre- and post-training. Increased pitch range and variability, decreased speaking rate, and decreased stress levels were reported post-training.

CHECK YOUR KNOWLEDGE

1. Describe four auditory-perceptual features of the hearing-impaired voice.
2. How does the voice change after cochlear implantation?

Transgender Patients

SLPs are seeing an increased number of transgender clients desiring to changing their past communication styles to match their new gender identities. Most are going through a male-to-female (MtF) transition, with a desire to develop a more feminine voice and communication style. The fewer female-to-male (FtM) clients wish to acquire a more masculine speaking style. The World Professional Association for Transgender Health (WPATH, 2012), working to improve the living conditions of persons with gender identity change, recognizes the benefits of changing one's speech, voice, and general communication style (Cohen-Kettenis and Plafflin, 2010). For a strict definition of changing one's gender to that of the opposite sex, the term *transsexual* (TS) is more accurate, but WPATH recognizes that the descriptive term *transgender* (TG) is now more commonly used.

The effectiveness of SLP services in enabling MtF transgender clients to produce their new gender speaking targets has been well-established in several studies described by Dacakis and colleagues (2012). SLPs working in less-dense population areas, compared to SLPs working in large cities, usually see fewer TG persons. An actual prevalence or incidence figure in the United States for the TG population in 2012 has not been established. One potential barrier to service delivery is the perception of bias of SLPs against TG individuals with communication impairments (Kelly-Campbell and Robinson, 2011). Clinicians may need to establish contact with the TG community in their area to understand how to meet their needs.

Though there is a growing literature base for speech/voice change in the TG patient (Adler and colleagues, 2012), much of what is done clinically is related to positive outcome data where the patient performs more like the target gender, and the TG patient is pleased by his or her therapy outcome (shown by comparing pre- and post-VHI scores, for example). Group-evidence-based practice data are difficult to generate because of the relative scarcity of TG patients in one clinical setting, costs, the fragility of the social-psychological situation emerging around the patient, the influence of other associated treatments (such as hormone therapy), and so on (Oates, 2006).

The ten communication behaviors listed below appear to be behaviors that are most different between the sexes:

language/lexicon	pitch
breathiness	pitch flexibility
facial expression	rate
gesture	volume and loudness
intonation	vowel prolongation

The language difference between the sexes can be quite striking. The female may use more adjective-adverb descriptors than her male counterpart does. Males tend to use more controlling direct sentences with less conditional words like I believe or maybe or perhaps (Hooper, 2006). Males tend to use shorter spoken sentences than do females. The breathiness heard in many female voices (Van Borsel and colleagues, 2009) can often be modeled and taught in MtF therapy. Facial expression needs to be increased for the MtF client, often developing a more consistent smile. A more feminine speaking pattern requires greater use of intonation, such as letting the pitch rise more toward the end of sentences (Wolfe and colleagues, 1990).

Elevating voice pitch is an obvious goal for the biologic male desiring to develop a feminine speaking style. Speaking pitch elevation in MtF clients has received extensive study (Mayer and Gelfer, 2008; McNeill and colleagues, 2008). In TG voice changes, the average F_0 shift in adult males is from 120 Hz (B2) to a desired female F_0 of approximately 170 Hz (F3) (Boone and Wiley, 2000). Biologic males show less pitch variability than do adult females. The SLP develops pitch variability lessons for the MtF client (Boone and colleagues, 2009). Prolongation of vowels is often a characteristic of female speech, which seems to result in a slower rate of speech. Both decreasing rate of speech and increasing volume and loudness appear to be useful in establishing a more feminine communication style (Boonin, 2006). Vowel prolongation appears to be the primary speaking characteristic for slowing down rate of speech when comparing biologic males and females with transgender females (Van Borsel and De Maesschalek, 2008).

These ten communication behaviors have been integrated into a graphic scale that portrays a visual display of the TG client's talking/voicing style (see Figure 8.1). The TG client and the SLP watch and listen to the playback. In our practices, we spend the balance of the time reviewing each of the ten variables, circling the variable

FIGURE 8.1 Gender Speech–Voice Presentation

Name: _____   Date: _____

	M				Target				F	Comments
Altered Lexicon	1	2	3	4	5	6	7	8	9	
Breathiness	1	2	3	4	5	6	7	8	9	
Facial Expression	1	2	3	4	5	6	7	8	9	
Gesture	1	2	3	4	5	6	7	8	9	
Intonation	1	2	3	4	5	6	7	8	9	
Pitch	1	2	3	4	5	6	7	8	9	
Pitch Flexibility	1	2	3	4	5	6	7	8	9	
Rate	1	2	3	4	5	6	7	8	9	
Volume and Loudness	1	2	3	4	5	6	7	8	9	
Vowel Prolongation	1	2	3	4	5	6	7	8	9	

Summary/Plan:

A rating scale used in an SLP private practice for documenting communication style for transgender clients (MtF) and (FtM).

performance number in black ink. The target value for each variable is in the middle of the scale, the 5 value. The MtF client is scored on the left side of the scale, 1 to 5; the FtM scale is on the right, 9 down to 5. For example, a very masculine client desiring to move toward femininity would score many 1 or 2 values in the beginning. With some therapy and much practice, TG clients move toward the 5 value. During selected future therapy sessions, the scale is readministered and values are circled in different ink colors. Thus, successful therapy outcome can be seen and heard, and also illustrated by visible changes on the rating scale.

The typical TG client is most concerned about his or her voice pitch. At the initial therapy session, clients may wish to demonstrate their self-taught attempts at changing pitch to better represent their new gender identity. Also, the typical listener to TG speech and voice identifies pitch as the biggest variable to change. The FtM client can lower voice pitch from taking male androgen hormones, causing other masculinizing effects like increased muscle definition, increased appetite, and increased body and facial hair. The estrogen hormones taken by the MtF have no effect on vocal folds, with no contributing changes to pitch or voice quality. Voice presents the "greatest challenge for up to 90% of transitioning MtF clients" (Bowers and colleagues, 2006, p. 96). In voice therapy for the MtF client, we concentrate on elevating voice pitch (often up to F3 or G3) and on increasing pitch variability and intonation, such as raising pitch at the end of a phrase or sentence (Gelfer and Schofield, 2000).

In initial therapy sessions, attention is given to pitch followed by speaking rate and voice volume, both of which have a primary gender-marking function in communication (Boonin, 2006). The adult female speaks at a slower rate than her male counterpart. In our therapy with the MtF client, we work to prolong vowels and take intra-phrase pauses to slow overall speaking rate slightly under the normal speaking rate of 145 to 175 words per minute (wpm) (Fitzsimmons and colleagues, 2001). A slightly faster rate is encouraged for the FtM client. Voice volume is slightly higher for adult males than for females. In our therapy with TG clients, we have success encouraging voice intensity levels that are consistent with the target gender (Oates and Dacakis, 1983).

We discuss in therapy how the overall gender presentation is affected by the language and gestures that the client uses in conversation, at work, and at play. The SLP interested in language differences (Hooper, 2006) between the sexes can identify some of the polarities that can be avoided or incorporated by persons in gender transition. Language pragmatics is accompanied by typical nonverbal behaviors that are somewhat different between the sexes, such as body posture, facial expression, eye contact, or hand gestures (Hirsch and Van Borsel, 2006).

Pre- and postadministration of the VHI (Jacobson and colleagues, 1997) can offer powerful data indicating the success of changing one's communication style to match one's new gender identity (Hancock and colleagues, 2011). The TG person in transition is usually experiencing difficult psychological and social problems. These problems often outweigh the patient's need for voice change. Accordingly, the SLP must look at the transgender patient from a counseling perspective, with the need to provide strong psychological support. When the patient is ready to change communication style to match his or her desired target gender, the SLP has much to offer with voice therapy (Adler and colleagues, 2012).

CHECK YOUR KNOWLEDGE

1. List five communication behaviors that differ between the sexes.
2. List four areas of speech–voice change with the MtF transgender client.

VOICE THERAPY FOR RESPIRATORY-BASED VOICE PROBLEMS

Respiratory problems often influence how a child or adult is able to use voice. Severe problems in respiration often require life-saving medical–surgical intervention. In milder breathing problems, the SLP can often play both a diagnostic and therapeutic role, working closely with the pulmonary medicine physician and the respiratory therapist. Let us consider a few respiratory problems and their overall management, including possible voice therapy.

Airway Obstruction

The voice clinician may encounter a number of children and adults with voice problems related to airway obstruction. Although obstructive airway problems require medical–surgical intervention and management, the SLP may play an important part in both identification and management of the disorder. Airway obstruction has two basic contributing causes (O'Hollaren, 1995): (1) structural and lesion mass airflow interference and (2) abnormal laryngeal movement interference.

Airflow Interference

Laryngeal-mass obstruction to airflow can have both infectious and noninfectious causes. Severe involvement of the epiglottis and supraglottal structures is almost always the result of a bacterial infection, treatable with appropriate antibiotic therapy. Depending on the size of the supraglottal swelling, inspiratory and expiratory breathing can be seriously compromised. Subglottal obstruction from disease is most often seen in croup, a viral disease that is usually characterized by inhalation stridor. Once croup is differentiated from problems such as paradoxical vocal fold dysfunction (which is often confused with asthmatic stridor), effective treatment includes "hydration, humidification, racemic epinephrine, and corticosteroids" (O'Hollaren and Everts, 1991). Airway obstruction can be caused by space-occupying lesions such as papilloma, granuloma, carcinoma, or large cysts—all described in Chapter 4. Once such lesions are identified as compromising the airway, effective medical management may include radiation therapy to reduce the lesion size, or surgical reduction or removal of the lesion. The obstructive lesion is watched closely; when it becomes too large, such as is often observed in juvenile papilloma, a surgical approach restores required airway competence. The voice clinician often plays an important role with the postsurgical, mass-lesion patient, establishing the best voice possible with voice therapy (despite a scarred and abnormal glottal margin).

Vocal Fold Paralysis

The most common laryngeal movement obstruction to air movement within the airway is laryngeal paralysis, unilateral or bilateral. In Chapter 5, we looked at the possible causes of vocal fold paralysis, and surgical and voice therapy management; thus, we will not repeat that information here. Suffice it to say that, while unilateral vocal fold paralysis contributes to some compromise of the open airway, bilateral abductor paralysis produces a life-threatening obstacle to air passage, requiring immediate surgical intervention.

Asthma

In asthma, the patient experiences a narrowing of airway tubes, particularly in the bronchi and bronchioles, which limits the free passage of air. Spasms of the airway can be caused by the external smooth muscles going into spasm, causing a narrowing of the opening (Berkow and colleagues, 1997). This causes the inner lining of mucosa tissue to become compressed and inflamed, resulting in some mucosal swelling and irritation, and causing some production of mucus (which further obstructs the passageway). The patient struggles to take in a breath. The asthmatic spasms can be triggered by stimuli such as pollens, dust mites, animal dander, cold air, smoke, and exercise. The asthmatic symptoms may be chronic (they come and go) or part of a sudden and severe reaction that may require immediate medical intervention.

The SLP does not usually encounter the patient during severe respiratory obstruction. Patients with asthma sometimes complain of voice symptoms, which are usually attributed to treatment with inhaled corticosteroids (Stanton and colleagues, 2009). Asnaashari and colleagues (2012) recently evaluated the quality of phonation in a group of 34 adults with untreated mild to severe persistent asthma and compared these participants to a group of nonasthmatic, age- and sex-matched healthy controls. These clinical researchers found that lower airway diseases such as asthma can impair voice quality. When dysphonia is chronic and interferes with quality of life, patients may seek the help of the voice clinician.

The SLP must first differentiate true subglottal asthma from parodoxical vocal fold movement (PVFM). In the asthmatic patient, the primary management step is treating the spasms and inflammation that interrupt the patient's natural breathing. Oral corticosteroids (Djukanovic and colleagues, 1997) appear to be the most effective treatment for asthma symptoms and airway inflammation; these authors concluded that "a moderate dose of oral corticosteroids leads to a marked reduction in airway inflammation . . . resulting in reduced airway hyperresponsiveness" (p. 831). Another form of steroid application is the use of aerosolized albuterol (Strauss and colleagues, 1997), which appears to reduce airway inflammation experienced by the asthmatic patient. Reduction of airway inflammation appears primary for increasing airway dilation and thus allowing a greater passage of air into and out of the lungs.

When respiratory symptoms are under some control, the voice clinician may help the patient develop and use a functional voice. Phonation can often be helped by reducing the number of syllables the patient says on one breath. A baseline measurement should be taken. The patient should then be instructed to cut the total number in half. For example, if a patient says 20 syllables on one expiration, the patient should be instructed to limit utterances to half that number, or 10 syllables per breath. This seems to prevent vocal fold squeezing, which makes the last words of the phrase or sentence sound squeezed or dysphonic. Help the person to develop methods of renewing breath while speaking. Good posture with the head not tilted upward or downward, the open-mouth approach, vocal hygiene, and the yawn-sigh approach have all been found helpful for the asthmatic patient who wishes to improve vocal efficiency (see Chapter 7).

Emphysema

Among various chronic pulmonary diseases experienced by the adult population, emphysema is the most common. Emphysema is a type of chronic obstructive pulmonary disease involving damage to the air sacs (alveoli) in the lungs. As a result, the body does not get the oxygen it needs. The primary cause of emphysema is smoking or from continuous exposure to smoke-laden dust. The continuous smoke exposure in the lungs causes the alveolar walls to lose their elasticity, collapsing on pulmonary expiration (Berkow and colleagues, 1997). This collapse of the alveoli in turn causes the bronchioles (the airway conduits to and from the alveoli) to collapse. The result of this alveoli-bronchiole collapse is difficulty in emptying the lung during expiration (Sataloff, 1997a). Consequently, the high residual air volumes preclude taking in adequate oxygen renewal on inspiration. The patient with moderate to severe emphysema struggles to get sufficient breath to sustain his or her life. Voice abnormality is of secondary concern.

Up to 30 million people in the United States suffer from an emphysema-related illness, making it the fourth largest cause of mortality in the United States (National Emphysema Foundation, 2007). Because the primary cause of emphysema is cigarette smoking, the first mandatory treatment step is to stop smoking. Mild emphysema can begin to show after only five or seven years of continuous, heavy smoking. It is the mildly involved patient, often a professional user of voice, whom we often see with a voice problem.

Voice management can begin only after the patient stops smoking. Formal respiratory therapy for these patients is better off left in the hands of the respiratory therapist or other pulmonary specialists. For example, the patient might be using prescribed bronchodilators, inhaled steroids, or even supplemental oxygen. The voice clinician often begins intervention by taking voice measurements specific to air volume and available pressures for voicing, measures of duration, and sound pressure level of the voice. Observation of the patient during speaking, oral reading, and singing tasks may also reveal some unnecessary postural-skeletal behaviors the patient is using to maintain breathing, movements that may be inefficient and counterproductive to good voice control.

Some directed practice in diaphragmatic-abdominal breathing in the sitting or standing (vertical) position may be useful, as well as practice in counting syllables per utterance in an attempt to become more aware of when to renew breath. Shortening the length of phonation can help the patient have more control over voice loudness. The emphysema patient can sometimes improve voice quality by speaking at a slightly higher voice pitch. Other VFAs, such as focus, gottal attack changes, masking, and pitch inflections, might be tried in the search for a stronger functional voice (see Chapter 7).

Faulty Breath Control

Many children and adults appear in the clinic with faulty breath control, either caused by some organic disease or from functional misuse, or both. That is, there may be a functional overlay to an organic respiratory disease that can be treated directly to improve overall respiratory function as well as provide better breath support for voice. There are an endless number of respiratory diseases, most of which may have some impact on voice. The SLP who works with voice patients soon learns to consult with physicians and therapists who work with patients with respiratory diseases.

What we do with voice problems related to respiratory problems must be consistent with the limitation imposed by various respiratory diseases and the treatments the patient may be receiving from other professionals. The clinician should not be preoccupied with the presenting disease problem, but face the patient more generically, as a person with a voice disorder that shows itself in various pitch-loudness-quality dimensions. In fact, faulty breath control may show itself more as a functional problem than as an organic one. For most patients, the voice clinician should assess respiratory-voice function following many of the evaluation procedures presented in Chapter 6. The voice evaluation should supplement any other respiratory assessment information. We use the management and therapy suggestions developed in the VFAs called respiration training for developing better breath support for patients with faulty breath control (see Chapter 7).

Paradoxical Vocal Fold Movement

Paradoxical vocal fold movement (PVFM) is inappropriate adduction of the vocal folds during inspiration. It can be seen in both children and adults. PVFM has been known as paroxysmal vocal cord dysfunction (PVCD), episodic laryngospasm, and irritable larynx syndrome (Maturo and colleagues, 2011). PVFM is recognized in the medical community as a disorder to consider when symptoms of respiratory distress do not respond to treatment for asthma (see Case Study 3 in Chapter 6). Trudeau (1998) suggested three possible etiologies of PVFM: (1) psychogenic, as in conversion reaction; (2) visceral, related to upper airway sensitivity; and/or (3) neurological, a form of laryngeal dystonia. These categories need not be mutually exclusive. A number of studies of PVFM strongly suggest a psychogenic basis, but others have reported no psychogenic basis in about one in four patients (Altman and colleagues, 2000; Forrest and colleagues, 2012); this suggests that the basis for PVFM may be multifactorial and is not strictly of a psychological origin.

As described by Vertigan and colleagues (2006), triggers for PVFM are classified as (1) inhaled (smoke, fumes, or steam), (2) temperature (cold air or high humidity), (3) activity (talking, laughing, deep breathing, swallowing, or exercise), and (4) intrinsic (throat sensations, shortness of breath, or stress). Chronic cough has been described in approximately 80% of patients with PVFM (Newman and colleagues, 1995) and is often the primary symptom (Murry and colleagues, 2004). PVFM often masquerades as asthma in young athletes (Sullivan and colleagues, 2001), with the prevalence as high as 5% in Olympic-level athletes (Rundell and Spiering, 2003). Therefore, it is helpful to monitor the patient during physical activity with flow-volume loop testing (Gallivan and colleagues, 1996). However, the patient is usually asymptomatic during the time of evaluation, so a good case history and interview is mandatory. With respect to the asymptomatic patient, Guss and Mirza (2006) have suggested that PVFM can be elicited and observed with methacholine challenge testing (MCT), that is, an aerosol that stimulates bronchoconstriction.

In the largest study to date on pediatric PVFM (Maturo and colleagues, 2011), 59 children with PVFM were evaluated. Speech therapy as an initial treatment resulted in a 63% success rate after four treatment sessions, and it was a more successful treatment than anti-reflux therapy. Eighteen of the children were diagnosed with a psychiatric condition. Children with inspiratory stridor at rest had a lower initial success rate with speech therapy; a higher rate of underlying psychiatric disorders; and a high rate of success after psychiatric treatment that required, on average, three sessions over a two-month period.

While most treatment regimens for PVFM employ voice therapy and intensive use of laryngeal videoendoscopic biofeedback, Altman and colleagues (2000) offer the use of Botox and video feedback as viable treatment options for the problem. The long-range efficacy of using Botox for the treatment of PVFM is not clearly determined, though it has been shown to be effective in patients with refractory cough (see the next section in this chapter).

Trudeau (1998), Blager (1995),Von Berg and colleagues (1999), Mathers-Schmidt (2001), Case (2002), and Murry and colleagues (2004) report good success in their respective laryngeal control programs that minimize the airway obstruction experienced by the patient with PVFM. Their programs place emphasis on helping the patient to become aware of aberrant and normal vocal fold positioning during both inspiration and expiration. Some of these programs use video feedback. We use extensive videoendoscopy of correct and abnormal vocal fold postures for both phonation and quiet respiration for the PVFM patient to both observe and produce. Patients become aware of how to produce vocal fold configurations in their own larynx, showing them what to do to "open the airway when you take in a breath." We have found the use of the yawn-sigh to be a useful technique for opening the vocal folds and creating a more open airway (see Chapter 7). Other therapy procedures described by Trudeau (1998) include nasal inspiration, working on /s/ duration (not to maximum levels), and the use of diaphragmatic-abdominal breathing. Murry and colleagues (2010) report successfully treating chronic cough in patients with PVFM with a combination of anti-reflux treatment (use of proton-pump inhibitors [PPIs]) and respiratory retraining.

CHECK YOUR KNOWLEDGE

1. List and describe three etiologies for PVFM.
2. List and describe four triggers for PVFM.

Chronic Cough

Chronic refractory cough is a significant clinical problem and a common reason for patients to present to ENT clinics. It may occur with PVFM, LPRD, and muscle tension dysphonia (MTD), or it may be independent of these conditions. Chronic cough has physical side effects, such as laryngeal trauma (Colton and colleagues, 2011); social consequences, such as embarrassment and negative impact on quality of life (Ma and colleagues, 2009); and financial consequences, such as expensive medications and lost work productivity.

Chu and colleagues (2010) report the use of Botox in successful treatment of patients with chronic cough in a small series of cases. Even with aggressive medical management by the ENT and/or pulmonologist, however, cough persists in approximately 20% of patients (Haque and colleagues, 2005). This group of patients, with refractory or idiopathic cough, may respond to treatment by the SLP. In their recent tutorial on the role of speech pathology in the management of patients with chronic refractory cough, Vertigan and Gibson (2012, p. 36) outline four components to speech pathology treatment for cough: education, cough control techniques, vocal hygiene training, and psycho-educational counseling. A handful of studies have reported the outcome of speech pathology treatment for cough (see Vertigan and Gibson [2012] for a summary). In general, it appears that there is a role for the SLP in the management of refractory cough. The goals of speech pathology intervention should be reduced cough reflex sensitivity, improved voluntary control of cough, and reduced laryngeal irritation (Vertigan and Gibson, 2011).

Tracheostomy

A tracheostomy, or external opening into the trachea, may be necessary when an individual experiences respiratory difficulties due to an obstruction of the upper airway, has problems with pulmonary toilet (managing secretions), or requires mechanical ventilation to maintain adequate respiration. A tracheostomy fundamentally alters the physiology of voice and swallow because the stoma is below the level of the larynx, thereby bypassing the upper airway. Decisions regarding the type and size of the tracheostomy tube will be made by the ENT, based on the individual's diagnosis, physical status, and medical needs. The SLP is also a core member of the evaluation team, with clearly established roles and responsibilities (Kazandijian and Dikeman, 2008).

Depending on the type of tracheostomy tube the individual receives, he or she may or may not be able to use a tracheostomy speaking valve, which is a one-way removable valve that is attached to the open end of the tracheostomy tube. Specific indications and therapy for children and adults with tracheostomy tubes are discussed by Mason (1993). In addition to providing direct services, SLPs are also responsible for patient and family counseling and investigation of support services. Several organizations provide support to specific tracheostomy and ventilator-dependent populations.

SUMMARY

In this chapter, we have presented voice disorders in children and adolescents, older adults, those with hearing impairment, those who are transgendered, and those with a variety of respiratory-based conditions. We also discussed the professional voice user and the management of dysphonia in this population of patients, whose numbers are increasing. While patients from the aforementioned groups may also have primary or concomitant functional, organic, or neurogenic contributors to their dysphonia, they each present unique management challenges (see Chapter 7 for case studies).

CLINICAL CONCEPTS

The following clinical concepts correspond with many of the objectives at the beginning of this chapter:

1. In the geriatric patient with dysphonia, the voice problems are sometimes due to normal age-related changes, while other times the voice problems are sometimes due to pathologic changes that are more a consequence of disease process. You may see a speaker with Parkinson's disease (PD) who has a soft voice (see Chapter 5); a speaker with weak respiratory muscles who has to take more frequent breaths during talking; a speaker with hearing loss who has difficulty monitoring and adjusting his or her voice, resonance, and speech output; and a speaker with dysarthria who cannot control the flow of air through the glottis, resulting in changes in pitch, loudness, and voice quality (see Chapter 5).

2. Many voice-disordered patients will come to you because of changes to the voice related primarily to youth. Some examples include a preschool-age child who is in a loud daycare center and has to raise his or her voice to be heard; an elementary-age child who participates in extracurricular activities such as cheerleading, glee club, or debate team and uses his or her voice excessively throughout and beyond the school day; and an adolescent in high school who

cannot participate in extracurricular activities such as being on a sports team because of his or her dysphonia and the social stigma that it brings.

3. Some voice-disordered patients will come to you because they are professional voice users. Some examples include a school teacher whose voice does not hold up throughout the day and who uses a lot of her sick days because of chronic dysphonia, a singer who overuses or misuses his voice and whose performances thus suffer, a call center operator whose dysphonia interferes with her effectiveness in helping callers and thus misses out on potential job advancement opportunities, a salesperson whose dysphonia is distracting and a barrier to closing deals successfully, and a minister whose "message is lost in the messenger" because of a distracting voice quality.

4. Some voice-disordered patients will come to you because of hearing impairment. They may be adults or children, and the hearing loss may have been prelingual or postlingual. Such patients will need counseling and intervention to learn how to make their voices sound more natural given their decreased auditory self-feedback. In some cases, voice therapy may occur after cochlear implantation, when auditory self-feedback has been improved.

5. Some voice-disordered patients will come to you because they suffer from paradoxical vocal fold movement (PVFM), with our without chronic cough. Voice therapy can be an important adjunct to medical management and may include the use of many of the VFAs outlined in Chapter 7.

GUIDED READING

Read the following articles.

Hazlett, D. E., Duffy, O. M., & Moorhead, S. A. (2011). Review of the impact of voice training on the vocal quality of professional voice users: Implications for vocal health and recommendations for further research. *Journal of Voice, 25*, 181–191.

Forrest, L. A., Husein, T., & Husein, O. (2012). Paradoxical vocal cord motion: Classification and treatment. *Laryngoscope, 122*, 844–853.

Using the information reported in the two articles, identify three clinical research questions that still need to be answered related to therapy interventions.

PREPARING FOR THE PRAXIS™

Directions: Please read the case studies and answer the questions that follow. (Please see page 319 for the answer key.)

Vivienne is a 77-year-old telephone receptionist at a busy state government office. She reports talking on the phone for at least 30 minutes out of each hour and talking in person to local citizens for 15 minutes out of the hour. Her chief voice complaints are harsh voice quality, poor voice durability, and laryngeal pain upon phonation. She saw an otolaryngologist (ENT), who diagnosed her with presbyphonia.

1. As the voice clinician, you review the ENT report and find that laryngoscopic examination most typically reveals:
   A. Space-occupying lesions at the anterior third of both vocal folds
   B. Mild bowing of the vocal fold margins
   C. Focal adductory dystonias of the true vocal folds
   D. A full unilateral vocal fold paralysis

2. You telephone Vivienne to schedule her for her first voice appointment. You are not surprised to hear speech and voice that are:
   A. Normal in pitch
   B. Normal in amplitude
   C. Breathy and hoarse
   D. Normal in number of words per phrase

3. Vivienne presents with no systemic diseases, and she is very willing to comply with your recommendations for increased vocal quality and amplitude. Suggested intervention techniques would include:
   A. A personal amplification system to use with patrons and co-workers at the office
   B. Complete voice rest for at least a week
   C. A rigorous vocal hygiene program only
   D. Exploring techniques to improve respiratory and vocal efficiency
   E. Both A and D

   Stefanie is a male-to-female transgender client who has been referred to you. She has begun hormone treatment and is seeking direction with respect to voice and pragmatic speech and language.

4. As a novice clinician in the area of transgender intervention, it is important for you to know that:
   A. Males typically show a slower rate of speech than females do
   B. Females tend to use fewer adjective-adverb descriptors than males do
   C. Males tend to generate greater inflection toward the ends of phrases
   D. Typical transgender voice client is very concerned about his or her pitch

   Marti is a female adolescent high school athlete who has been referred to the emergency room (ER) on several occasions for respiratory distress. A well-informed ER physician makes the diagnosis of paradoxical vocal fold movement.

5. As the SLP who received the consult for voice therapy with Marti, it is important for you to know that PVFM is best managed through:
   A. Botox
   B. Surgery
   C. Behavioral intervention
   D. Asthma intervention

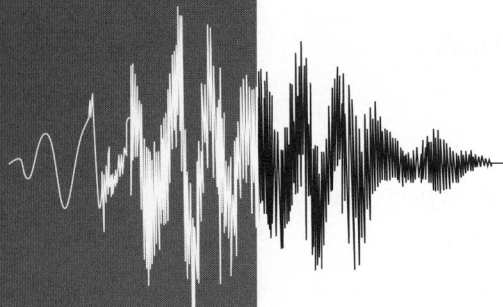

CHAPTER 9

Management and Therapy Following Laryngeal Cancer

Head and neck cancer strikes at some of the most basic human functions, including verbal communication, eating, and breathing. In this chapter, we review the risk factors and epidemiology of head and neck cancer. We also provide a historical and contemporary review of medical–surgical management. Case examples demonstrate the intervention approaches taken by the speech-language pathologist (SLP).

RISK FACTORS, INCIDENCE, AND DEMOGRAPHICS IN HEAD AND NECK CANCER

Head and neck (H&N) cancer is the fifth most common cancer worldwide (Parkin and colleagues, 2002). Global cases of laryngeal cancer are approximately 160,000. The highest rates of H&N cancer occur in Southeast Asia and central and southern Europe (Boyle and Levin, 2008). H&N cancers account for approximately 3 percent of all cancers in the United States (Jemal and colleagues, 2010). More than 50,000 men and women in this country are expected to be diagnosed with H&N cancers in 2013 (American Cancer Society, 2011). In terms of costs, H&N cancers are responsible for $3.2 billion dollars in healthcare expenditures and approximately 4.4% of all cancer treatment expenditures each year (Jemal and colleagues, 2010).

In the United States, the risk for a man developing cancer over his lifetime is one in two; for a women, it is one in three (American Cancer Society, 2011). H&N cancer is diagnosed most often in people over the age of 50. Alcohol and tobacco (including chewing tobacco) account for approximately 75% of oral, oropharyngeal, hypopharyngeal, and laryngeal cancers (Gandini and colleagues, 2008). The combined effects of these two agents substantially increase this risk. The human papilloma virus (HPV) has been more recently linked to the development of oropharyngeal cancers (tonsillar and base of tongue) in younger and younger Americans (Chaturvedi and colleagues, 2011). Over 90% of H&N cancers fall under the category of squamous cell carcinoma (Sano and Myers, 2009).

CHECK YOUR KNOWLEDGE

1. Why are men more likely than women to develop H&N cancer?
2. Why are older adults more likely than younger adults to develop H&N cancer?

HISTORICAL REVIEW

A surgeon by the name of Billroth performed the first total laryngectomy in 1873. Even at that time, there were concerns about the rehabilitation of communication. The artificial larynx (AL), invented in 1874 by Gussenbauer, has seen numerous changes and technologic advances over the years. Versions of these instruments are used in rehabilitation today.

Remarkably, the first tracheal puncture, a precursor to the present-day prosthetic voice restoration (Blom and Singer, 1979), was performed by a patient on himself in 1932. This interesting individual used a hot ice pick to create a tract between the trachea and hypopharynx, thus facilitating sound production within the oral cavity and allowing the production, by report, of a good voice (Guttman, 1932).

Laryngeal transplant surgery's first success came in 1969 with a physician named Kluyskens. His patient had a cancer history but survived for eight months before a second tumor took his life. It has been surmised that immunosuppressive therapy predisposed this patient to the second cancer. Laryngeal transplant surgery must overcome four major hurdles in order to prove successful: resolving blood supply, resolving reinnervation issues, preventing transplant rejection, and justifying the procedure. The first successful transplant of the larynx was performed in 1998 at the Cleveland Clinic on a patient who sustained extensive laryngeal trauma in years prior (Strome and colleagues, 2001). This patient survives after 15 years (Knott and colleagues, 2011). In 2010, successful laryngotracheal transplantation was performed at the University of California at Davis in a patient who had sustained complete stenosis of her larynx and proximal trachea 12 years prior to her transplant. According to one of the surgeons, D. Gregory Farwell (personal communication), she still presents with an excellent voice and enjoys a normal diet. She also remains tracheotomy-dependent despite an attempt at selective reinnervation of her left vocal fold. Her endoscopy demonstrated a normal-appearing larynx with vocal folds in the midline position and with little volitional movement but intact motor and sensory reinnervation. At last follow-up, she had no evidence of rejection and an excellent quality of life. In spite of these successes, full laryngeal transplants remain rare. Current guidelines suggest that laryngeal transplantation should be considered a viable option for those with laryngeal trauma that cannot be surgically repaired, for those with bulky benign laryngeal lesions who would otherwise require a total laryngectomy, for those who have had other organ transplants and a current advanced-stage laryngeal cancer, and for those who are cancer-free for five years postlaryngectomy. More recently, scientists have been exploring the development of a bioengineered human larynx (Baiguera and colleagues, 2011).

MODES OF CANCER TREATMENT

Each cancer treatment mode—radiation therapy (RT), surgery, and chemotherapy (CT)—presents some complications to the voice. For example, irradiation can cause swelling of the mucosa in the early stages of treatment, followed by dryness and stiffness of the vocal fold cover weeks and even months after treatment. The long-term effects of radiation therapy involve the fibrosis of soft tissue, which limits the normal range of muscle motion (Leonard and Kendall, 1997).

When surgery is among the treatment options, the extent and location of the tumor dictates the extent of surgery. If the tumor crosses the midline, then total or near-total (or subtotal) laryngectomy may be indicated; if the tumor is located on only one side of the larynx, then hemilaryngectomy or other partial laryngectomy may be an option. Surgery can leave a tissue deficit following tumor removal, and stiffness due to scarring may follow healing. The tissue deficit may also leave a gap in the glottal area when the folds approximate. This gap may cause air wastage and a breathy vocal quality, and may result in inadequate vocal loudness and short phonation times. In addition, the gap in tissue and the stiffness of the surrounding tissue may lead to irregular vocal fold vibration due to impaired mucosal wave motion. Many individuals experience moderate to severe side effects with chemoradiation intervention. In sum, dryness, inadequate tissue mass, irregular vocal fold edges, and stiffness can all make vibration of the vocal fold cover extremely difficult or impossible. This will render the voice abnormal in one or more vocal parameters.

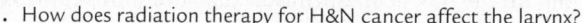

CHECK YOUR KNOWLEDGE

1. How does radiation therapy for H&N cancer affect the larynx?
2. How does radiation therapy for H&N cancer affect the voice?

CASE EXAMPLES

The picture of a larynx in Figure 9.1 shows a lack of tissue mass due to surgery for removal of a laryngeal cancer. There is a gap between the vocal folds even in full adduction. The voice is breathy, low in loudness, and rough in quality. The breathy quality results from the air wastage through the glottal gap, while the low loudness level is due to inadequate medial compression required for louder voice production. The rough vocal quality is due to two factors: (1) unequal mass between the right and left vocal folds, and thus an irregular vocal fold vibrator pattern, and (2) an attempt to compensate for the excessive glottal gap by hyperactivity of the false vocal folds, which weight the vocal folds unequally. A third factor, for which the effect is difficult to estimate, is the scarring following surgery. On laryngostroboscopy, the vocal folds appear unevenly stiff, likely due to scarring that produces adynamic segments in the vocal folds in the area where tissue has been excised. In

**FIGURE 9.1 Lack of Tissue Mass in Right Vocal Fold After Surgical Removal of Laryngeal
Cancer**

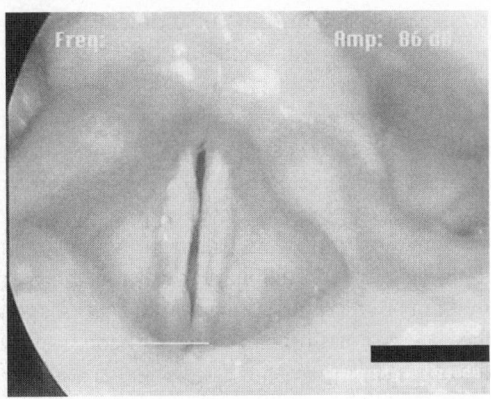

voice therapy for this patient, we need first to eliminate the excessive vocal effort, thus reducing the false fold activity. We began with the VFA of inhalation phonation, which retracts the false folds (see Chapter 7). We gradually shifted from inhalation to exhalation phonation using the /i/ vowel because it is produced with the root of the tongue elevated and out of the hypopharynx. The next step in voice therapy was to use an upward pitch shift to slightly increase vocal fold tension and gain slightly better approximation (reducing the glottal gap) of the postsurgical vocal folds. The upward pitch could be only slight due to some vocal fold scarring. Greater shifts upward produced too much tension of the vocal folds, and phonation breaks occurred due to stiffness of the vocal fold cover. A shift of 20 to 25 Hz was desirable in this case. The improved approximation from increased vocal fold tension during pitch shift increased vocal loudness. Subglottic air pressure was increased slightly as well. This case demonstrates how the treatment (surgery) for cancer produced a dysphonia as a by-product of treatment for the disease. Voice therapy was based on achieving the necessary vocal adjustments using VFAs that would alter the effects of postsurgical anatomy and physiology of the larynx and also counter the inappropriate compensatory behaviors the patient had developed.

The second case addresses voice therapy for stiffness of the vocal fold cover due to fibrotic changes secondary to radiotherapy. For this case, we instructed the patient to shift his pitch downward to take advantage of the greater mucosal wave that occurs in lower pitches and also to decrease subglottic air pressure so the folds were not overdriven. We used this therapy approach in a patient who had irradiation treatment for a superficial bilateral cancer of the vocal fold cover. He was able to return to teaching with a much improved voice and a voice that would last throughout the teaching day. The pre-therapy voice was very weak, extremely breathy, and of very short duration of phonation. This was due to a more or less uniform bilateral stiffness of the entire vocal fold area. The effect is very much like that produced by surgical stripping of the vocal fold to remove vocal fold cancer.

A third case illustrates another role of the SLP in the follow-up and management of patients treated for laryngeal cancer. A 26-year-old female was seen for evaluation of voice following surgical removal of superficial squamous cell cancer. The

Inhalation Phonation is a helpful Voice Facilitating Approach for any patient presenting with ventricular dysphonia. This section of the text applies inhalation phonation to a voice user who presents with uneven vocal fold edges due to surgery; however, other patients featured on the **video** present with supralaryngeal hyperfunction due to a number of functional and neurogenic reasons. Inhalation phonation helps encourage elongation of the true vocal folds and discourages the medialization of the false vocal folds. Grand Rounds: Why is inhalation phonation best facilitated with the phoneme /i/?

We use Glottal Fry as a diagnostic probe for patients who need to reduce laryngeal hyperfunction and increase the opportunity for relaxed vocal fold vibration. In the case of irregular vocal fold vibration due to scarring, Glottal Fry encourages easy and relaxed vibration while reducing demands on breath support. Note on the **video** segment that Glottal Fry is used as a probe for patients presenting with vocal hyperfunction for reasons ranging from vocal overuse to spasmodic dysphonia (see Differential Diagnosis of a Complex Voice Disorder, Chapter 6). Grand Rounds: What is the average frequency of glottal fry?

patient is a nonsmoker, does not use alcohol, and is a vegetarian and marathon runner. She is in excellent shape but has cancer of the larynx. The cancer has returned three times in less than two years and has been removed three times. The decision of a team of ENT physicians is to continue to monitor the return of the cancer and remove it before it becomes deeply embedded in the vocal folds. The speech pathology clinic is to evaluate the patient every four to six months, along with evaluations by the ENT team. The SLP provides videostroboscopic monitoring of the larynx and acoustic evaluation of the voice as a means of tracking the cancer regrowth. Figure 9.2 is a picture of the larynx of this young adult female patient with laryngeal cancer. In addition, the SLP provides ongoing voice management so the patient is using the larynx optimally and does not engage in vocal abuse, which may make the voice poorer in quality and contribute to edema, a condition that can make obtaining an accurate status of the cancer more difficult. While this is a very unusual case, the monitoring role of the SLP is not unusual and has been applied in cases of contact ulcer, papilloma, and polyps and polypoid cord degeneration.

We cannot overstate the important role of laryngeal endoscopy in the case of differentially diagnosing laryngeal cancer. For example, a 72-year-old man was referred to our clinic for voice therapy to treat hypophonia because of Parkinson's disease. Because this patient had been diagnosed with PD years before, he was referred to our clinic without an imaging study of the larynx. Instead of revealing bowed vocal folds bilaterally, rigid endoscopy at our clinic revealed a unilateral space-occupying lesion that was whitish and irregular at the edges. A referral to an ENT physician and subsequent biopsy rendered a diagnosis of T1 glottic cancer; this patient was successfully treated with laser surgery and radiation.

VOICE FACILITATING APPROACHES

Our clinical experience with postsurgical and postradiotherapy treatment of dysphonia has demonstrated some success using the following approaches, which were discussed in Chapter 7:

FIGURE 9.2 Four Views of the Larynx of a 26-Year-Old Female with Recurring Squamous Cell Carcinoma, Followed over a Two-Year Period

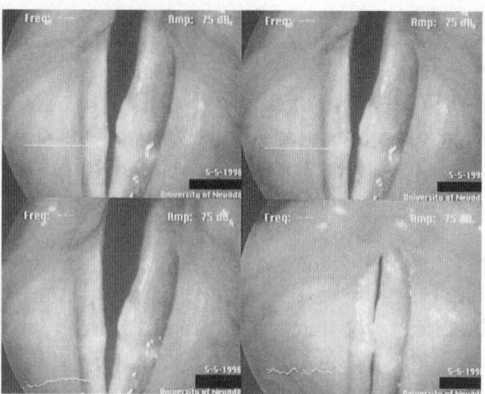

1. Inhalation phonation using the vowels /i/, /u/, and /o/.
2. Pitch shifts upward and downward based on the patient's vocal response.
3. Glottal fry if vocal fold stiffness is not too great.
4. Nasal-glide stimulation.
5. Head turned to the side and lateral digital pressure applied to the thyroid cartilage.
6. Loudness change, usually lower.
7. Tongue protrusion /i/.
8. Glottal fry to tone.

Patients with postsurgical and/or postirradiation dysphonia are a challenging vocal population. The critical factor in success with voice therapy is the degree to which the mucosal wave has been preserved. More often than not, we have been able to improve the voice of these patients through voice therapy, but we have not always been successful due to too much vocal fold stiffness or scarring or the absence of tissue (postsurgically), creating irregular vocal fold medial edges. These patients may also have difficulty swallowing and thus may benefit from swallowing therapy (Logemann, 1998).

VOCAL HYGIENE

In addition to the techniques listed above to improve the voice, we have also noted the need for additional attention to vocal hygiene, such as avoiding excessive strain when trying to talk over noise and increasing water intake. Increased hydration is a key component in these often dry patients. Reduction of alcohol intake, which also is dehydrating, and substitution of silent cough and sniff swallow (Zwitman and Calcaterra, 1973) for voiced coughing and throat clearing, respectively, are crucial for these patients. Because their anatomy and physiology is often altered by treatment of the disease, these patients have less latitude or tolerance for vocal abuse and their mode of vocal fold vibration is less robust.

LARYNGECTOMY

The anatomic and physiologic changes involved in a total laryngectomy are described well in the literature (Blom and colleagues, 1998; Keith and Darley, 1994). In short, the laryngeal and hypopharyngeal cartilages are removed, along with the hyoid bone, all extrinsic and intrinsic muscles of the larynx, and the upper rings of the trachea. The uppermost portion of the trachea is brought forward and fit flush with the neck. An external stoma (mouth) is created, which permanently serves as the patient's new airway. Figures 9.3 and 9.4 show pre- and postlaryngectomy head and neck anatomy.

 Tongue Protrusion /i/ appears pretty bizarre on the **video**, but it is an effective voice technique. When protruded, the back of the tongue is pulled out of the oral pharynx, and the pharynx and laryngeal additus are open to produce easy, clear voice. The production of the voice with the tongue protruded is sufficiently novel to break maladaptive (bad) vocal habits often associated with hyperfunction.

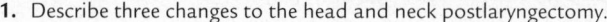

CHECK YOUR KNOWLEDGE

1. Describe three changes to the head and neck postlaryngectomy.
2. What changes in lifestyle do you think occur as a result of having a stoma?

FIGURE 9.3 Normal Vocal Tract Anatomy

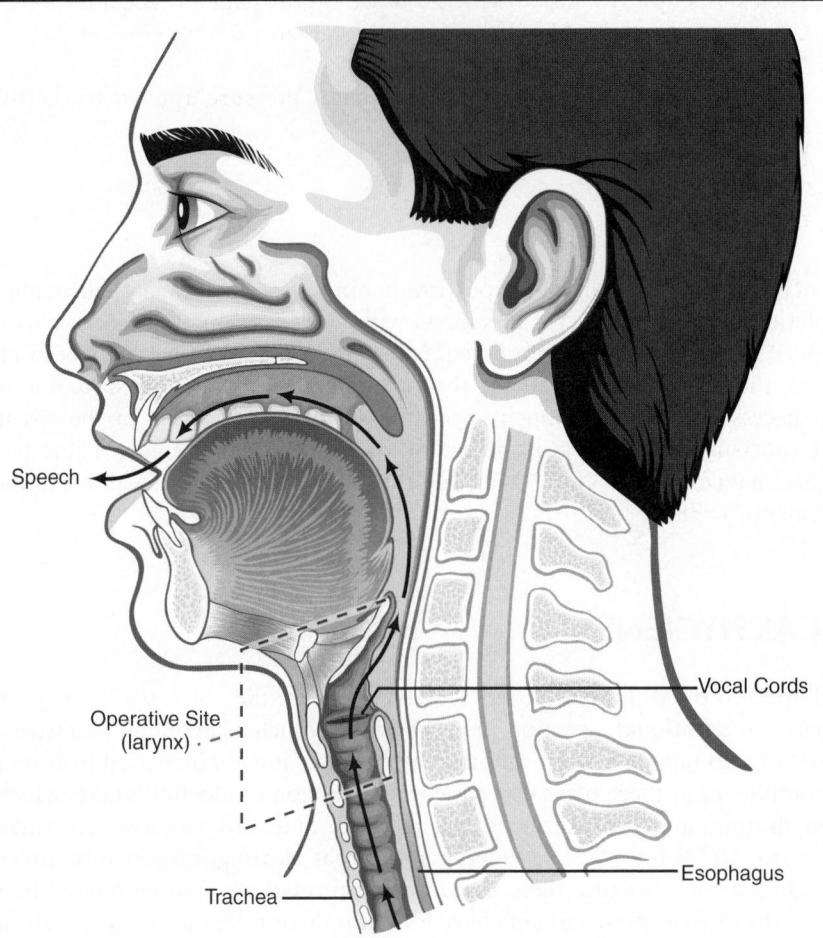

Speech

Operative Site
(larynx)

Trachea

Vocal Cords

Esophagus

TUMOR STAGING

The tumor, node, metastasis (TNM) clinical staging system defines the extent of disease, with variations depending on the location of the cancer (breast, colon, lung, liver, prostate, and head and neck). This section will focus on H&N disease and its TMN staging criteria. Tumor staging is critical for establishing the disease status and patient prognosis, and for selecting the most effective treatment paradigm. When staging an H&N tumor, information gleaned from the physical examination, radiographic studies (CT scans, MRIs, PET scans), and operative and pathologic findings are included in this process. The SLP should have an understanding of the TNM criteria in order to appreciate patient management implications. Correct staging is critical for optimizing treatment and maximizing outcome. TNM staging in the H&N may encompass tumors involving the nasal cavity; nasopharynx; paranasal sinuses; oral cavity; salivary glands; oropharynx; hypopharynx; and supraglottic, glottic, and subglottic larynx (American Joint Committee on Cancer, 2010). The

FIGURE 9.4   Vocal Tract Anatomy After a Total Laryngectomy

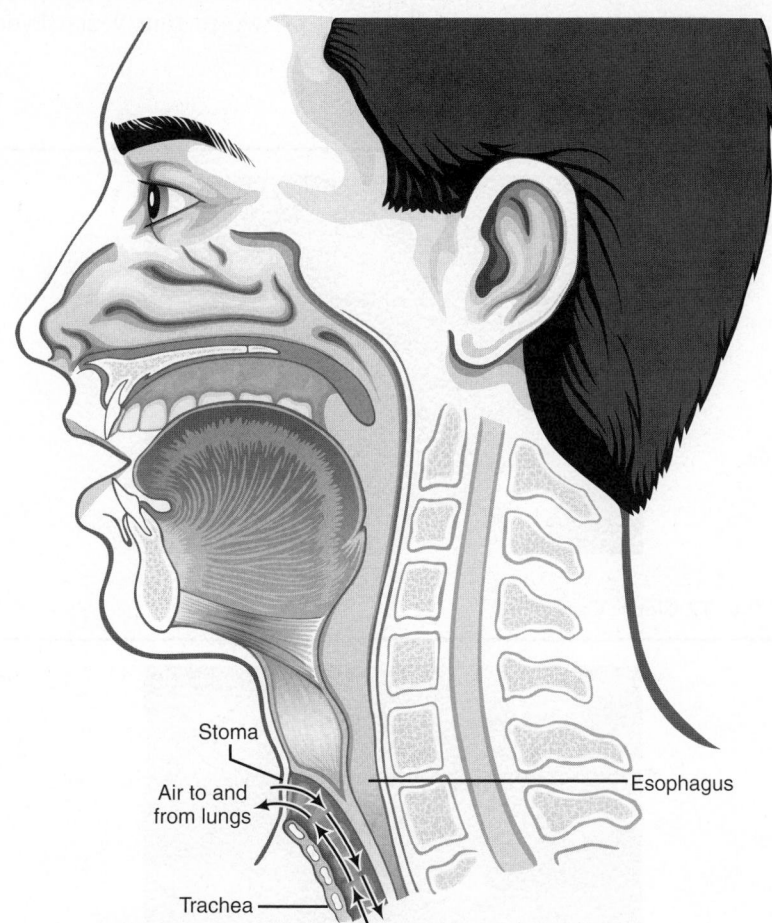

Stoma

Air to and
from lungs

Esophagus

Trachea

presenting stage of the cancer is the most important prognostic indicator for patient
survival.

- T (primary tumor: extent, size, invasiveness):Tis = "in situ" small surface lesion,
  noninvasive, dysplasia. T1 = small tumor very localized. T2 = more penetrating
  and larger tumor. T3 = penetrating lesion of muscle and possibly cartilage, movement of a vocal fold is impaired because of cartilaginous invasion. T4 = very
  large, highly invasive and penetrating tumor. The size and extent of the primary
  tumor increases from Tis through T4. The higher the corresponding number, the
  greater the risk for local, regional, and distant spread (see Figures 9.5 to 9.8).
- N (regional lymph node involvement):N0 = no spread to the neck lymph
  nodes. N1 = spread to one lymph node (ipsilateral). N2 = spread to one lymph
  node ipsilateral measuring more than 3 cm, or multiple contralateral or bilateral neck lymph nodes. N3 = spread to one or more lymph nodes measuring
  more than 6 cm. Regional spread equates to a poorer prognosis, and the site of
  the primary tumor is a major determining factor in this metastasis.
- M (distant spread):M0 = no evidence of distant spread. M1 = distant spread.

Distant spread of the cancer from the primary tumor in the H&N to other organ sites (lung, bone, liver). This is more common in late stage, advanced cancers and carries a survival expectancy of two to four years (Lyden and colleagues, 2011).

FIGURE 9.5 T1 Glottic Cancer

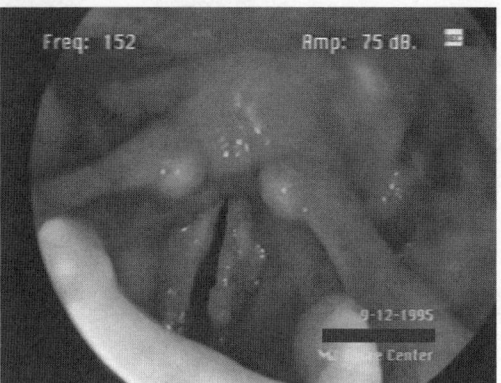

FIGURE 9.6 T2 Glottic Cancer

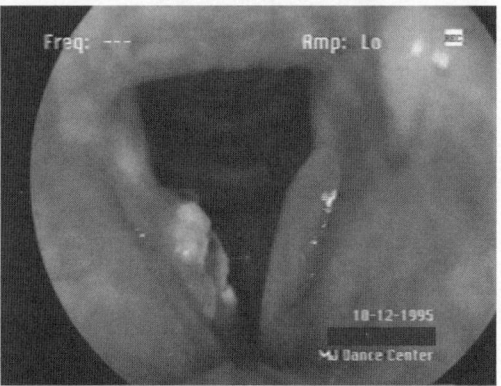

FIGURE 9.7 T3 Glottic Cancer

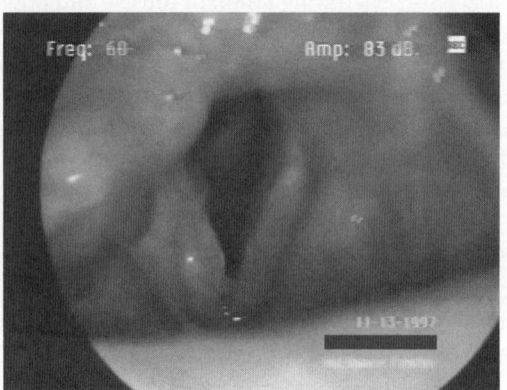

FIGURE 9.8 T4 Supraglottic and Glottic Cancer

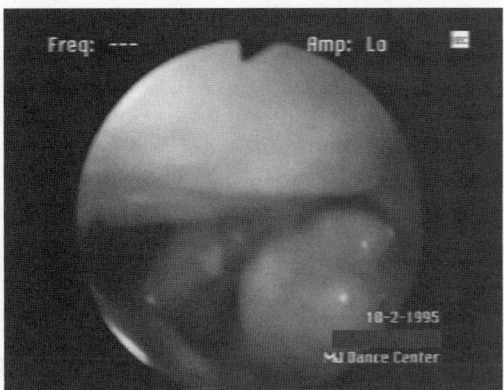

SURGICAL ADVANCES AND ORGAN PRESERVATION PROTOCOLS

The surgical management of head and neck cancer is evolving secondary to the introduction of robotic assisted surgery, less invasive endoscopic procedures, and laser microsurgery (Xu and Fung, 2012). These techniques preserve surrounding healthy tissue by approaching an organ transorally or through a small incision rather than the more traditional open procedures (partial or total laryngectomy). The desire to reduce the need for major surgical resections without compromising oncologic control is possible with advances in both radiation therapy (RT) and chemotherapy (CT). Preserving an organ without sacrificing survival is changing the landscape in head and neck cancer management (Haigentz and colleagues, 2010). Organ preservation, which on the surface may be an exciting alternative, does *not* guarantee a functional organ and is *not* without toxic side effects (Xu and Fung, 2012). Despite treatment advances, the total laryngectomy is the most common procedure for advanced laryngeal cancer.

PREOPERATIVE COUNSELING

Because laryngectomy alters respiration, swallowing, and speech, it is essential that the patient understand the concept of laryngectomy and details about the surgery and speech rehabilitation. Therefore, a presurgical counseling session is recommended for the patient and his or her family. Typically, in larger medical or teaching institutions, counseling would involve an interdisciplinary team. Members of such a team may include ENT physicians, nurses, social workers, SLPs, oncologists, prosthodontists, and dentists. In a smaller or more rural environment, the SLP may be the sole provider of information. Regardless of the setting or facility, the SLP should illustrate and describe the changes that occur in the speech mechanism as a result of laryngectomy. Written information, illustrations, and films about various alaryngeal communication options should be provided. The SLP should also demonstrate artificial larynges and address patient concerns and questions. Information may be accessed through the Internet from organizations such as the International Association of Laryngectomees (IAL) or WebWhispers. The booklet *Self-Help for the*

Laryngectomee (Lauder, 2001) can be reviewed with the patient. Whenever possible, it is recommended that a laryngectomized patient-visitor, one who has successfully completed medical–surgical treatment and speech rehabilitation, be included. This provides a unique opportunity for personal contact with an experienced mentor.

Over the years, we have observed, and it is well reported in the literature, that laryngectomees have psychological profiles similar to amputees. Naturally, their primary concern is their immediate health prognosis. We address these concerns by explaining that surgical and ancillary intervention are state of the art, and that head and neck cancers are among the more curable cancers. A checklist for pre- and post-operative consultation is found in Keith and Darley (1994, pp. 144–145) and in Doyle and Keith (2005, pp. 372–373).

POSTLARYNGECTOMY COMMUNICATION OPTIONS

The laryngectomee has three general communication options, none of which is mutually exclusive. In esophageal speech (ES), air is "inhaled" into the pharyngoesophageal segment (PE) and then expelled, setting the tissue of the PE segment into vibration for a voice source. The second option is the electrolarynx, which falls under the general category of artificial larynx (AL). This method introduces sound for speech through an instrument externally placed against the throat or oral structures, or through a fitted prosthetic electrolarynx inserted into the mouth while speaking. The third option is tracheoesophageal (TEP) voice restoration surgery, which may be performed at the time of the total laryngectomy (primary) or sometime after surgery (secondary). An opening or puncture is made through the posterior wall of the trachea, extending through the anterior wall of the esophagus. A prosthesis inserted into the puncture shunts pulmonary air into the esophagus, causing the upper esophageal sphincter and surrounding tissues to vibrate. This creates the sound that can be used for TE speech.

Numerous studies have reviewed patterns of vocal rehabilitation preferences and use among laryngectomees. A study by Hillman and colleagues (1998) revealed that a small percentage of laryngectomees developed usable ES (6%) or remained nonvocal (8%). The predominant method of choice was an AL (55%), while 31% opted for TEP speech. These patterns of use are quite different from the findings of Ward and colleagues (2003), who followed 55 total laryngectomees over a five-year period. Although an electrolarynx was introduced as the initial communication mode directly after surgery, 74% of the patients developed TEP speech as their primary mode of communication. Compared with electrolarynx users, TEP speakers reported significantly lower levels of disability, handicap, and distress. ES was not an option in this study. Researchers in Japan (Koike and colleagues, 2002) reported outcomes of speech therapy for 65 laryngectomees who were offered ES and AL options only. Forty-two percent of the patients acquired practical ES and 91% acquired both ES and AL speech. On the flip side, 151 experienced SLPs ranked their preference for voice rehabilitation methods for laryngectomy patients. TEP speech was the most preferred method and the AL was the least preferred (Culton and Gerwin, 1998). Laryngectomy patients were asked to rate levels of satisfaction with their method of alaryngeal communication (Clements and colleagues, 1997). Patients were divided into four groups, by method of communication: tablet writers, ES, AL, and TEP speech. Compared with the other groups, the TEP speakers expressed more satisfaction with their speech quality, ability to communicate over the phone, and ability to interact with others. Similar to the Ward and colleagues (2003) study, TEP speakers also rated their overall quality of life higher. These findings are of interest because, unlike previous studies focusing on the intelligibility of speech judged by listeners (Doyle and colleagues, 1988; Max and colleagues, 1997; Sedory and colleagues, 1989), this study polled patients on their own perceptions of speech. The remaining sections in this chapter address these three communication modes—the artificial larynx (AL), traditional esophageal speech (ES), and tracheoesophageal puncture (TEP) speech—for the postlaryngectomy patient.

THE ARTIFICIAL LARYNX

We frequently encourage the use of an AL during the first few days, weeks, or months following surgery. When healing is still incomplete and swelling may be significant, we may introduce the patient to a Cooper-Rand intraoral AL, commonly used in years past and still available. This device is shown in Figure 9.9 with other ALs. Any intraoral AL such as the Cooper-Rand or orally adaptable neck instrument does not require pressure to the neck and thus works when fistulae or swelling are problems. Older models such as the Western Electric and Aurex (also presented in Figure 9.9) have been superseded by technologically more advanced options such as the Servox Digital, Servox Inton, NuVois, SolaTone, and TruTone. Their operational concept remains unchanged, and familiarity with both older models and current versions is beneficial for any practicing clinician. Currently available ALs and a review of features are easy to find online through the IAL website, WebWhispers, or specific manufacturer sites.

FIGURE 9.9 Seven Artificial Devices

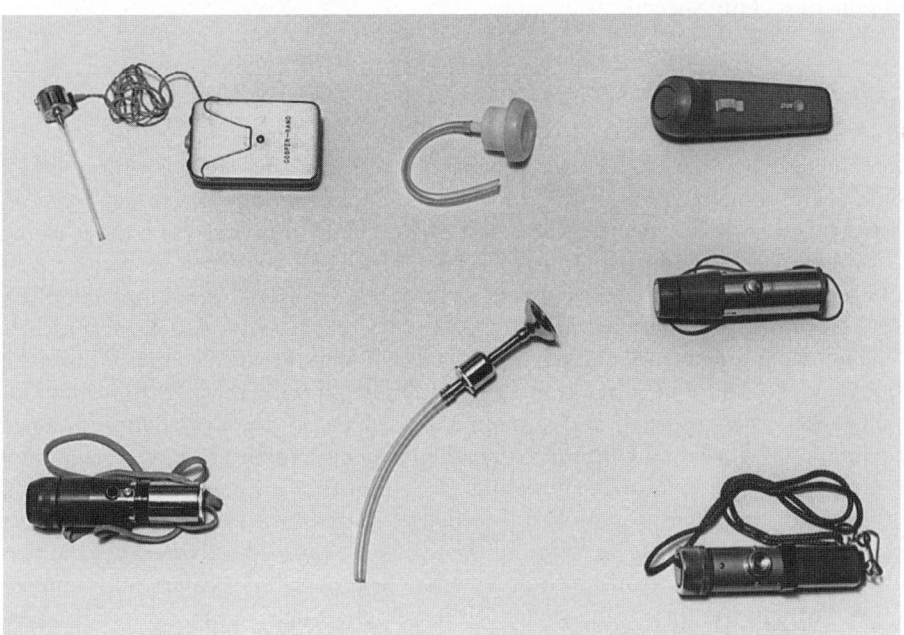

Top left: Cooper-Rand electrolarynx. Top center: Memacon artificial larynx DSP8 pneumatic. Top right: Western Electric neck device. Bottom left: Park Jed-Com electrolarynx. Bottom center: Tokyo reed-type pneumatic artificial larynx. Center right: Servox neck device. Bottom right: Aurex neck-held electrolarynx NeoVox.

Watterson and colleagues (1998) investigated the speech intelligibility (for vowels and sentences) of four different electronic neck ALs. Among other findings, the vowel /a/ was most intelligible and /u/ was the least intelligible. On a scale of 1 to 5 (5 being highly intelligible), the mean sentence intelligibility rating for all ALs combined was found to be 2.98. Even if the laryngectomee uses TEP speech, the use of an AL is a good alternate mode of phonation should the other mode fail or the external environmental factors (e.g., background noise) dictate a shift to another mode of speech.

In looking at alternative types of ALs, one should not overlook the various pneumatic types of artificial devices. (Two examples of pneumatic types may be seen in Figure 9.9.) These devices are simple and easy to use, and remain quite affordable. One end of the device is placed over the stoma, and the other end has a mouthpiece that contains a diaphragm sound generator that is activated when the user exhales through the stoma. They produce a satisfactory form of alaryngeal speech. Indeed, we have had professional voice users such as a preacher and athletic coach who used the pneumatic type of AL quite successfully. In our experience, this category of device has seen a dramatic decline in use over the years in the United States. Today, the pneumatic typically is not even presented as a postoperative option. Even though cost effectiveness and good intelligibility are afforded by these instruments, their visual appearance seems prohibitive. Obviously, patient choices appear to be driven by more than just cost and speech intelligibility (Ik and colleagues, 2009).

In the course of rehabilitation and beyond, a patient often chooses more than one communication method. Typically, an AL is the initial option and by choice may be used exclusively. Conversely, the AL may be abandoned altogether or relegated as a backup to another method such as esophageal speech (ES) and/or tracheoesophageal puncture (TEP) speech.

ESOPHAGEAL SPEECH (ES)

While the development of TEP speech has made the use of ES less frequent, the SLP should know something about this form of speech and how to teach it if the need arises. At the very least, one needs to know where to find information on the teaching of ES. We provide this information in this chapter based on our experience with teaching hundreds of laryngectomees. Also, many of the techniques for development of ES are good principles to follow in the development of other types of alaryngeal speech.

Following a conventional laryngectomy, two methods of teaching ES may be employed: injection and inhalation. We usually begin with the injection method, which is the easiest to teach and is quite compatible with the articulation practice the patient may have used with the artificial larynx. Both methods, however, employ the same basic principle of compressing air within the oropharynx and injecting this denser air into the more rarefied (less dense) space of the esophagus. Denser air within a body moves in the direction of the less dense body of air whenever the two bodies are coupled. Some of the compressed air within the oral cavity undoubtedly escapes through the lips, some through the velopharyngeal port, and some (particularly if the esophagus is open) into the esophagus. Both methods for ES bring compressed air into the esophagus; once the air is in the esophagus, external forces compress the air within it and expel it. It is hoped that the esophageal expulsion sets up a vibration of the pharyngoesophageal (PE) segment, and the patient experiences an eructation or "voice." We consider separately the procedures for teaching the injection method and the inhalation method (sometimes combined with injection).

The Injection Method

Certain consonants appear to have a facilitating effect in producing good ES. Individuals may have their own favorite facilitating sounds, but more often than not these are plosive consonants (/p/, /b/, /t/, /d/, /k/, and /g/) or affricatives containing plosives (/t/ or /d/). Hudgins and Stetson (1937) reported many years ago that /p/, /t/, and /k/ were the easiest sounds for the new laryngectomee to use; Moolenaar-Bijl (1953) reported that the same phonemes produced esophageal speech faster in most patients than the traditional swallow method of teaching. Specific steps for teaching injection might include the following:

1. Discuss with the patient the dynamics of airflow, explaining that compressed, dense air always flows in the direction of less dense, rarefied air. Explain how the movements of the tongue in the injection method increase the density of the air within the mouth, enabling the air to move into the esophagus. Then demonstrate how the whispered articulation of a phoneme, such as a /t/ or a /k/, is the kind of tongue movement that produces the injection of air into the esophagus. After producing the whispered /t/, demonstrate for the patient an esophageal voice for words such as *tot* or *talk*.

2. Now ask the patient to produce the phoneme /p/ by intraoral whisper. Care must be taken that the sound is made by good firm compression of the lips, with no need for stoma noise. Make sure that the patient avoids pushing out the pulmonary exhalation or using tongue and palatal-pharyngeal contact as the noise source. The intraoral whisper can be taught effectively by having the patient hold his or her breath and then attempt to "bite off" a /p/ by compressing the air caught between his or her abruptly closed lips. The patient should continue practicing this until true intraoral articulation is clearly grasped. This is demonstrated when he or she is consistently able to produce a precise /p/. Once the patient can do this, he or she should move to the next voiceless plosive, /t/. Here, the tongue tip against the upper central alveolar process is the site of contact, and practice should be continued until the patient can produce a precise, clear /t/. The same procedure should be repeated for /k/, again first demonstrating for the patient the different site of contact.

3. When good intraoral voiceless plosives have been produced, the patient is ready to add the vowel /a/ to each plosive. With /p/, for instance, he or she makes the plosive, and then immediately attempts to produce an esophageal phonation of /a/, producing in effect the word *pa*. If this is successful, the patient may combine the /p/ with a few other vowel combinations before going on to the /t/ and /k/. If the patient fails to produce the esophageal voice at this point, he or she should go back and work for even crisper articulation of the plosive sounds. If the patient is still unsuccessful after increased practice in articulation, he or she should attempt the inhalation method as the primary means of air intake.

4. Introduce the words *pat, pip, pack, pot,* and *pop.* The task is now to say each word, one at a time, renewing the esophageal air supply as the patient speaks, which is an obvious advantage of using the injection method. It is through the mere process of articulation that the patient takes in air. After the patient has demonstrated success with these phonemes, introduce their voiced cognates, /b/, /d/, and /g/.

5. Additional phonemes, such as /s/, /z/, /ʃ/, /t/, /z/, and /d/, may be introduced for practice. As the patient gains phonatory skill with each new consonant, he or she must spend extra time learning to improve both the quickness and the quality of production. Too many patients err in trying to develop functional conversation too

early. Considerable time should be spent at the monosyllabic word level practicing one word at a time and making constant efforts to produce sharp articulation and a good-sounding voice.

6. Practice with basic control techniques is essential for developing successful and fluent esophageal speech. Therefore, we have the patient practice several skills directly in each speech session:

    a. Rapid production (one-half second or less) of esophageal phonation can improve response. If we call for ten productions of the /a/ vowel, the patient must respond with ten productions.

    b. Ability to sustain a tone for two and a half to three seconds or longer.

    c. Ability to interrupt the tone into three or four segments.

    d. Ability to stress the first or second syllable on command, such as in the word *chipper* (for first-syllable stress) and *above* for (second-syllable stress).

    e. Ability to make a soft or loud tone on command.

7. At this point, if the patient has been successful, the inhalation method can be introduced to improve air intake and esophageal phonation. The patient should produce a normal inhalation and, at the initial moment of exhalation, produce the consonant and say the word. Beyond the single words alone, we often couple the words together in phrases, such as *bake a cake, stop at church, park the black cart,* and so on. Once plosive-laden phrases are mastered, we then use the oral reading materials from voice and diction books, including, when possible, the facilitative consonants we have been using.

The Inhalation Method

The flow of air in normal respiration is achieved by the transfer of air from one source to another because of the relative disparity of air pressure between the two sources. For example, when the thorax enlarges because of muscle movement, the air reservoir within the lung increases in size, rarefying (decreasing) the air pressure within the lung. Because the outside atmospheric air pressure is now greater, the air rushes in until the pressure within equals the outside pressure. The flow of air is always from the more dense to the less dense air body, and the flow continues until the two bodies are equal in pressure. By this same airflow mechanism, the esophagus inflates in the inhalation method of air intake. The patient experiences a thoracic enlargement during pulmonary inhalation, which reduces the compression on all thoracic structures, including the esophagus. If the cricopharyngeus opening into the esophagus is slightly open at the time of the slight increase in the size of the esophagus, air from the hypopharynx flows into the esophagus. During the exhalation phase of pulmonary respiration, when there is a general compression of thoracic structures, the esophagus also experiences some compression, which aids in the expulsion of the entrapped air. As this air passes through the approximated structures of the PE segment, a vibration is set up, producing esophageal phonation. The advantage of the inhalation method of esophageal air intake is that it follows the patient's natural inclination pulmonary inhalation followed by exhalation-phonation. Simply to take a breath and then talk is the most natural way of speaking, and for this reason the inhalation method offers the patient learning esophageal speech some early advantages.

The following steps for teaching the inhalation method are best used in combination with the injection method:

1. Explain and demonstrate to the patient some aspects of normal respiration. Many normal speakers, for example, have never thought much about normal respiration, and many do not know that their voicing has always been an exhalation event. Explain to the patient that when the chest is enlarged by muscle action, the air flows into the lungs; in the laryngectomee's case, the air comes through the stoma opening in the trachea and down into the lungs. Point out that the chest enlarges by muscle action, not by air inflation; thus, the air comes in as the chest enlarges. When the laryngectomee's chest enlarges, a concomitant enlargement of the esophagus usually takes place. When the esophagus is enlarged, there is a greater chance for air to flow in. When the chest becomes smaller, the pulmonary air is forced out, and the air within the esophagus is also more likely to be expelled. If possible, demonstrate esophageal voice using this method.

2. Before attempting to produce voice, the patient should practice conscious relaxation and correct breathing methods. He or she should become aware of thoracic expansion and abdominal distention on inhalation and of thoracic contraction on exhalation. Respiration practice should only be long enough to permit the patient to develop this kind of breathing awareness because patients do not seem to benefit much from extended breathing exercises per se.

3. Now the patient should attempt to add air into the esophagus during his or her pulmonary inhalation. Diedrich and Youngstrom (1966) recommended that "the patient be told to close his mouth and imagine that he is sniffing through his nose, and to do so in a fairly rapid manner" (p. 112). Even though the sniff is basically a constricted inhalation, it is frequently accompanied by esophageal dilation (the normal person often swallows what he or she sniffs). As an extension of the sniff, the patient should be asked to take a fairly large breath (through the stoma, of course). When his or her lungs appear to be about half inflated, the patient should say "up" on exhalation. This procedure can be repeated until the patient experiences some phonatory success.

4. For the patient who does not experience success in step 3, the following variation of the inhalation method sometimes produces good esophageal air. Ask the patient to take a deep breath, and, as he or she begins the inhalation, to cover the stoma. While the muscular enlargement of the thorax continues (despite the patient's lack of continuing inhalation), there will be a corresponding enlargement of the esophagus, perhaps permitting air to flow into the esophagus. For the patient who can get air into the esophagus but cannot produce the air escape necessary for phonation, the same mechanism applies in reverse. Here, the patient takes a deep inhalation and, as he or she begins to exhale, occludes the stoma. As the thorax begins to decrease in size, pressure increases on the esophagus, which might well result in expulsion of esophageal air (and phonation).

5. If esophageal phonation is achieved by either of the last two steps, the patient should proceed from his or her "up" response to single monosyllabic words beginning and ending with voiceless plosives. Time should be spent practicing at this single-word level until the technique is mastered in terms of loudness, quality of sound, and articulation. The patient who masters the basic techniques of air intake and phonation at the single-word level may become the best esophageal speaker.

TRACHEOESOPHAGEAL PUNCTURE (TEP)

Today, most laryngectomees are candidates for the tracheoesophageal puncture (TEP) and the prosthetic approach to alaryngeal speech rehabilitation. In many patients, the TEP will be performed at the same time as the total laryngectomy (Hamaker and Hamaker, 1995), which is called a primary TEP. Also, a cricopharyngeal myotomy (weakening the PE segment by surgically cutting all the muscle fibers) is often performed at the time of laryngectomy. This is done to create a PE (pharyngoesophageal) segment that does not present excessive resistance to the outward flow of air during phonation and allows for adequate vibration of the PE segment during alaryngeal voice production.

A number of researchers have described candidacy requirements for successful TE speech regardless of the timing of the procedure. First, the patient must have adequate pulmonary support to shunt air from the lungs and trachea to the esophagus (Panje, 1981). Therefore, individuals with lung cancer, asthma, or other severe lung disease may not be appropriate candidates for this mode. Second, the patient must possess the necessary cognitive and sensorimotor skills to occlude the stoma for speech (or manipulate a tracheostoma valve) and to remove and clean the prosthesis (Bosone, 1994). These two criteria have been superseded in importance, however, secondary to the introduction of low-pressure prostheses options requiring reduced pulmonary support, and the advent of indwelling prostheses that are placed by either an ENT physician or an SLP. The patient must have a PE segment that vibrates adequately to generate a sound source for speech. This is performed via insufflation testing, a diagnostic procedure that transfers air from the stoma site to below the PE segment through a transnasally placed catheter. If the PE segment does not adequately vibrate via insufflation testing, alternative intervention techniques may be applied. Techniques currently include Botox injections, myotomy, and pharyngeal plexus neurectomy. For details of these techniques, see American Speech-Language-Hearing Association (2004a).

Research by Knott and Lewis (2012) report that the traditional TEP guideline hierarchy should be restructured to include the following: severe dysphagia, radiation fibrosis, stoma and or tracheal stenosis, esophageal stricture, and extensive flap reconstruction. All of these factors carry a substantial risk to limit TEP candidacy.

Consensus appears to support no substantial outcome differences between primary versus secondary TEP placement (Boscolo-Rizzo and colleagues, 2008; Chone and colleagues, 2005). The obvious advantages of the primary procedure are more rapid communication rehabilitation and the elimination of a second surgical procedure. If the TE prosthesis has not been inserted at the time of the primary or secondary puncture, the patient will be ready for prosthesis insertion five to seven days after fistula creation. It is important to understand that there are two major types of prostheses: those that the patient can insert and manipulate (traditional) and those that are inserted and removed by the physician or the SLP (indwelling). Although a variety of prostheses are available, they have in common a silicone tube, a one-way valve, and a tracheal flange (Keith and Darley, 1994). The fistula is dilated and the prosthesis is inserted. A good description and pictures of these procedures is provided by Blom (1995) and McFarlane and Watterson (1995b). The fitting of the correct length of the prosthesis is critical for the best TE voice result. A prosthesis that is too short may be expelled during forceful coughing, and there is a substantial risk for distal tract closing even if the prosthesis remains in place. One that is too long makes contact with the posterior esophageal wall, thus interfering with voice production and causing a leak due to malfunction of the one-way valve or fistula enlargement. The correct length is determined by placing the measuring device (Figure 9.10) into the stoma and through the punctured fistula. This procedure allows one to gauge the distance from the posterior wall of the trachea to the posterior wall of the esophagus. When the correct prosthesis is selected, the TE puncture fistula must be dilated with the dilator (Figure 9.11). With an inserting device and a gel cap for an indwelling prosthesis in this case, constant firm pressure is applied until the prosthesis slips into place. The gel cap eases the insertion of the prosthesis by reducing friction and providing lubrication for the surrounding skin. The stoma is then occluded by the thumb or the finger and voice production is tested. If the prosthesis is in place and the back wall of the esophagus is not in contact with the prosthesis, then the air is shunted into the esophagus and the PE segment is set into vibration.

The patient who is a TEP speaker is generally able to develop good esophageal voice more quickly than the patient with a conventional laryngectomy. On expiration, by shutting off the open stoma with a finger or by using a one-way stoma valve, the patient can divert tracheal air directly into the esophagus. Being able to do this negates the need for teaching the patient to trap air in the esophagus by either the injection or the inhalation method. In addition, the TEP speaker has a much larger

FIGURE 9.10 Measurement of Tracheoesophageal Puncture Tract Length Using the Blom-Singer Measurement Device

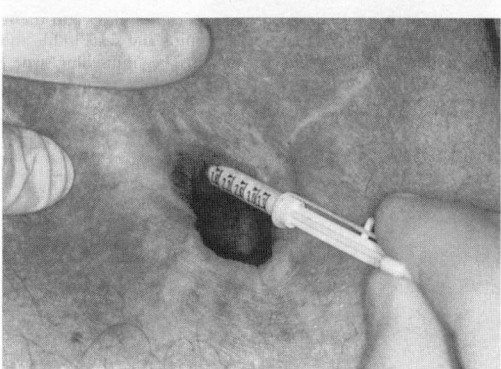

FIGURE 9.11 A Blom-Singer Tracheoesophageal Dilator Is Inserted Through the Stoma into the Esophageal Puncture

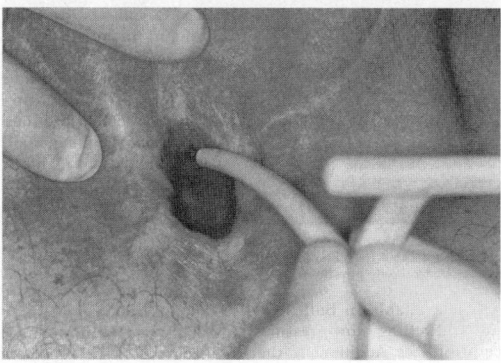

air reservoir with which to speak (up to 3,000 cc of pulmonary air versus approximately 80 to 100 cc of air trapped in the top of the esophagus).

Two types of TE prostheses are shown in Figure 9.12. The patient may also wish to wear a one-way valve fastened over the stoma. This valve permits air to come in from the outside on inspiration but shuts off on expiration, allowing air to travel through the shunt into the esophagus (Blom and colleagues, 1998; Lewin and colleagues, 2000). Fujimoto and colleagues (1991) looked at the effect of the valve on developing good voice as opposed to using finger closure of the stoma and found that there were no real differences in quality of voice between the two methods. The patient who must use his or her hands in work might profit from wearing the stoma valve; otherwise, occluding the open stoma when one wants to speak might be best achieved by using one's finger. It appears that research favors the low-pressure prosthesis (see Figure 9.13) over the duckbill prosthesis for developing the best speaking voice (Pauloski and colleagues, 1989).

FIGURE 9.12 Insertion of a Blom-Singer Low-Pressure Voice Prosthesis on a Safety Lock Inserter

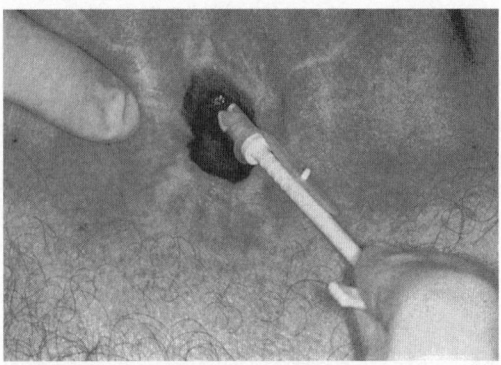

FIGURE 9.13 Two Blom-Singer Prostheses

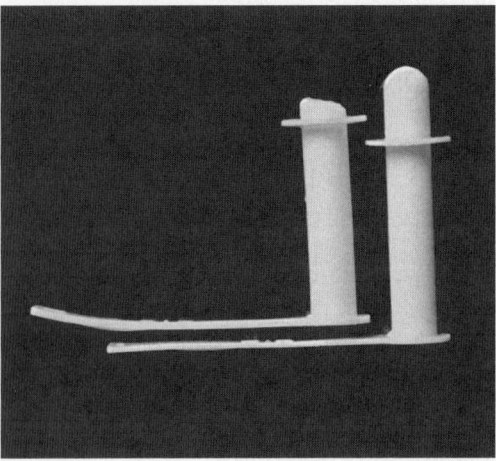

The top larger prosthesis is a modification of the original duckbill prosthesis inserted via a shunt through the trachea into the esophagus. The lower slightly smaller prosthesis is the newer low-pressure voice prosthesis.

The teaching steps below are designed for the patient with a tracheoesophageal shunt and who uses finger occlusion of the stoma to speak:

1. The SLP should review the procedures the patient has had. The article by Hamaker and Hamaker (1995) is helpful because it summarizes most of the surgical procedures available.

2. A review of how normal voice is produced is helpful for the patient who may never have realized, for example, that all speech in English is produced on pulmonary expiration.

3. Practice should be given to producing precise articulation. The patient should be encouraged to practice intraoral whispers so that the words are distinct and clearly understandable to listeners.

4. The patient is asked to take in a normal breath, occlude his or her stoma with a thumb or finger, and say a monosyllabic word on expiration. It is important that the patient be counseled to use the thumb or finger only as a diverting body to the airstream. Sending the air through the shunt (or the appliance in the shunt) does not require heavy finger pressure. Only a very light touch is required to divert the air from the stoma on expiration. If voice is achieved on the single word, the patient can proceed to the next step. If not, the patient should practice the timing of inspiration (open stoma) and expiration (closed stoma) in synchrony with saying one word. Trial-and-error repetitions may be needed here. Most patients can produce an effortless esophageal voice with very little difficulty. It has been our observation that patients who cannot successfully divert tracheal air through the shunt are pushing too hard with their fingers. Only light touch on the stoma opening is needed. Because many patients undergo a cricopharyngeal myotomy to weaken the muscle of the PE segment, only modest air pressure is required to set the segment into vibration.

5. Move from single words to phrases as soon as the patient is able. It is important to keep the inspiratory breath a normal one. The patient needs no more breathing effort than he or she ever did. It takes some practice to time the inspiratory–expiratory phonation to match the words or phrases one is attempting to say.

6. Once the patient can say phrases, it has been our observation that, by using natural articulation, he or she begins injecting air into the esophagus from above and using the pulmonary air passing out through the esophagus. Therefore, some patients can speak some words and phrases without occluding their stomas, obviously renewing the air reservoir within the esophagus by injection. Extended daily practice of several hours for a week or two is required before a patient with a TE shunt is able to use his or her new esophageal voice conversationally.

7. Review with the patient that the best voice seems to be produced with the least amount of effort; that is, a normal speaking breath, light finger touch, and so on.

8. The patient should be instructed in how to change, clean, maintain, and care for his or her own prosthesis(Blom, 1995; Blom and colleagues, 1998).

Anyone who is attempting to assist a patient to develop TEP speech should become thoroughly familiar with the devices, procedures, and materials involved. Blom (1995) provides guidance in patient selection, esophageal insufflation testing, indwelling prostheses, and prosthetic fitting. This information is updated occasionally (ASHA,2004a).

OVERVIEW OF THE PHARYNGOESOPHAGEAL (PE) SEGMENT

When discussing alaryngeal speech, it is just as important to appreciate the anatomy and physiology of the PE segment as it is to understand the larynx when learning about voice. The name of the PE segment essentially defines its location. This segment is also known as the neoglottis (or new glottis); following a total laryngectomy, it is bounded by the pharynx superiorly and the esophagus inferiorly. It is comprised of three distinct muscles: the inferior pharyngeal constrictor (IPC), cricopharyngeus (CPM), and uppermost esophageal muscle (UES). This segment is highly variable in location, length, shape, and tone among individuals (Lundström and colleagues, 2008); it is tonically contracted at rest and relaxes only during swallowing, vomiting, and burping.

When discussing the PE segment, the following are true:

- The PE segment is typically visible through an endoscope.
- There are numerous shapes (circular, triangular, split side to side, split anterior to posterior, irregular) as defined by its open phase configuration.
- This segment is capable of vibration (vibration is defined by site, e.g., posterior wall, anterior wall, left or right wall, or all walls).
- Saliva may be visible (none, slight, moderate, severe).
- A traveling wave may be seen.
- Vibration may be regular or irregular.
- There is a predominating phase (open, closed, equal).

These descriptors are similar to observation made in true vocal fold vibration using stroboscopy or high-speed digital imaging (HSDI). Because this PE segment is surgically created at the time of the total laryngectomy, understanding its shape, configuration, and vibratory characteristics may promote optimal alaryngeal voice in the future. This advancement appears likely only through future research utilizing HSDI of the PE segment.

To afford the reader a better understanding of the PE segment and how and why it is capable of producing sound, three distinct images of PE segment vibration during stroboscopy are presented in Figures 9.14, 9.15, and 9.16.

FIGURE 9.14 Vibrating Neoglottis During Stroboscopy in TEP Speech

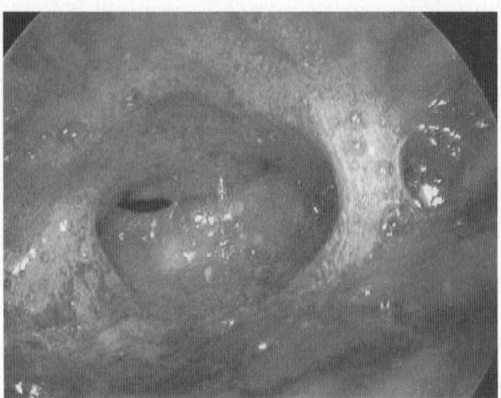

FIGURE 9.15 Vibrating Neoglottis During Stroboscopy in TEP Speech

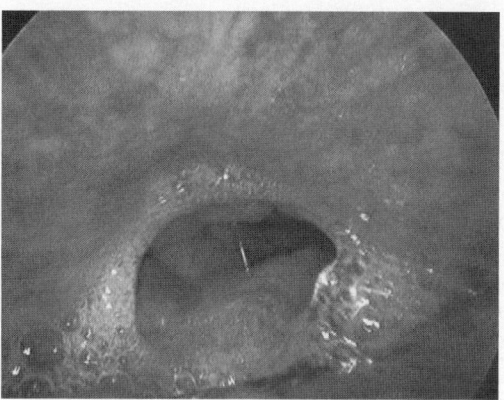

FIGURE 9.16 Vibrating Neoglottis During Stroboscopy in TEP Speech

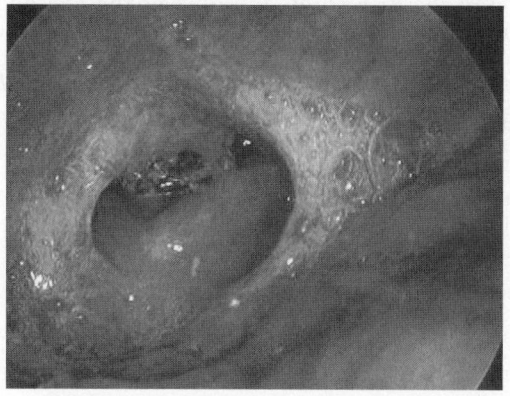

SUMMARY

In this chapter, we considered the types or modes of cancer treatment (radiation, surgery, and chemotherapy) and their effect on the voice. Some case examples that demonstrate the voice treatment approach used with patients undergoing each method of treatment were considered. Factors such as vocal fold dryness and stiffness as well as absence of tissue post-treatment were discussed. Voice Facilitating Approaches, which have been successful in producing vocal improvement in patients who have been treated for laryngeal cancer, were listed.

The importance of topics such as vocal hygiene and preoperative teaching for patients who have been diagnosed with laryngeal cancer was presented. The treatment approaches for patients who underwent total laryngectomy were also provided. The methods used and references for further information on these approaches were covered. A variety of ALs both past and present were presented. Methods of ES, and TEP speech production were provided in detail.

GUIDED READING

Read the following articles.

> D'Alatri, L., Bussu, F., Scarano, E., Paludetti, G., & Marchese, M.R. (2012). Objective and subjective assessment of tracheoesophageal prosthesis voice outcome. *Journal of Voice*. Epub ahead of print. doi:10.1016/j.jvoice.2011.08.013

> Bussian, C., Wollbrück, D., Danker, H., Herrmann, E., Thiele, A., Dietz, A., & Schwarz, R. (2010). Mental health after laryngectomy and partial laryngectomy: A comparative study. *European Archives of Otorhinolaryngology, 267*, 261–266.

Describe four ways in which the information reported in the articles might influence your clinical practice.

PREPARING FOR THE PRAXIS™

Directions: Please read the case study and answer the five questions that follow. (Please see page 319 for the answer key.)

> *Mr. O presents with a squamous cell carcinoma tumor of the larynx that is described by his ENT physician and oncologist as large and penetrating. In addition, CT scans have identified multiple lymph node involvement.*

1. This cancer would be described as:
   A. T1, N3
   B.. T2, N1
   C. T4, N3
   D. T2, N2

2. Due to the advanced stage of the CA, the gold standard for intervention is:
   A. Radiation only
   B. Laryngectomy
   C. Hemilaryngectomy
   D. Chemotherapy only

3. Preoperative laryngectomy counseling should:
   A. Include the patient and his or her family, and provide contact with an experienced laryngectomee mentor
   B. Provide illustrations and films about the respiration, phonation, and swallowing changes post-surgery
   C. Provide all postlaryngectomy communication options
   D. All of these

4. Which of the following statements is true concerning the three major communication options available to Mr. O postlaryngectomy?
   A. They are mutually exclusive.
   B. Research has found that ES is easy to learn and use by most laryngectomees.
   C. Only ES employs the PE segment.
   D. TEP employs lung air.

5. The attribute that would render Mr. O a likely candidate for successful TEP use would be:
   A. Little to no fibrosis
   B. A history of multiple radiation interventions
   C. Extensive flap reconstruction
   D. Esophageal stricture

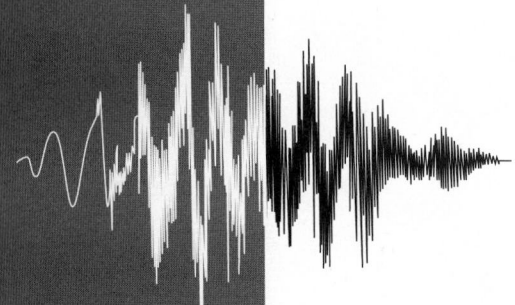

CHAPTER 10

Resonance Disorders

─ ▪ ▪ ▪ ▫ ─────────────── **LEARNING OBJECTIVES** ─────────────── ▫ ▪ ▪ ▪ ─

After reading this chapter, one should be able to:

- Describe the differences among hyper-, hypo-, and assimilative nasality.

- Define two clinical probes that can be used to assess hypernasality, and explain physiologically what is occurring during these probes.

- Discuss why stimulability testing is so important.

- Explain what can be determined regarding velopharyngeal function during an oral examination.

- Describe the various instrumental assessments of velopharyngeal function, and cite their advantages and disadvantages.

- Explain what kinds of testing can differentiate between hyper- and hyponasality.

- Explain why the Voice Facilitating Approach of yawn-sigh is effective for reducing stridency.

Using a source-filter approach, we treat the disorders of resonance in this text separately from the disorders of voice that result from the larynx being misused or from laryngeal lesions. Many of the neurological disorders discussed in Chapter 5 have a nasal resonance component; these disorders are treated separately in that chapter. The nasal resonance disorders of hypernasality, hyponasality, and assimilative nasality, and the oral-pharyngeal resonance disorders of stridency, thin voice quality, and cul-de-sac voice are the focus of this chapter.

RESONANCE DEFINED

Resonance may be defined as selective amplification and filtering of the complex laryngeal tone by the cavities of the vocal tract after that tone has been produced by the vibration of the vocal folds. Stated another way, vocal resonance is the perceptual increase in loudness of the laryngeal tone due to the concentration and reflection of sound waves by the oral, pharyngeal, and nasal cavities during voice production. The vocal folds provide the source of vibration that gives rise to the complex sound waves. These periodic vibrations, characteristic of the normal voice, are filtered in the supraglottal space of the pharyngeal, oral, and nasal cavities, or the upper airway. Our discussion of resonance in Chapter 2 showed that the *F*-shaped upper airway amplifies and filters the sounds coming into it from the larynx, depending on the frequency of the sound waves and the shape and size of the particular cavity. The pharyngeal cavities constantly change their horizontal and vertical dimensions by active movement of muscles, which in turn alters the overall configuration (Kent and Read, 2002; Pershall and Boone, 1986; Watterson and McFarlane, 1990). The open coupling between the pharyngeal cavity and the oral cavity (particularly when the velopharyngeal [VP] mechanism is closed) enables the traveling sound wave to be filtered even more by the continuous modifications of oral cavity size that occur during speech by the movements of the tongue and jaw. What emerges as voice resonance is the fundamental frequency (laryngeal vibration) modified by the natural resonant frequencies occurring at the various supraglottal sites (above the vocal folds), within the pharynx, and through the oral cavity. When the VP port is open, the pharyngeal-oral coupling with the nasal cavity is then possible so that sound waves are further absorbed and filtered as they pass through the chambers of the nasal cavity (for example, for the production of /m/, /n/, and /ŋ/ in English). For the remaining sounds of English, however, the VP port is closed, or nearly so, and the impedance is high for the transmission of sound waves into the nasal cavities (McWilliams and colleagues, 1990).

DISORDERS OF NASAL RESONANCE

There are three types of nasal resonance disorders: hypernasality, hyponasality, and assimilative nasality. Although individuals listening to speakers with these disorders might only be able to say, "The voices all sound nasal," distinct differences among the three types call for differential diagnosis and management and different voice therapy approaches. As a prelude to our discussion of separate approaches, let us define hypernasality, hyponasality, and assimilative nasality.

Hypernasality

Hypernasality is an excessively undesirable amount of perceived nasal cavity resonance during the phonation of normally non-nasal vowels and non-nasal voiced consonants. Voiced consonants and vowel production in the English language are primarily characterized by oral resonance, with only slightly nasalized components being acceptable. If the oral and nasal cavities are coupled to one another by lack of VP closure (for whatever reason), the periodic sound waves carrying laryngeal vibration receive heavy resonance within the nasal cavity. Velopharyngeal dysfunction (VPD) is the term for inappropriate transmission of the sound wave into the nasal cavities. VPD may be caused by impaired motion of the VP mechanism (incompetence), a tissue deficiency (insufficiency), or a mixture of both (inadequacy). The speech characteristics of VPD are audible nasal air emission, reduced intraoral air pressure, and hypernasality.

Hyponasality

Hyponasality is reduced or completely lacking nasal resonance for the three normally nasalized English phonemes: /m/, /m/, and /ŋ/. Hyponasality is usually the result of anatomical obstructions within the nasal cavity. Hyponasality can be categorized as an articulatory substitution disorder for which the nasal consonants are usually perceived as their voiced, non-nasal cognates (/b/, /d/, /g/). Hyponasality may be associated with abnormally large adenoids and tonsils, a deviated nasal septum, an obstructed naris, choanal atresia, nasal turbinate swelling, or allergic rhinitis. In a study by Andreassen and colleagues (1994), 14 children were seen prior to adenoidectomy and at intervals of one, three, and six months following surgery. Aerodynamic, acoustic, and perceptual measures were obtained at each visit. Andreassen and colleagues reported (p. 263) a significant reduction in nasal airway resistance, coupled with a significant increase in nasalance values, following surgery. Perception of hyponasality did not change significantly, however. This underscores the fact that nasal resonance (in this case, hyponasality) is a phenomenon of auditory perception.

Assimilative Nasality

With the case of assimilative nasality, the speaker's vowels or voiced consonants sound nasal when adjacent to the three nasal consonants. The VP port is opened too soon and remains open too long, so that vowel or voiced consonant resonance preceding and following nasal consonant resonance is also nasalized. Dworkin and colleagues (2004) report that this type of nasality may be a result of exposure to faulty speech models or exaggerated regional dialect patterns that may normally have subtle nasal (twang) characteristics. This type of voice disorder is considered functional, and speech and voice intervention is warranted and very effective.

Normal English consonants are produced with high intraoral pressures (3 to 8 cm H_2O) with essentially no nasal airflow except for the three nasal consonants, which have low intraoral pressures (0.5 to 1.5 cm H_2O) and high rates of nasal airflow (100 to 300 cc sec), as reported by Mason and Warren (1980). Aerodynamic studies of cleft palate speakers and speakers with resonance imbalance have provided some needed quantification to help differentiate patients with excessive nasal resonance from patients lacking sufficient nasal resonance (Warren, 1979). From his studies of air pressures and airflow patterns, Warren has estimated the size of the VP port for various speaking activities. Although most normal speakers demonstrate tight VP closure with no air leakage, speakers with VP openings as small as 5 mm or less may still have voice quality that is perceived by listeners as normal (Mason and Warren, 1980). Patients with nasal voices who produce high nasal airflow rates are *perceived* (we stress *perceived* because hypernasality is a perceptual phenomenon that can only occur on voiced sounds) as having hypernasality, whereas hyponasality is perceived as a speaker with a cold or stuffed-up nose and is accompanied by low nasal airflows due to an occluded nasal passage (e.g., nasal polyps or swollen turbinates) or a closed VP mechanism. Probably no area of voice therapy is more neglected or more confusing than therapy for nasal resonance problems.

EVALUATION OF NASAL RESONANCE DISORDERS

There are more similarities than differences between patients with resonance disorders and those with phonation disorders. For this reason, many of the evaluation procedures outlined in Chapter 6 are equally relevant here. In addition to obtaining the necessary medical data (such as what treatment has already been provided), clinicians must pursue case history information (description of the problem and its cause, description of daily voice use, variations of the problem, onset and duration of the problem, and so on). Clinicians must observe closely how well the patients seem to function in and outside the clinic. Considering how subjective our judgments of resonance disorders are, it is crucial that clinicians know how their patients perceive their own voices. A mild resonance problem, for example, can be perceived by a patient and/or others as severe, but a severe resonance problem, at times, may be ignored. We have known of adults with unrepaired clefts of the palate that had markedly severe hypernasality and had come to accept their vocal quality as normal. Indeed, some consider the legendary country and western singers Willie Nelson and George Jones as hypernasal, whereas others think that they sing with an "authentic regional twang."

Perceptual Analysis of Speech

An obvious way to begin the evaluation of someone with a nasal resonance disorder is to listen carefully to his or her voice during conversation. This can provide a gross indication of what the problem may be (assimilative nasality, hypernasality, or hyponasality). The perceptual aspect of nasal resonance disorders is extremely important. It is difficult, however, to make a clinical judgment about nasality by listening to someone as he or she speaks; in fact, such a judgment is likely to be wrong. For example, Bradford and colleagues (1964) found that neither a group of four experienced judges nor a group of four inexperienced judges could reliably judge the recorded voice samples of children producing /a/ and /i/ with nares open and closed (by digital pressure). This may not be too surprising because both vowels are basically non-nasal in English. The judges were similarly unreliable when judging nasality from conversational speech samples. Although the casual judgment that "something is nasal about the speech" is usually correct, not all examiners can quickly and reliably differentiate the type of nasality (hypernasality, assimilative nasality, hyponasality) on the basis of such a conversational sample alone. Voice quality judgments are more accurate if made on the basis of recorded samples of a patient's conversational speech, his or her vowels in isolation, and his or her sentences (some with only oral phonemes and some loaded with nasal phonemes). Loading sentences with nasal phonemes is helpful for making judgments of hyponasal speech. By carefully structuring the test samples, rather than relying on conversation, one can control the phonemes used and their order, which is helpful in detecting assimilated nasality. The recorded sample also allows the clinician repeated playback. Focusing on a specific parameter (loudness, pitch, quality, hypernasal versus hyponasal) on each playback may increase the clinician's objectivity. To counter the "halo" effect—the influence of a speaker's articulation on the judgment of his or her nasality—Sherman (1954) developed a procedure of playing the connected speech sample backward on the tape recorder, thus precluding the identification of any articulation errors. Reverse playback is most helpful in differentiating between hypernasality and hyponasality. Spriestersbach (1955) found that the reverse playback of speech samples of cleft palate subjects reduced the correlations between articulation proficiency-pitch level and judgments of nasality.

We have found that asking patients to repeat or read aloud passages that are totally free of nasal consonants, such as "Betty takes Bob to the show" (Boone, 1993), or passages that are loaded with nasal consonants, such as "many men in the moon" (Boone, 1993), helps us differentiate hypernasality, hyponasality, and assimilative nasality from one another. It is important to note that hypernasality occurs only on vowels, semivowels, and voiced consonants. Phrases loaded with nasal consonants are used only to demonstrate hyponasality. The absence of normal nasal resonance on these nasally loaded phrases is diagnostic of hyponasality.

We have also found that if we use the following simple screening procedures, we get a good, quick clinical classification of the type of resonance disorder present. These quick tests are simple and require no instruments to perform.

We begin the screening by having the patient say these two sentences while gently pinching the nares: "My name means money" and "Mary made lemon jam." If these sound "plugged" both when the nares are pinched and when the nares are released, the problem is hyponasality. In other words, if there is no difference between the nose-held and nose-released conditions, the problem is hyponasality. If there is a big difference between the nose-held and nose-released conditions, then the problem is likely hypernasality.

Another simple clinical technique is called the snap release /s/. We have the patient sustain a loud /s/ while the nares are pinched and then quickly released. If a "snap" is heard on releasing the nares, this means the VP mechanism is partially open and the problem is probably hypernasality. The snap is actually nasal air emission, but it gives a clue of the status of the VP mechanism. While hypernasality is a phenomenon of voiced sounds only, this technique uses a nonvoiced sound /s/ to test the adequacy of closure of the VP mechanism. This is done because there is more intraoral breath pressure required for a voiceless consonant, /s/, than a voiced consonant, and this greater pressure is a better test of the adequacy of the VP mechanism.

Next, we have the patient say, "This horse eats grass" and "I see the teacher at church." If we hear any "snorting" back in the pharynx, we can assume that it is probably due to inadequate closure of the VP port and that the problem with this speaker's voice is hypernasality. We next ask the patient to say, "Maybe baby, maybe baby." If there is no difference between the /m/ in *maybe* and the /b/ in *baby*, and both sound like *maybe*, the problem is hypernasality; however, if both words sound like *baby*, the problem is hyponasality. Finally, we ask the patient to sustain the /i/ and the /u/ vowels while we gently flutter the nose (*nasal flutter test*) by rapidly pinching and releasing the nares with the thumb and forefinger. If we hear a pulsing change in the acoustic signal, the problem is hypernasality.

Hoarseness

It would seem that individuals with hypernasality are at increased risk for hoarseness associated with vocal hyperfunction. McWilliams and colleagues (1969) endoscopically evaluated 32 children with cleft palate and hoarseness and reported that 84% of the children had vocal fold abnormalities. The most common problem was bilateral vocal fold nodules. In a follow-up study, McWilliams and colleagues (1973) reevaluated 27 of the original subjects. Seventy percent continued to present with their original vocal fold abnormalities, and it was suspected that the hoarseness was associated with VP dysfunction. Indeed the authors reported that surgical removal of the vocal nodules was not effective unless attention was also given to the faulty underlying VP mechanism. In light of these and later findings (see Lewis and colleagues, 1998; D'Antonio and colleagues, 1988), the clinician must not only make judgments about resonance, but he or she must also listen closely to and make observations about vocal quality for problems of hoarseness, loudness, and breathiness.

Simple Clinical Instrumental Assessment

For testing beyond these clinical techniques, we recommend a few additional strategies to assess nasal air emission and hypernasality using some relatively inexpensive but effective instruments. Place a fogging mirror (a mirror capable of being fogged) under a naris and instruct the client to repeat a non-nasal sentence, such as, "Buy baby a bib." Ensure that the mirror is deflected away from the naris when the client is quietly breathing and at the ends of productions. Also, the mirror must not touch the nose or face of the patient. The mirror will fog if the VP mechanism is open during non-nasal productions. The mirror is also effective for detecting nasal energy during sustained non-nasal phonemes, such as /s/.

Another effective low-tech instrument is a listening tube, or what we call an octopus. By fitting nasal olives at the ends of hollow rubber tubing, the clinician is able to detect puffs of nasal emission or hypernasality by placing one olive at the patient's naris and the other at the clinician's ear. The See-Scape™ (Pro-Ed Inc., Austin, Texas) device has a small Styrofoam disk encased in a clear plastic tube that floats when a patient demonstrates nasal airflow. The airflow is detected in much the same manner as with the listening tube. A nasal olive is placed at the patient's naris. If the patient exhibits nasal energy during non-nasal sentences, the float rises from the bottom toward the top of the tube.

Perhaps the most inexpensive instrument is a simple straw. As described by Kummer (2011), placing the short end of the bending straw at the tip of the child's nostril and the other end near the examiner's ear can help detect even mild hypernasality and emission of air.

The SLP may also be able to "feel" hypernasality as vibrations on the side of the nose. Nasal emission of air can often be felt by placing the index fingers lightly in the area of the cartilage.

These simple instruments, while diagnostic, are also used for feedback during therapy for hypernasal individuals, with or without excessive nasal air emission.

Stimulability Testing

Originally, stimulability testing was designed for use with problems of articulation; however, it is also effective for use with problems of voice. The basic purpose of stimulability testing, as first described by Milisen (1957), was to see how well the patient can correctly produce a sound made in error when he or she is repeatedly presented with the correct sound through both auditory and visual stimuli. One way of distinguishing between true problems of VP insufficiency (the mechanism is incapable of adequate closure) and VP inadequacy (the mechanism has the capability of closure) is to determine whether the patient can produce oral resonance under stimulability conditions (Morris and Smith, 1962). Obviously, the patient's success in producing oral resonance is a strong indication that VP closure is possible. Shelton and colleagues (1968) have observed:

> If repeated stimulation consistently results in consonant productions which are distorted by nasal emission and vowels which are unpleasantly nasal, the inference can be drawn, at least tentatively, that the individual is not able to change his speaking behavior because of VP incompetence (p. 236).

Another simple stimulability test is to elevate the patient's velum with a tongue depressor while fluttering the nose during the patient's production of a sustained /i/ vowel. Next, remove the tongue depressor and repeat the process listening for a difference in resonance. If the difference is dramatic, the patient will likely not be able to benefit from voice–speech therapy alone but will require a palatal lift, speech obturator, or surgical management. Watterson and McFarlane (1990) describe five classes of VP function based on videoendoscopic observations during speech testing: (1) normal VP function, (2) consistent VP incompetency (VPI), (3) task-specific VPI, (4) irregular VPI, and (5) abnormal resonance without VPI.

Articulation Testing

Articulatory proficiency can provide a good index of a patient's VP closure. *Nasal emission of air,* the escape of air through the nose, is a common articulation error on plosive affricate and fricative phonemes among subjects with VPD. Even though a patient may have his or her articulators in the correct position (place of articulation) in relation to their lingual-alveolar-labial contacts, the error occurs because increased oral pressure escapes nasally through the VP port. The presence or absence of nasal emission, therefore, is an important diagnostic sign of VP adequacy. It is important in articulation testing to distinguish between errors that result from faulty articulatory positioning and errors related to dysfunction of the VP structure.

An excellent articulation test for assessing competency of VP closure is found in the 43 special test items from the *Templin-Darley Tests of Articulation* (Templin and Darley, 1980), known as the *Iowa Pressure Articulation Test* (IPAT). This subtest of the *Templin-Darley Test* is particularly sensitive for identifying the presence of nasal emission during the production of certain consonants. However, any standardized articulation test is useful for determining those phonemes that are distorted because of inadequate VP closure. The clinician must closely assess the identified errors to determine if lingual placements are adequate to make the target phoneme correctly. Many younger children with VP problems exhibit sound substitutions and omission errors (compensatory articulation) in addition to the nasal emission and nasal snort distortions. Older children and adults with nasal emission problems may well have correct articulatory lingual placements, and their distortions are products of posterior nasal escape of the airstream. Following successful pharyngeal flap surgery or the proper fitting of a speech appliance, nasal emission and compensatory errors sometime continue until they are addressed through speech remediation. This is why therapy aimed at correct place of articulation is usually appropriate for children with cleft palate. General intervention strategies for compensatory articulation have been reported by Trost-Cardamone (1990), Kummer and Lee (1996), and Golding-Kushner (2001).

The so-called pressure consonants provide the best test of the adequacy of the VP mechanism. These 16 consonants—/p/, /b/, /k/, /g/, /t/, /d/, /f/, /v/, /s/, /z/, /ʃ/,

/ʒ/, /dʒ/, /tʃ/, /θ/, /ð/—should be included in any testing of the adequacy of the VP port mechanism because these sounds require the greatest degree of VP closure and the greatest intraoral air pressure. On the other end of the spectrum, hyponasality, in its purest and most overt form, would be exhibited on an articulation test with these oral substitutions for the nasal phonemes: /b/ → /m/, /d/ → /n/, and /g/ → /ŋ/. The sentence "My name means money" would be produced, for example, as "By dabe beads buddy." Assimilative nasality would be observable only for vowels or voiced consonants in words containing nasal phonemes.

CHECK YOUR KNOWLEDGE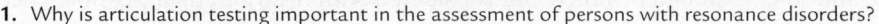

1. Why is articulation testing important in the assessment of persons with resonance disorders?
2. List one commercially available articulation test that might be clinically useful in assessment of persons with resonance disorders. Without the benefit of a commercially available articulation test, describe how you would test for hypernasality versus hyponasality.

THE ORAL EXAMINATION

As important as the oral examination is in patients with articulation disorders, it is less so for most patients with VP disorders. Oral examination provides a limited amount of information about the strength, range of motion, and degree of VP function because the anatomic point of closure is superior to the lower border of the velum. That is, the clinician cannot actually see the nature of velar and pharyngeal function simply by viewing the mechanism through the oral cavity. For example, poor uvular-tip contact with the posterior pharyngeal wall does not indicate lack of closure more superiorly in the pharynx, where closure may actually occur. Conversely, the contact of the uvula to the posterior pharyngeal wall is not necessarily an indication of adequate VP function. A markedly short, sluggish, or flaccid soft palate can certainly be noted on direct inspection of the oral cavity, and such a notation is a diagnostically important indicator for further evaluation of VP function. To truly determine the degree, speed, accuracy, and range of motion of the velopharynx, however, direct observation of the entire system is necessary.

By direct visualization of the oral structures, the clinician can make a gross observation of the relationship of the velum to the pharynx; note the relative size of the tongue; make a judgment about maxillary–mandibular occlusion; view the height and width of the palatal arch; survey the general condition of mucosa, faucial arches, and dentition; and determine if there are any clefts, open fistulas, or evidence of submucous cleft. Oral inspection of the tongue is critical because some problems of functional nasality may be related to inappropriate size of the tongue in relation to the oral cavity, poor or posterior tongue carriage, or irregular tongue movement due to an upper or lower motor neuron lesion.

The clinician should make a thorough search for any openings of the hard or soft palate that might contribute to an articulation distortion or to some problem of nasal resonance. Some patients have small openings (fistulas) or lack of fusion around the border of the premaxilla, particularly in the area of the alveolar ridge. In some individuals, such fistulas may produce airstream noises, creating articulatory distortion (by loss of intraoral air pressure), but almost never do such isolated openings this far forward on the maxilla produce nasal resonance. The more posterior the palatal fistula, the greater its effect on nasal resonance.

The absence or presence of soft-palate and hard-palate clefts should be noted; if such clefts have been previously corrected surgically, the degree of closure should be noted. In the case of a bony-palate defect, for example, sometimes the bony opening has been covered by a thin layer of mucosal tissue that is not thick enough to prevent oral cavity sound waves from traveling into the nasal cavity. This same observation applies to the occasional submucosal cleft at the midline of the junction of the hard and soft palates. The major signs of a submucosal cleft are bifid or split uvula, inverted A-shape defect in the velum, lack of a palpable posterior nasal spine, or a thin soft palate (which may appear darker in color) in the midline portion. Any other structural deviations—of dentition, occlusion, labial competence, tongue control, and so on—should be noted and considered with regard to their possible effects on speech production and nasal resonance.

LABORATORY INSTRUMENTATION

Many instruments available today can help the clinician evaluate various aspects of nasal resonance. These instruments can also be valuable in the process of managing the patient with a nasalization problem. We consider separately instruments that provide aerodynamic data, acoustic information, radiographic visualization, and visual information.

Aerodynamic Instruments

Pressure transducers and pneumotachometers are instruments of choice for measuring the relative air pressures and airflows emitted simultaneously from the nasal and oral cavities during speech (Leeper and colleagues, 1998; Warren, 1979). Other instruments are available that measure pressure and flow. As mentioned in Chapter 6, the Phonatory Aerodynamic System™ (PAS) (KayPENTAX Corp., Montvale, New Jersey) is a good instrument for airflow measures and can be used with a tube in the mouth or with a face mask. The PAS is a device that combines airflow and air pressure measurement capabilities. Pressure and flow data are measured from the two channels simultaneously, which permits relative comparisons. Normal speakers, except during the production of nasal consonants, exhibit relatively no nasal pressure or flow. Speakers with nasality problems show deviations in the relative amount of nasal and oral flows, as is well documented in the work of Mason and Warren (1980) and Warren (1979). The aerodynamic procedures basically provide the clinician information about possible leakage through the nose when the VP mechanism should be closed. Manometers have also been useful for measuring relative nasal-oral airflow. Manometers measure the amount of pressure of the emitted airstream and do not measure resonance per se. Manometers are discussed in Chapter 6.

Nasometry

The Nasometer™ II (KayPENTAX Corp., Montvale, New Jersey) is a noninvasive microcomputer-based system that developed from earlier work by Fletcher (1978) to measure the relative amount of oral-to-nasal acoustic energy in an individual's speech. An adaptation of the original Tonar II (Fletcher, 1972), the Nasometer collects oral and nasal sound intensity simultaneously using two microphones located on either side of a nasal separator. The sound separator rests against the upper lip of the subject and is held in place by headgear (see Figure 10.1). The Nasometer computer digitizes, filters, and then compares the separated signals in a ratio. The product, called *nasalance,* increases as nasal intensity increases relative to oral intensity. In addition to providing nasalance data, the Nasometer provides visual feedback on a computer screen for the patient. The feedback allows the clinician to set a predetermined level of acceptable nasalance. This feature adds another feedback dimension in real time to the client when attempting to alter oral-nasal ratios in therapy sessions.

Three passages are commonly used to obtain nasalance scores: the Zoo Passage, which contains no nasal phonemes; the Rainbow Passage, which contains 11% nasal phonemes; and the Nasal Sentences, which contain approximately 35% nasal phonemes. Each of these passages can be easily accessed at the ASHA website (www.asha.org). Fletcher and colleagues (1989) obtained nasalance scores from 117 children with no history of resonance disorders. The mean nasalance scores for each stimulus were significantly different from the others, indicating that nasalance scores are sensitive to the proportion of nasal phonemes in each speech sample.

Using the Nasometer in a study of 20 children with normal VP function and 20 children at risk for VP insufficiency, Watterson and colleagues (1996) constructed and tested two novel stimuli for obtaining nasalance measures from young children in an attempt to establish a cutoff score between normal and excessive nasalance. The new passages constructed and studied were the Turtle Passage and the Mouse Passage. The Turtle Passage contained no normally nasal consonants; the Mouse Passage contained about 11% nasal consonants. They concluded that "[c]linicians

FIGURE 10.1 The Nasometer™ II in Clinical Use

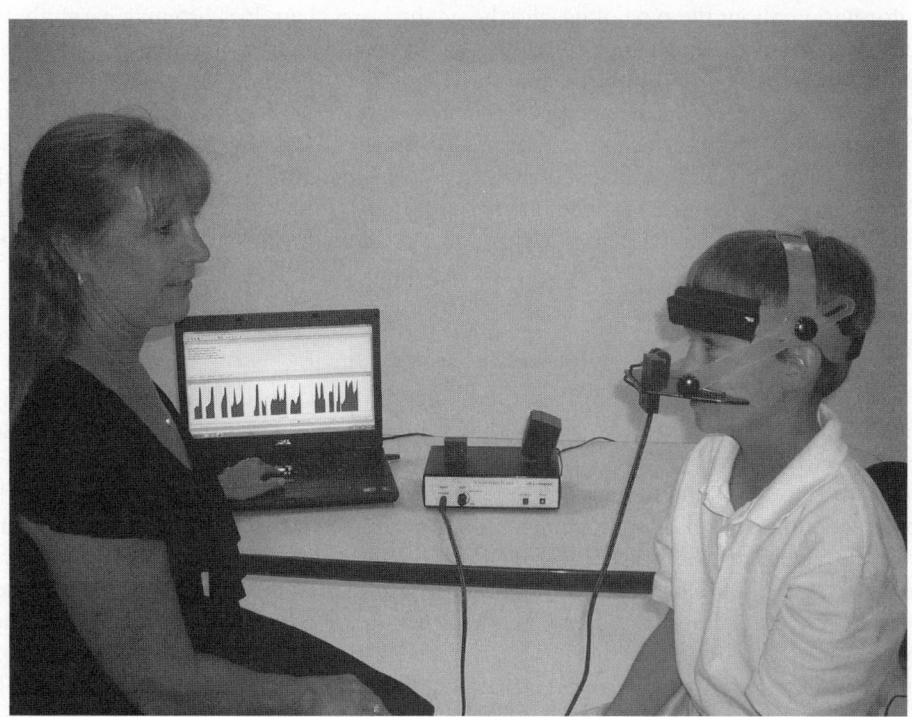

Source: Courtesy of KayPENTAX®.

should have least confidence in nasalance scores for patients who are borderline normal. Because borderline normal patients are difficult to classify, however, absolute nasalance cutoff scores may never be a reality" (p. 72). Watterson and colleagues (1998) used the Nasometer to study nasalance in low- and high-pressure speech. They concluded from their study of 20 children with managed clefts and five children without clefts that "[s]ensitivity and specificity scores indicated that the Nasometer™ was reasonably accurate in distinguishing between normal and hypernasal speech samples."

The NasalView™ (Tiger DRS, Inc., Seattle, Washington) is another microcomputer-based system that measures oral-nasal resonance. Lewis and Watterson (2003) compared nasalance scores from the Nasometer and NasalView via five sentences produced by 50 elementary school children with no history of resonance disorders. They found that the speech stimuli weighted with different vowel types were differentially affected by the different acoustic filtering used in the Nasometer and the NasalView. They suggested that the two instruments provide different information and that scores are not interchangeable.

Spectrography

It has been demonstrated spectrographically that speakers with increased nasalization demonstrate more prominent third formants with an increase in formant bandwidth, accompanied by a rise in fundamental frequency. In his acoustic study of nasality using the spectrograph, Dickson (1962) concluded that there was no way to "differentiate nasality in cleft palate and non–cleft palate individuals either in terms of their acoustic spectra or the variability of the nasality judgments" (p. 111). It is doubtful that the visual printout provided by the spectrograph can provide the clinician with any more information about the type of nasality he or she hears than does listening carefully to the same samples. This is not surprising because nasalance is a perceptual phenomenon. The spectrograph and the Computerized Speech Lab™ (CSL) (KayPENTAX Corp., Montvale, New Jersey) can help identify the aperiodic noise of nasal emission, but differentiating between spectrograms of speakers with hypernasality and those with hyponasality or assimilative nasality is most difficult and not clinically practical. As clinicians learn to use the spectral analyses provided by the spectrograph and CSL, however, these instruments may well become most useful tools for studying various parameters of nasality. (The CSL was discussed in Chapter 6.)

Radiography

Radiographic studies of the VP mechanism during speech provide ready information about structural and physiological limitations of the mechanism in those patients who demonstrate VP incompetence. For example, through a lateral-view film, we can determine the relative amount of VP opening during speech, the length of the velum and relative movements of the velum, and the posterior pharyngeal wall (Bowman and Shanks, 1978). There are limitations to the use of lateral views attempting to view closure, however, because lateral wall movement of the pharynx, which may contribute heavily to VP closure, cannot be visualized. Sometimes the patient is asked to swallow barium and, as the barium passes through the pharynx, measurements are made of the relative pharyngeal opening as it relates to the VP closing mechanism (Skolnick and colleagues, 1980). The most useful radiographic views of VP closure require the patient to make some speech utterances, including phrases and sentences that include high-pressure consonants. The SLP needs to work closely with the radiologist, presenting the speech tasks as the films are made and "reading" the films when they are completed. Sometimes a radiographic display can demonstrate a problem in VP closure that cannot be detected by any other method except for nasoendoscopy. Exposure to radiation is still a concern that must be considered in risk-benefit decisions.

Endoscopy

Shelton and Trier (1976) have written that direct measures of VP competence through the use of "endoscopes, nasopharyngoscopes, and ultrasound apparatus" offer some advantages in making treatment decisions. The oral endoscope (Zwitman and colleagues, 1976) has been a useful instrument for determining the degree and type of VP closure, as shown in Figure 10.2. The body of the oral endoscope is extended above the tongue within the oral cavity so that the lighted tip and viewing window lie just below the uvula and within the oropharyngeal opening. By turning the viewing window up toward the VP area, the velum, the lateral pharyngeal walls, and the posterior pharynx may be visualized. Two views of varying degrees of VP closure in the same subject are shown in Figure 10.2. One important disadvantage of the oral endoscope is that one can observe only vowel or limited consonant and vowel combinations such as /pa/ or /ba/. This is due to the unnatural introduction of the oral endoscope into the oral cavity and its effect on articulation and connected speech (McFarlane, 1990).

For many of us who work in the area of cleft palate or who work with those who have VP inadequacy due to structural defects (such as postcancer surgery) or neurological defect (such as one of the dysarthria subtypes discussed in Chapter 5), the use of video nasoendoscopy of the VP mechanism has become the gold standard. For example, with a nasal fiberoptic endoscope, which places a small flexible scope through the nose and down into the pharynx, the clinician can observe VP closure (during connected speech) from above the closure site (Miyazaki and colleagues,

FIGURE 10.2 Velopharyngeal Closure
········

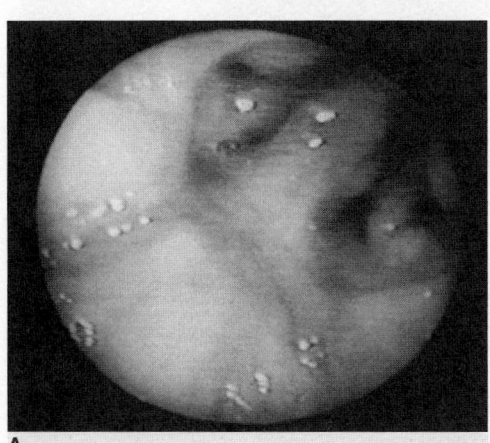 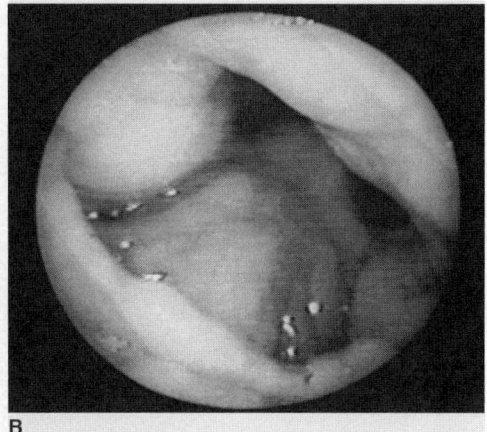

A   B

This oral videoendoscopic view of velopharyngeal closure demonstrates two degrees of closure in a sequence, from an open velopharyngeal mechanism in (A) through the bulging of Passavant's Pad with posterior and lateral pharyngeal wall movement and the velar movement in (B).

1975; Watterson and McFarlane, 1990) and the dynamics of VP function can be studied. The primary advantage of the flexible endoscope is that it is not invasive to the oral cavity and consequently does not impede tongue, lip, or jaw movements during dynamic articulation (a limitation of the oral endoscope). The oral and nasal endoscopic probes are effective instruments for assessing VP competence in patients with nasal resonance problems because they offer direct observation of velar length and movement, degree of lateral and posterior pharyngeal wall movement, and the type of VP closure the patient is using. Perhaps most important, this examination allows the clinician and the patient to see the various types and degrees of VP closure during a variety of phonetic contexts.

Watterson and McFarlane (1990) discuss in detail the use of transnasal videoendoscopy of the VP port mechanism. They discuss the use of sustained vowels, sustained consonants, single words and sentences, and phrases as speech stimuli in speech testing for VP competency. The use of high vowels such as /i/ and /u/ as well as stops (/p/, /k/, /t/), fricatives, and affricates allows the examiner to make important statements about the ability of the VP mechanism to manage complex speech tasks successfully. The information gained by using such stimuli guides therapy and management decisions. For example, it is important to know whether the patient consistently experiences nasal air escape on a particular phoneme, such as /s/; if there is a breakdown of VP function only at the phrase level; or if the particular phoneme, such as /s/, occurs in the context of a blend.

As McFarlane (1990) and Boone and McFarlane (1994) have shown, even children can be examined with nasoendoscopy without the use of any topical anesthetics. Figure 10.3 shows a patient being examined with rigid endoscopy, and Figure 10.4

FIGURE 10.3 Oral Videoendoscopy

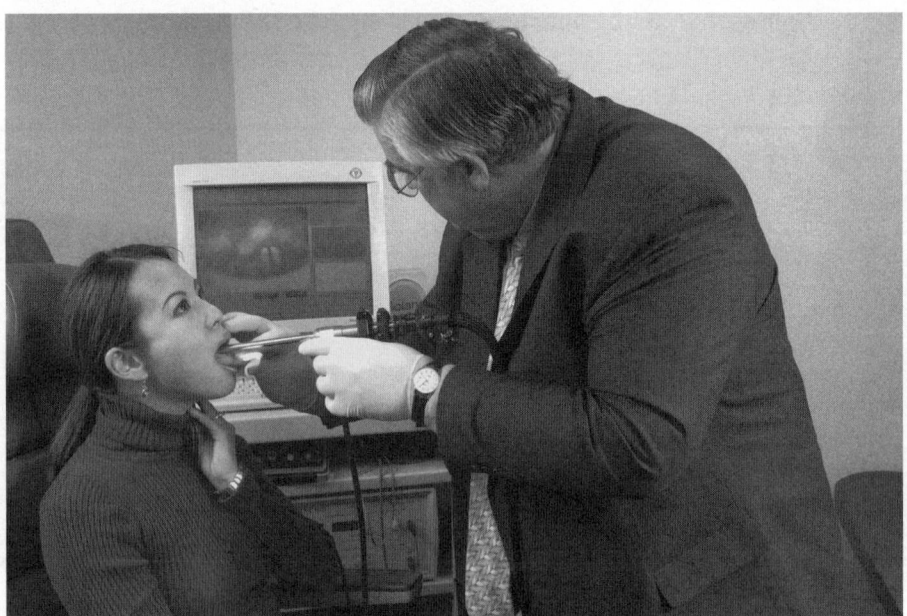

This patient is examined by oral videoendoscopy. Children and adults are routinely evaluated in this manner without the use of any topical anesthetic.

FIGURE 10.4   Nasoendoscopy of a Child with a Voice Disorder

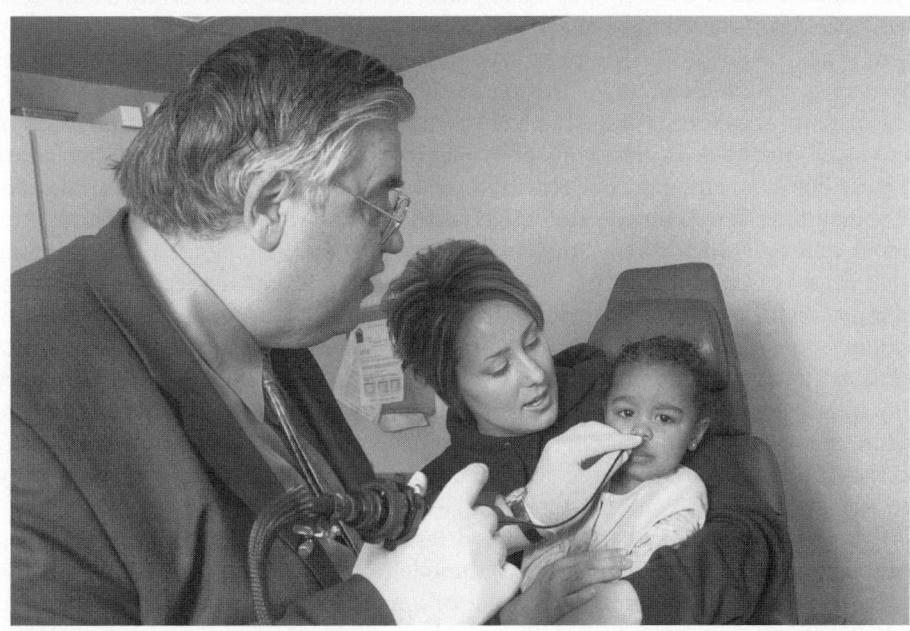

shows a child being examined with nasoendoscopy, both without the aid of topical anesthesia. Indeed, in a prospective, double-blind study, Leder and colleagues (1997) concluded that "speech-language pathologists can perform independent and comfortable transnasal endoscopy without administration of any substance to the nasal mucosa" (p. 1352).

Distinct variations in patterns of VP closure have been demonstrated by Zwitman and colleagues (1974) and Zwitman (1990). Some subjects have only velar movement without associated pharyngeal wall movement, some subjects primarily have lateral and posterior pharyngeal wall constriction, and some achieve closure by a combination of velar and pharyngeal movements. Watterson and McFarlane (1990) have described five useful classes of VP function and provide a basis for making recommendations for clinical treatment.

TREATMENT OF NASAL RESONANCE DISORDERS

Hypernasality

The presence of excessive nasal resonance (hypernasality) is relatively dependent on the judgment of the listener. That is, some languages and regional dialects require heavy nasal resonance and therefore consider pronounced nasalization of vowels to be normal. Others, however, such as Standard U.S. English, tolerate little nasal resonance beyond the three nasal consonants. Thus, a native New Englander with a nasal twang exhibits normal voice resonance in Portland, Maine, but when he or she travels to New Knoxville, Ohio, the people there may perceive his or her voice as excessively nasal. Variations do exist in the degree of nasality among the voices of the people in Ohio, of course, but a certain amount of resonance variability can exist among any particular population without anyone being bothered by it. If, however, a particular voice in Ohio (or any other place) stands out as "excessively nasal," then that voice is considered to have a resonance disorder. The judgment of hypernasality, then, is as dependent on the speech-language milieu of the speaker and his or her listeners as it is on the actual performance of the speaker.

The speaker who is judged to be hypernasal increases the nasalization of his or her vowels and voiced consonants by failing to close his or her VP port. This failure to close the VP opening may be related to neurological or structural-organic defects, or it may have a functional etiology. Hypernasality frequently accompanies unrepaired cleft palate and the accompanying short palate (inadequate tissue). Among other causes of the disorder are surgical trauma (e.g., postadenoidectomy), accidental injury to the soft palate, and impaired innervation of the soft palate as a result of poliomyelitis or some other form of upper or lower motor neuron disease or traumatic brain injury(incompetent movement). Sometimes temporary hypernasality may follow surgical removal of the adenoids and tonsils as the patient attempts to minimize the pain by not moving his or her VP mechanism. But when hypernasality persists for two or three months or more following adenoidectomy or tonsillectomy, the adequacy of the VP mechanism must be suspected and evaluated.

Some people speak with hypernasal resonance for purely functional reasons, perhaps to maintain a lingering internal model of a previously acceptable form of resonance, or perhaps to imitate the voice of someone they admire (such as a famous political figure or performer). Although the majority of people with hypernasal voices probably have some structural or neurological basis for their lack of VP competence, the ease of imitating a hypernasal voice tells us that it could be relatively easy to become hypernasal with perfectly adequate and normal VP anatomy and physiology. Hypernasality is one voice problem in which the distinction must be made between organic and functional causes because the treatment recommended is quite specific to the diagnosis.

If there are any indications of physical inadequacy of the VP closure, the primary role of the SLP is to refer the patient to a specialist who can provide the needed physical management: a plastic surgeon, say, or a prosthodontist. The SLP makes the determination of the mechanism's adequacy for speech purposes, and the patient and other professionals together determine the best corrective approach. If surgery is selected, the SLP shares the results of the speech–voice evaluation to aid with the selection of an appropriate surgical procedure. Postsurgically, the SLP evaluates the repaired VP mechanism to determine its adequacy for speech-language production.

If dental appliances are to be selected, the SLP suggests the type of appliance, lift, or prosthesis with a bulb, and assists with the design and fitting of the appliance. If a prosthetic form of management is used, then the SLP is involved in the initial fabrication and fitting of the velar lift or obturator. Subsequent modifications of these devices are directed by the SLP based on the results of his or her speech testing and the patient's response to clinical speech stimulation.

There is no evidence that voice therapy to improve resonance has any positive effect in the presence of physical inadequacy. In fact, there is some indication that voice therapy to improve the oral resonance of patients with palatal insufficiency (those who lack the physical equipment to produce closure) usually fails; in addition, such attempts are usually interpreted by the patient as his or her own fault—as a defeat indicating low personal worth—and thus take an obvious toll on the patient's self-image. An example of the ineffectiveness of speech therapy in the presence of a severe inadequacy of VP closure is provided by this case of a teenage girl with VP dysfunction who had received speech therapy for both articulation and resonance for a period of seven years:

> Barbara, age 14, had received seven years of group and individual speech therapy in the public schools and in a community speech and hearing clinic for "a severe articulation defect characterized by sibilant distortion, and for a severely nasal voice." Barbara's mother became upset because of Barbara's continued lack of progress and her tendency to withdraw from social contact with her peers, which, the mother felt, was related to her embarrassment over her continued poor speech. Barbara was evaluated by a comprehensive cleft palate team, which, after reviewing her history, found that her nasality dated from a severe bout of influenza when she was six years old. The influenza had been followed immediately by a deterioration of speech. Subsequent speech therapy records were incomplete, although the mother reported that the therapy had included extensive blowing drills, tongue-palate exercises, and articulation work. Physical examination of the velar mechanism found that Barbara had good tongue and pharyngeal movements, but bilateral paralysis of the soft palate; even on gag reflex stimulation, only a "flicker" of palatal movement was observed. Lateral cinefluorographic films confirmed the relatively complete absence of velar movement. The examining speech pathologist found that Barbara had normal articulation placement of the tongue for all speech sounds, despite severe nasal emission of airflow for fricative and affricate phonemes. Low back vowels were relatively oral in resonance, whereas middle and high vowels became increasingly nasal. It was the consensus of the evaluation team that, with the presenting movement incompetency that Barbara was (and had been) a poor candidate for speech therapy. It was recommended that she receive a pharyngeal flap and be evaluated again several weeks after the operation. The surgery was successful and had an amazingly positive effect on Barbara's speech. Although hypernasality disappeared, some slight nasal emission remained. Barbara was subsequently enrolled in individual speech therapy, where she experienced total success in developing normal fricative-affricate production.

Barbara's case dramatically shows the futility of continued speech therapy when real VP dysfunction exists. Without the operation, Barbara could have received speech therapy for the rest of her life, with no positive effect whatsoever on her voice.

VP dysfunction has two primary alternatives for treatment: surgical or dental. When structural adequacy is achieved, the remediation services of the SLP can produce further changes in the patient's speech and resonance.

Surgical Treatment for Hypernasality

The evaluation of the oral and VP mechanism may reveal the existence of structural inadequacies such as open fistulas, open bony and soft tissue clefts, submucosal clefts, and short or relatively immobile or stiff soft palates. The plastic surgeon is usually the medical specialist most experienced in making decisions about when and if surgical closure of palatal openings is required based on the recommendation of the SLP. The SLP is best able to assess the adequacy of the VP port mechanism during speech. Usually, the major reason (often the only reason) for surgical or prosthetic treatment in these patients is to improve speech, but swallowing almost always improves, too.

When the diagnostic tests have been completed, the SLP and surgeon must arrive at the plan for management. The SLP should be familiar with available options for anatomic correction and should participate in the decision for surgery. "The surgeon must know the alternative treatments and anticipated results of his operations. The timing of surgery can be a mutual decision" (Grace, 1984, p. 152). For those individuals who have cleft palate, the primary surgical procedure usually involves closing the cleft and still maintaining adequate palatal length. Most patients with cleft palate, however, require multiple secondary surgical procedures at later times, such as rebuilding structures or eliminating earlier surgical scars (Peterson-Falzone and colleagues, 2001). Many patients with hypernasality have a velum that is too short for closure or a velum that does not move adequately for closure. Such patients often profit from a surgically constructed pharyngeal flap.

In the procedure for surgically constructing the pharyngeal flap, the surgeon takes a small piece of mucosal tissue from the pharynx and uses it to bridge the excessive VP opening, attaching the tissue to the soft palate. This tissue acts as a substitute structure for an inadequate velum by deflecting both airflow and sound waves into the oral cavity and allowing the walls of the pharynx to close adequately onto the lateral margins of the pharyngeal flap. Bzoch (1989), discussing the physiological and speech results for 40 patients who had received pharyngeal flap surgery, reported that the procedure was most effective in reducing both hypernasality and nasal emission (if present) in most of the subjects. Although pharyngeal flap surgery, or any other form of palatal surgery, must not be considered a panacea for all resonance problems, it often helps align oral-nasal structures (allowing open or closed coupling of the nasal and oral cavity) so that, for the first time, speech and voice therapy can be effective.

Regarding the use of surgical methods to correct speech problems, Grace observed:

> Postoperative speech testing is mandatory to objectively evaluate the results of surgery and reassess speech goals. The surgeon may profit from observing a postoperative evaluation, much as the speech pathologist would profit from seeing surgery. All too often there is a tendency for the surgeon to divorce the patient when the surgery is completed, with the expectation that the battle will be won or lost by the speech pathologist. (Grace, 1984, p. 154)

When speaking of surgery in cleft palate patients, Grace went on to say, "In truth, the success of surgery varies widely from patient to patient, and it cannot be assumed that anatomy is restored to normal upon completion of the operation" (p. 154). This reality is reflected in the ongoing exploration for improved surgical techniques in pharyngoplasty, such as sphincter pharyngoplasty (Witt and colleagues, 1999), and covering the exposed muscular surface of the flap with nasal mucosa (Stoll and colleagues, 2001).

Dental Treatment of Hypernasality

Both orthodontists and prosthodontists can play important roles in treating individuals with hypernasality, particularly those with cleft palate. The orthodontist may have to expand the dental arches so that the patient can experience more normal palatal growth and dentition. The prosthodontist, by constructing various prosthetic speech appliances and obturators, may be able to help the patient preserve his or her facial contour and, by filling in various maxillary defects with prostheses, may cover open palatal defects such as fistulas and clefts. The prosthodontist may also be able to build speech-training appliances to provide posterior VP closure. In evaluating 21 adults with acquired or congenital palate problems, Arndt and colleagues (1965) found that both groups made significant "articulation and voice gains with obturation." These findings have subsequently been confirmed by Tachimura and colleagues (2000) and by Konst and colleagues (2003). These researchers found that children with unilateral cleft lip and palate who used a prosthesis during the first year of life followed a more normal path of phonological development between two and three years of age. Many cleft palate subjects are fitted with appliances featuring acrylic bulbs that are fitted into the VP port space. If the bulbs are well positioned near the posterior and lateral pharyngeal walls, there is often a noticeable reduction of both nasality and air escape. Articulation, which depends on adequate intraoral air pressure and normal resonance, may be achieved with speech–voice therapy in conjunction with a properly fitted speech appliance such as an obturator or palatal lift. Two lateral views of obturators are shown in Figure 10.5. Figure 10.6 shows a palatal lift prosthesis designed for an adult male with a paralyzed palate following traumatic brain injury in an accident.

When commenting on the role of the SLP in the prosthodontic management of patients with VP inadequacy, Ahlstrom (1984), a prosthodontist, stated, "One of the primary diagnostic services that an SLP can offer is the determination of VP competence in patients; this helps the prosthodontist in determination of what type of

FIGURE 10.5 Obturators

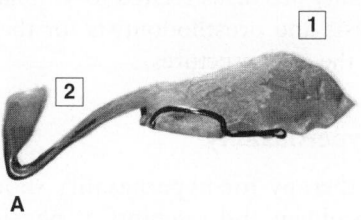

A

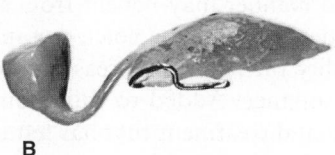

B

This photo features two different sizes of obturators. The obturator in (A) was made for an adult: (1) is the palatal part and (2) is the pharyngeal part. The obturator in (B) was made for a five-year-old girl with structural (cleft palate) hypernasality and with an extremely short velum following surgical repair.

FIGURE 10.6 Palatal Lift Device

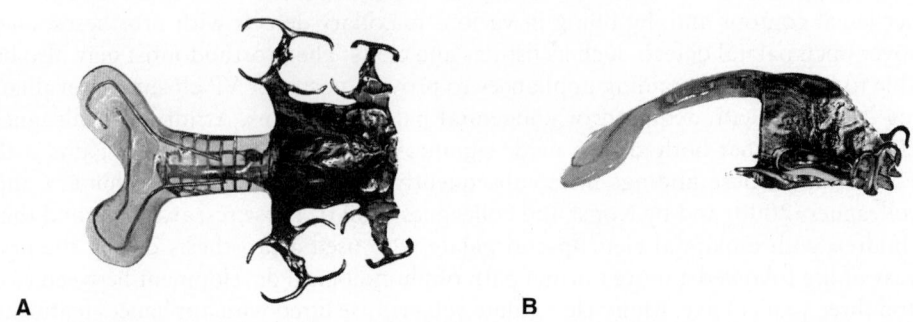

A   **B**

A superior or top view is shown in (A); a lateral or side view is shown in (B). This palatal lift was designed for an adult with a neurogenic (dysarthria) problem of hypernasality (velopharyngeal incompetency). Note the fluke-shaped lift that elevates the palate, which is quite different from the obturator in Figure 10.5 and is designed to occlude part of the velopharyngeal port for velopharyngeal insufficiency.

appliance or procedure may be necessary" (p. 150). Many patients with dysarthria, which may include a hypernasality component, have an immobile velum and thus lack sufficient velar movement to achieve closure. Such patients, who experience weakened or paralyzed soft palates, might well profit from consulting a prosthodontist about being fitted with a lift appliance to hold the immobile palate in a higher position so that some pharyngeal contact is possible (Mazaheri, 1979). The palatal lift in Figure 10.6 was made for just such a patient, who now has normal resonance with the device. For nasality problems related to VP inadequacy, SLPs should freely consult both orthodontists and prosthodontists for their ideas on how to achieve adequate functioning of the oral structures.

Voice Therapy for Hypernasality

Any attempts at voice therapy for hypernasality should be deferred until both the evaluation of the problem and attempts at physical correction (surgical or prosthodontic) have been completed. The primary requirement for developing good oral voice quality is the structural adequacy of the VP closing mechanism. Ruscello (2008) clearly advises that any attempts to improve VPI using exercises such as blowing, sucking, or other nonspeech activities are ineffective. Articulation therapy for children who present with pharyngeal fricatives and glottal stops or other errors of place and manner may benefit from such instruction (Golding-Kushner, 2001). Without adequate closure, voice therapy is futile. For individuals who speak with hypernasality for functional reasons, however, voice therapy can help develop more oral resonance. Added to this group are occasional patients who have had surgical or dental treatment that has left them with only a marginal VP closing mechanism; in voice therapy, this mechanism may be trained to work more optimally. Watterson and colleagues (1994) studied nasalance in the speech of 30 normal young adults and found that, while there was no statistical difference in nasalance scores under three different loudness levels, there was a strong systematic trend for the lowest nasalance scores to occur in the loudest conditions, while the highest nasalance scores occurred under the softest conditions.

Patients appreciate learning about their voice problems in language they can understand. Counseling the voice patient, including direct explanations of the voice problem, may be more effective with the patient than applying various symptomatic voice therapy techniques. Watch this **video** to appreciate how each counseling approach is handled a little differently. Grand Rounds: Describe how you might help a child understand the consequences of continued abuse and emphasize what can be expected (a better voice) if he or she reduces or eliminates such abuses.

The implication is to experiment with increased loudness levels in cases of minimal or borderline VPI.

The Nasometer computer display gives the patient instant feedback information about the peak nasalance level, the target level of oral-nasal ratio, and the moment-to-moment level of nasalance. If the patient is capable of developing greater oral resonance, he or she works incrementally, using the Nasometer feedback system, toward goals of acceptable oral resonance. Various Voice Facilitating Approaches (described in Chapter 7) may be used successfully with the Nasometer, nasal listening tube, See-Scape™ (Pro-Ed, Inc., Austin, Texas), nasal mirror, or stethoscope. They can even be used with a digital recorder or the unaided ear. Kuehn (1997) has experimented with the use of continuous positive airway pressure (with sleep apnea equipment) as a possible means to reduce hypernasality. To date, studies of the approach seem to indicate that the levator veli palatini muscle works harder and contracts with more force when presented with positive airway pressure. This seems to be true for both normal people and those with repaired cleft palates.

Here are some approaches that have been helpful clinically:

1. **Altering tongue position.** A high, forward carriage of the tongue sometimes contributes to nasal resonance. Efforts to develop a lower, more posterior carriage may decrease the perceived nasality.
2. **Change of loudness.** A voice that has been perceived as hypernasal is sometimes perceived as more normal if some other change in vocalization is made. One change that often accomplishes this is an increase in loudness; by speaking in a louder voice, the patient frequently sounds less hypernasal (Watterson and colleagues, 1994). One should try both increased and decreased loudness levels with each patient to determine which condition best reduces nasality.
3. **Auditory feedback.** If the patient is motivated to reduce his or her hypernasality, a great deal of therapy time should be spent learning to hear the differences between his or her nasal and oral resonances.
4. **Establishing new pitch.** Some patients with hypernasality speak at inappropriately high pitch levels, which contribute to the listener's perception of nasality. Speaking at the lower end of one's pitch range seems to contribute to greater oral resonance.
5. **Counseling.** No voice therapy should ever be started without first explaining to the patient what the problem seems to be and the general course of therapy that is being planned.
6. **Feedback.** Developing an aural awareness of hypernasality with some oral-pharyngeal awareness of what hypernasality "feels" like is a most helpful therapeutic device.
7. **Open mouth.** Hypernasality is sometimes produced by an overall restriction of the oral opening. In such cases, efforts to develop greater oral openness may reduce the listener's perception of excessive nasality.
8. **Focus.** For some patients, focusing on the facial mask area seems to increase nasality; for other patients, however, particularly those whose hypernasality is of functional origin, doing so noticeably improves resonance.
9. **Respiration training.** Increased loudness is often achieved by respiration training.

These techniques achieve their results by altering the speech production, for example, by pitch modification, increased or decreased airflow, reduced air pressure on the VP port, or enhanced feedback to the patient by using mirror fogging, acoustic changes,

Regardless of the causal factor of the disorder (organic, neurogenic, or functional), we find that patients' voices improve with feedback, be it auditory or visual or both. **Video 1** and **Video 2** show that when patients are provided with immediate feedback, they are likely to alter and adapt voice behaviors. Grand Rounds: Describe how biofeedback is supported by what we know about motor learning theory.

or changes in the location of vibratory patterns. We find these methods very successful with patients who have resonance disorders or whose VP ports are "borderline adequate" or better. When the VP mechanism is less adequate, surgical or prosthetic management is in order prior to initiating voice therapy techniques. When the degree of VP mechanism adequacy is in serious question, a period of intensive trial voice and articulation therapy may determine the need for other management approaches. This trial therapy should be intensive (three sessions per week minimum) but of short duration (three weeks), and it should be conducted with the understanding that it is a trial to determine if further therapy is indicated or if some other management approach is required. Under no circumstances should voice therapy for resonance disorders be continued when success is not forthcoming. Long periods of time without any progress are poor for motivation and the patient's self-image.

CHECK YOUR KNOWLEDGE

1. List three approaches to the treatment of hypernasality.
2. Are the approaches you listed mutually exclusive?

Hyponasality

Except for the nasal resonance required for /m/, /n/, and /ŋ/, vowels in Standard U.S. English require only slight nasal resonance. In severe cases, lack of nasal resonance produces actual articulatory substitutions for the three nasal phonemes as well as slight alterations of vowels. Hyponasality is characterized by the diversion of sound waves and airflow out through the oral cavity, which permits little or no nasal resonance. As discussed earlier in this chapter, this problem is related to some kind of nasal or nasopharyngeal obstruction, such as excessive adenoidal growth; severe nasopharyngeal infection, as in head colds; large polyps in the nasal cavity; and so on. Some patients who are hypernasal before surgical or prosthetic management emerge from such treatment with complete or highly excessive VP obstruction. Perhaps the pharyngeal flap is too broad and permits little or no ventilation of the nasopharynx, or perhaps an obturator bulb fits too tightly (the bulb can be reduced easily) and results in no nasal airflow or nasal resonance. Some kind of obstruction is the usual reason for a hyponasality problem, and the search for it must precede any attempt at voice therapy. We have seen a few cases, however, where hyponasality was caused by psychological or other functional factors such as reaction to stress or faulty learning.

Nasal airflow competence can be tested simply as part of an overall resonance evaluation: Ask the patient to take a big breath, close his or her mouth, and exhale through the nose. Then test the airflow through each nostril separately, compressing the naris of one nostril at a time with a fingertip. If there is any observable decrement in airflow, the nasal passage should be investigated medically. Appropriate medical therapy (medications, reduction of turbinates surgically, septal repair) should precede any voice therapy for hyponasality. Only rarely do patients have markedly hyponasal voices for wholly functional reasons, although we have seen a few such patients. Even though their hyponasal resonance may originally have had a physical cause, that cause may no longer be present, and the hyponasality may remain as a habit, a "set." One television news anchor with whom we worked had a hyponasal voice quality after many years of suffering from allergies. After moving to a new area of the country where the allergies were no longer a problem, he maintained his hyponasal voice by strength of habit until voice therapy produced a normal voice quality.

Occasionally a patient has chosen a hyponasal voice as a model, for whatever reason, and has learned to match its hyponasality with some consistency. We once had a patient who would use a marked hyponasal voice quality when he was challenged at work. Voice therapy was helpful in both these cases.

Voice therapy for increasing nasal resonance might include the following:

1. *Auditory feedback.* Considerable effort must be expended in contrasting for the patient the difference between the nasal and oral production of /m/, /n/, and /ŋ/. Oral and nasal resonance of vowels can also be presented for listening contrast. Audio feedback mentioned in Chapter 6 can be helpful with this technique.

2. *Counseling.* The resonance requirements for normal English must be explained to the patient, and his or her own lack of nasal resonance, particularly for /m/, /n/, and /ŋ/, pointed out. If the patient's problem is wholly functional, this explanation is of primary importance.

3. *Feedback.* Emphasis must be given to contrasting what it sounds like and "feels" like to produce oral and nasal resonance. The patient should be encouraged to make exaggerated humming sounds both orally and nasally, concentrating on the "feel" of the two types of productions.

4. *Nasal-glide stimulation.* This approach is one of the most powerful for hyponasality treatment. The phrases listed under this approach in Chapter 7 are very helpful (for example, "Momma made lemon jam," etc.).

5. *Focus.* Direction of the tone into the facial mask is usually successful.

6. *Visual feedback.* A fogging mirror or other airflow monitoring devices may be helpful in directing the patient's attention to normal nasal airflow in speech production of /m/, /n/, and /ŋ/.

Assimilative Nasality

The nasalization of vowels and voice consonants immediately before and after nasal consonants is known as *assimilative nasality*. Performance on stimulability testing provides a good clue about whether such nasal resonance is related to poor velar functioning or is functionally induced. A few neurological disorders, such as bulbar palsy, multiple sclerosis, and spastic dysarthria prevent the patient from moving the velum quickly enough to facilitate the movements required for normal resonance. The velar openings begin too soon and are maintained too long, lagging behind the rapid requirements of normal speech and nasalizing vowels that occur next to nasal phonemes. Any patient who presents with sudden onset of hypernasality or assimilative nasality should be suspect for a neurological disorder or disease until proven otherwise, and referral to a neurologist is in order. Most cases of assimilative nasality are of functional origin, however, and the patient shows good oral resonance under special conditions of stimulability.

Remember that in connected speech, all sounds are interdependent; as one sound is being produced, articulators are positioning for the next sound. This phonemic coarticulation allows for a certain amount of assimilation, even in normal speech. Assimilative nasality, therefore, is another perceptual problem: Whether the speaker's nasalization of vowels adjacent to nasal phonemes is excessive or not depends on the perception of the listener. The perception of assimilative nasality is, of course, related to the perception of excessive nasality; a normal, minor amount of nasality in the vowels following nasal phonemes would not be perceived, and increased amounts of nasal resonance would be judged quite differently by different listeners, according to their individual standards and experience. Therapy for assimilative nasality is likewise highly variable. It is, in fact, largely related to the locale (in some areas such resonance is a normal voice pattern), the standards of the speaker or clinician, their motivations, and so on.

The Nasometer is a useful therapy instrument for the patient who wants to reduce his or her assimilative nasality. The clinician and the patient can predetermine oral-nasal ratio goals that favor orality and then work incrementally toward eliminating the assimilative nasal resonance. The listening tube and See-Scape, discussed previously in this chapter, may also be effective feedback strategies. Voice therapy for assimilative nasality is best attempted only by those patients who are strongly motivated to develop more oral resonance. VFAs (see Chapter 7) might include the following:

1. *Auditory feedback.* Ear training should help patients discriminate between their nasalized vowels and their oral vowels. Patients should listen to recordings of their own oral/consonant/vowel/oral/consonant words as contrasted with their nasal consonant/vowel/nasal consonant words, such as these pairs: *bad–man, bed–men, bead–mean, bub–mum,* and so on. Voice and diction books often contain word pairs matching monosyllabic words using /b/, /d/, and /g/ with those using /m/, /n/, and /ŋ/. Once the patient can hear the differences between oral and nasal cognates, determine whether he or she can produce them.
2. *Counseling.* Because nasal assimilations are difficult to explain verbally, any attempt at explanation should be accompanied by demonstration. The best demonstration is to present the contrast between oral and nasal resonance of vowels that follow or precede the three nasal phonemes.

THERAPY FOR ORAL-PHARYNGEAL RESONANCE PROBLEMS

During speech, both the oral and pharyngeal cavities are constantly changing in size and shape, but the oral cavity is the most changeable resonance cavity. Speech is possible only because of the capability for variation of oral structures such as the lips, mandible, tongue, and velum. The most dramatic oral movements in speech are those of the tongue, which makes various constrictive-restrictive contacts at different sites within the oral cavity to produce consonant articulation. Vowel and diphthong production are possible only because of the size and shape adjustments of the oral cavity, which require a delicate blend of muscle adjustment of all oral muscle structures. Although many individuals display faulty positioning of oral structures for articulation, and thus articulate "badly," fewer individuals are recognized to have problems positioning their oral structures for resonance. Slight departures in articulatory proficiency are much more easily recognized than are minor problems in voice resonance. Even though an articulation error may be viewed consistently as a problem, faulty oral-pharyngeal resonance is usually accepted as "the way he or she talks," or as a regional dialect. Nasality problems are more likely to be recognized by lay and professional listeners as requiring correction than are oral-pharyngeal resonance departures. Any judgment of resonance is heavily influenced by the appropriateness of pitch; the degree of glottal competence, as heard in the periodic quality of phonation; and the degree of accuracy of articulation. Because quality of resonance appears to be basically a subjective experience, the goal in resonance therapy must be to achieve whatever voice "sounds best."

Singing teachers have long been aware of the vital role that the tongue plays in influencing the quality of the voice, and they devote considerable instructional and practice time to helping singing students develop optimum carriage of the tongue (Coffin, 1981). Although the postures needed to produce various phonemes attract the tongue to different anatomic sites within the oral cavity, with noticeable changes of oral resonance, more objective evidence of the role of the tongue in oral resonance may be obtained through instrumental analysis. In the spectral analyses afforded by the spectrograph, we can study the effects of tongue positioning and the distribution of spectral formants. The second formant seems to "travel" the most, changing position up and down the spectrum for various vowel productions. Boone and McFarlane (1993) demonstrate this in their study of the yawn-sigh technique (Chapter 7). The primary oral shaper for production of vowels appears to be the tongue.

Quality judgments cannot be made from the visual study of oral movements alone but depend primarily on hearing the sound of the voice. By using both the pitch and intensity readings at the same time on the Visi-Pitch (KayPENTAX Corp., Montvale, New Jersey), we have found that the real-time tracings on the monitor give useful information specific to better resonance. Often the resonance that sounds better to the ear is represented on the scope as less aperiodic (the frequency printout has less scatter) and more intense (greater amplitude of the intensity curve). The "better-sounding" voice often comes quite unexpectedly as the clinician and the patient use various facilitating approaches in their search for good oral resonance. Once the "good" voice is achieved, the Visi-Pitch offers useful feedback for the patient, often confirming by improvement in the scope tracings the subjective judgments the clinician and patient have made.

Reducing the Strident Voice

One of the most annoying oral-pharyngeal resonance problems is the strident voice. We use the term *stridency,* which means the unpleasant, shrill, metallic-sounding voice that appears to be related to hypertonicity of the pharyngeal constrictors (walls of the pharynx). Fisher (1975) described the strident voice as having brilliance of high overtones sounding "brassy, tinny, and blatant." Physiologically, stridency may be produced by the elevation of the larynx and hypertonicity of the pharyngeal constrictors, which decrease both the length and the width of the pharynx. The surface of the pharynx becomes taut because of the tight pharyngeal constriction. The smaller pharyngeal cavity, coupled with its tighter, reflective mucosal surface, produces the ideal resonating structure for accentuating high-frequency resonance.

Stridency may be developed deliberately, for example, when an actor develops a character or when a carnival barker or a store demonstrator uses it for its obvious attention-getting effects, or it may emerge when a person becomes overly tense and constricts the pharynx as part of his or her overall response to stress. A person who has this sort of strident voice—and who wants to correct it—can, in voice therapy, often develop some relaxed oral-pharyngeal behaviors that decrease pharyngeal constriction (increasing the size of the pharynx) and lessen the amount of stridency. Anything that an individual can do to lower the larynx, decrease pharyngeal constriction, and promote general throat relaxation usually reduces stridency.

The VFAs listed below (and described in Chapter 7) are most helpful in greatly reducing stridency.

We have had patients who presented themselves for voice therapy because their strident voice quality makes listeners feel they are angry, bossy, impatient, overly demanding, and so forth. One such patient, a 38-year-old female, reported problems in interpersonal interaction in the office and on the telephone. These problems were resolved with a course of eight voice therapy sessions using the following VFAs:

1. *Inhalation phonation.* Inhalation phonation tends to increase the size of the pharynx, relax the walls of the pharynx, and open the laryngeal aditus.
2. *Auditory feedback.* Explore various vocal productions with the patient, with the goal of producing a nonstrident voice. When the patient is able to produce good oral resonance, contrast this production with recorded strident vocalizations using loop recording feedback devices and following the various ear-training procedures.
3. *Establishing new pitch.* The strident voice is frequently accompanied by an inappropriately high voice pitch. Efforts to lower the pitch level often produce a voice that sounds less strident. We have found that a piano keyboard, an inexpensive electric keyboard, and the CSL are valuable tools in helping patients find and establish a new pitch level or range that produces a much less strident-sounding voice.
4. *Counseling.* Although it is difficult to explain problems of resonance to someone else, sometimes such an explanation is essential if the patient is ever to develop any kind of self-awareness about the problem.
5. *Glottal fry.* The glottal fry produces two beneficial effects. First, the fundamental frequency is somewhat lower following production of the glottal fry; second, the resonating cavity of the laryngeal aditus is enlarged following the production of the glottal fry (especially on ingressive glottal fry). The relaxation of the folds and the opening of the laryngeal aditus effectively reduce strident vocal quality.
6. *Hierarchy analysis.* For the individual whose voice becomes strident whenever he or she is tense, it is important to try to isolate those situations in which his or her nonstridency is maintained.
7. *Open mouth.* Because stridency is generally the product of excessive constriction, oral openness is an excellent way to counteract these tight, constrictive tendencies.
8. *Relaxation.* It is difficult to produce strident resonance under conditions of relaxation and freedom from tension. Either general relaxation or a more specific relaxation of the vocal tract is helpful in reducing oral-pharyngeal tightness.
9. *Tongue protrusion* /i/. This VFA increases the length and width of the pharynx (the whole throat cavity).
10. *Yawn-sigh* Because the yawn-sigh approach produces an openness and relaxation that is completely the opposite of the tightness of pharyngeal constriction, it is perhaps the most effective approach in this list for reducing stridency.

Improving Oral Resonance

Two problems of oral resonance are related to faulty tongue position: a thin type of resonance produced by excessively anterior tongue carriage, and a cul-de-sac type produced by posterior retraction of the tongue. The thin voice lacks adequate oral resonance, and its user sounds immature and unsure of him- or herself. This problem, which is somewhat common among both men and women, is characterized by a generalized oral constriction with high, anterior carriage of the tongue and only minimal lip-mandibular opening. The user of such a voice appears to be holding back psychologically, either withdrawing from interpersonal contact by demonstrating all the symptoms of withdrawal, or retreating psychologically to a more infantile level of behavior by demonstrating a babylike vocal quality. The first type, the one who withdraws from interpersonal contact, employs his or her thin resonance in certain situations, particularly when he or she feels most insecure; the second type uses the thin voice, the babylike resonance, more intentionally, in situations in which he or she wants to appear cute, to get his or her own way, and so on.

The following VFAs (described in Chapter 7) have been useful in promoting a more natural adult oral resonance:

1. *Change of loudness.* When the resonance problem is part of a general picture of psychological withdrawal in particular situations, efforts to increase voice loudness are appropriate for overall improvement of resonance.
2. *Digital manipulation.* This approach is especially helpful when the pitch of the voice is too high or the quality is breathy and the larynx is higher than normal.
3. *Establishing new pitch.* The thin voice is perceived by listeners to be drastically lacking in authority. Frequently, the pitch is too high. Efforts to lower the voice pitch often have a positive effect on resonance.
4. *Focus.* In Chapter 7, we looked at tongue position and its influence on voice quality. The babylike voice may disappear with greater posterior tongue carriage.
5. *Glottal fry.* The larger pharyngeal adjustment produced by glottal fry is generally helpful in improving resonance.
6. *Hierarchy analysis.* Symptomatic voice therapy is based on the premise that it is often possible to isolate particular situations in which we function poorly, with maladaptive behavior, and other situations in which we function comparatively well. By isolating the various situations and their modes of behavior, we can often introduce more effective behavior into "bad" situations in place of the maladaptive behavior. For those individuals who use a thin voice in specific situations, particularly during moments of tension, hierarchy analysis may be a necessary preliminary step to eliminate the aberrant vocal quality.
7. *Open mouth.* The restrictive oral tendencies of a thin-voiced speaker may be effectively reduced by developing greater oral openness.
8. *Relaxation.* If the thin vocal quality is highly situational and the obvious result of tension, relaxation approaches may be helpful, particularly when used in combination with hierarchy analysis.
9. *Respiration training.* Sometimes direct work on increasing voice loudness requires some work increasing control of the airflow during expiration.
10. *Visual feedback.* Patients whose anterior resonance focus is related to situational tensions may use feedback apparatuses to become aware of their varying states of tension. Feedback is best used with relaxation and hierarchy analysis.
11. *Yawn-sigh.* The yawn-sigh approach is an excellent way of developing a more relaxed, posterior tongue carriage.

Patients with a thin voice are often judged by listeners as immature, young, or lacking in authority. We have provided successful voice therapy to several attorneys, managers, and executives who suffered from thin voice quality, which was ineffective in their work.

The cul-de-sac voice is found in individuals from various etiologic groups: patients with oral apraxia; cerebral palsied children, particularly the athetoid type, who have a posterior focus to their resonance added to their dysarthria; some patients with bulbar or pseudobulbar-type lesions, who have a pharyngeal focus to their vocal resonance; and Deaf or severely Hard of Hearing children. The cul-de-sac voice, regardless of its initial physical cause, is produced by the deep retraction of the tongue into the oral cavity and hypopharynx, sometimes touching the pharyngeal wall and sometimes not. The body of the tongue literally obstructs the escaping airflow and the periodic sound waves generated from the larynx below. Although such a voice is often found in individuals with neural lesions who cannot control their muscles, and among Deaf children and adults, it is also produced in certain situations by individuals for wholly functional reasons. Such posterior resonance is very difficult to correct in patients who have muscle disorders related to various problems of innervation, particularly dysarthric patients. Resonance deviations in the Deaf may be changed somewhat in voice therapy, as described in Chapter 8, by dealing with special problems. For individuals who produce cul-de-sac resonance for purely functional reasons (whatever they are), the following VFAs from Chapter 7 are useful:

1. *Auditory feedback.* If, in the search for a better voice, the patient is able to produce a more forward, oral-sounding one, this should be contrasted with his or her cul-de-sac voice by listening to auditory feedback.
2. *Focus.* The forward focus in resonance required to place the voice in the facial mask makes the approach a useful one for patients with a cul-de-sac focus. High front vowels and front-of-the-mouth consonants are particularly good practice sounds to use with the focus approach.
3. *Glottal fry.* The production of the glottal fry opens the pharynx and the laryngeal aditus, thus enlarging the resonance cavity and adding to the openness of the whole vocal tract. The whole pharynx is relaxed, eliminating the cul-de-sac resonance.
4. *Hierarchy analysis.* If cul-de-sac resonance occurs only in particular situations, perhaps when the individual is tense and under stress, the hierarchy approach may be useful. If the individual can produce good oral resonance in low-stress situations, he or she should practice using the same resonance at levels of increasing stress, on up the hierarchy.
5. *Nasal-glide stimulation.* This approach helps to get a forward placement of the tongue and the sound, and can be used in conjunction with focus.
6. *Relaxation.* Posterior tongue retraction during moments of stress is often a learned response to tension. The patient who can learn a more relaxed positioning of the overall vocal tract may be able to reduce excessive tongue retraction.
7. *Tongue protrusion* /i/. With this approach, the tongue is extended outside the mouth and the pitch is elevated, and thus the base of the tongue is pulled forward and out of the oral pharynx, which is emphasized with the /i/ vowel. This eliminates the retracted tongue position that produces the back quality.
8. *Visual feedback.* For some patients, posterior focus of voice resonance may be situationally related to tension. Feedback is often useful for helping these patients monitor their varying tension states.

SUMMARY

Resonance disorders often result from produced by physical problems of structure or function at various sites within the speech tract. Primary efforts must be given to identifying any structural abnormalities and correcting these problems by dental, medical, or surgical intervention. Speech-language pathologists play an important role in the early evaluation and diagnosis of a resonance problem, as well as in providing needed voice therapy to correct the problem. Voice therapy is often necessary and very effective following surgical and dental prosthetic treatments. For both organic and functional resonance problems, specific Voice Facilitating Approaches are listed throughout this chapter to help patients develop better nasal and oral resonance.

GUIDED READING

Read the following articles.

> Kummer, A. W. (2011). Perceptual evaluation of resonance and velopharyngeal function. *Seminars in Speech and Language, 32,* 159–167.

> Hamilton, S., Husein, M., & Dworschak-Stokan, A. (2008). Velopharyngeal insufficiency clinic: The first 18 months. *Journal of Otolaryngology—Head & Neck Surgery, 37,* 586–590.

Describe four ways in which the information reported in the articles might influence your clinical practice.

PREPARING FOR THE PRAXIS™

Directions: Please read the case studies and answer the questions that follow. (Please see page 319 for the answer key.)

> *Leonardo is a second-grade student referred to you by his homeroom teacher, who asks you to look into his "strange vocal quality" that "comes and goes." The teacher mentions that he sounds "nasal." A quick screen using the key phonemes described in this chapter reveals that Leonardo produces the /b/, /d/, and /g/ in place of the /m/, /n/, and /ŋ/.*

1. This type of resonance disorder is most likely:
   A. Hyponasality
   B. Hypernasality
   C. Cul-de-sac
   D. Assimilative nasality

2. Concomitant sequelae would probably also include:
   A. Rhinorrhea
   B. Otitis media
   C. A history of allergies
   D. All of these

> *Clara is a third-grade transfer student who is referred to you with teacher and administrator observations of a "nasal voice." Clara has moved from*

three different school districts in a year and a half. There is no medical history available at the moment, but you go ahead and initiate a brief screen. You inspect the oral cavity, making clinical observations of the lips, tongue, teeth, and hard and soft palates, among other structures. You observe soft palate structure but do not focus on soft palate movement.

3. The soft palate movement is not a major area of clinical testing because it:
   A. Takes an extensive amount of time
   B. Provides little to no information about true velopharyngeal function
   C. Relies on tasks that are difficult for children to perform
   D. Requires a special test protocol

4. You ask Clara to count from 62 to 66. As she does so, you place a fogging mirror beneath the nares. The mirror fogs throughout the entire production, and you perceive moderate nasal resonance throughout. This type of resonance disorder is most likely:
   A. Hyponasality
   B. Hypernasality
   C. Cul-de-sac
   D. Assimilative nasality

5. The task of counting from 62 to 66 was used because it:
   A. Is comprised of high-pressure phonemes
   B. Is comprised of low-pressure phonemes
   C. Gives a quick look at articulation and the acquisition of any compensatory errors
   D. Both A and C

Answer Key

CHAPTER 1

1. C. 11 to 15%
2. B. 5 to 10%
3. B. 5 to 10%
4. C. 11 to 15%
5. E. More than 20%

CHAPTER 2

1. A. Superficial layer of the lamina propria
2. C. Irregular vocal fold vibration
3. E. Both A and B
4. B. Increased mass of the vocal folds
5. A. Poor respiratory support

CHAPTER 3

1. E. All of these
2. A. Swelling and redness of the vocal folds and arytenoid mucosa
3. E. All of these
4. D. Both A and B
5. B. Her voice remained consistent across speaking tasks

CHAPTER 4

1. B. Contact granuloma
2. A. Located on the nonvibrational portion of the glottis
3. C. Granulated tissue at the posterior aspect of the glottis
4. D. All of these
5. B. Continued anti-reflux regimen and intervention for reduced hard glottal attack

CHAPTER 5

1. B. X
2. C. Maladaptive behavior adopted to try to compensate for the irregular vocal fold arrests

3. D. Move voiced energy from the larynx to the face
4. C. Adductor SD
5. A. BTX-A injections

CHAPTER 6

1. C. Severely deviant
2. A. B2
3. E. Both B and C
4. B. Below the mean MPT for normal speakers his age
5. C. His hoarse voice interferes with his ability to participate in daily educational opportunities

CHAPTER 8

1. B. Mild bowing of the vocal fold margins
2. C. Breathy and hoarse
3. E. Both A and D
4. D. The typical transgender voice client is very concerned about his or her pitch
5. C. Behavioral intervention

CHAPTER 9

1. C. T4, N3
2. B. Laryngectomy
3. D. All of these
4. D. TEP employs lung air
5. A. Little to no fibrosis

CHAPTER 10

1. A. Hyponasality
2. D. All of these
3. B. Provides little to no information about true velopharyngeal function
4. B. Hypernasality
5. D. Both A and C

References

Abdel-Aziz, M. (2008). Palatopharyngeal sling: A new technique in treatment of velopharyngeal insufficiency. *International Journal of Pediatric Otorhinolaryngology, 72,* 173–177.

Abitbol, J., Abitbol, R., & Abitbol, B. (1999). Sex hormones and the female voice. *Journal of Voice, 13,* 424–436.

Adler, C. H., Bansberg, S. F., Hentz, J. G., Ramig, L. O., Buder, E. H., Witt, K., Edwards, B. W., Krein-Jones, K., & Caviness, J. N. (2004). Botulinum toxin Type A for treating voice tremor. *Archives of Neurology, 61*(9), 1416–1420.

Adler, R. K., Hirsch, S., & Mordaunt, M. (2012). *Voice and communication therapy for the transgender/transsexual client—a comprehensive clinical guide* (2nd ed.). San Diego, CA: Plural.

Agency for Healthcare Research and Quality. (2002). Criteria for determining disability in speech-language disorders. *AHRQ Publication No. 02-E010. Rockville, MD: Agency for Healthcare Research and Quality.*

Ahlstrom, R. H. (1984). Speech pathology: Views from medicine and dentistry. In S. C. McFarlane (Ed.), *Coping with communicative handicaps.* San Diego, CA: College Hill Press.

Ahmad, K., Yan, Y., & Bless, D. (2012). Vocal fold vibratory characteristics of healthy geriatric females: Analysis of high-speed digital images. *Journal of Voice, 26,* 239–253.

Akif Kilic, M., Okur, E., Yildirim, I., & Guzelsoy, S. (2004). The prevalence of vocal fold nodules in school-age children. *International Journal of Pediatric Otorhinolaryngology, 68,* 409–412.

Allegro, J., Papsin, B. C., Harrison, R. V., & Campisi, P. (2010). Acoustic analysis of voice in cochlear implant recipients with post-meningitic hearing loss. *Cochlear Implants International, 11,* 100–116.

Alliance for Gender Awareness. (2008). *1st national transgiving.* Bloomsbury, NJ: Author.

Altman, K. W., Atkinson, C., & Lazarus, C. (2005). Current and emerging concepts in muscle tension dysphonia: A 30-month review. *Journal of Voice, 19,* 261–267.

Altman, K. W., Mirza, N., Ruiz, C., & Sataloff, R. T. (2000). Paradoxical vocal fold motion: Presentation and treatment options. *Journal of Voice, 14,* 99–103.

Altman, K. W., Prufer, N., & Vaezi, M. F. (2011). The challenge of protocols for reflux disease: A review and development of a critical pathway. *Otolaryngology—Head and Neck Surgery, 145,* 7–14.

Altman, K. W., Schaefer, S. D., Yu, G-P., Hertegard, S., Lundy, D. S., Blumin, J. H., et al. (2007). The voice and laryngeal dysfunction in stroke: A report from the Neurolaryngology Subcommittee of the American Academy of Otolaryngology—Head and Neck Surgery. *Otolaryngology—Head and Neck Surgery, 136,* 873–881.

American Cancer Society. (2011). *Cancer Facts and Figures 2011.* Atlanta, GA: American Cancer Society. Retrieved October 3, 2011, from http://www.cancer.org/acs/groups/content/@epidemiologysurveilance/documents/document/acspc-029771.pdf

American Heart Association. (2012). *Heart disease and stroke statistics—2012 update.* Dallas, Texas: American Heart Association. *Circulation, 125,* e2.

American Speech-Language-Hearing Association. (1991). Amplification as a remediation technique for children with normal peripheral hearing. *ASHA, 33,* 22–24.

American Speech-Language-Hearing Association. (1998a). *The roles of otolaryngologists and speech-language pathologists in the performance and interpretation of strobovideolaryngoscopy* [Relevant Paper]. Retrieved from www.asha.org/policy

American Speech-Language-Hearing Association. (1998b). *Training guidelines for laryngeal video-endoscopy/stroboscopy* [Guidelines]. Retrieved from www.asha.org/policy

American Speech-Language-Hearing Association. (2001). *Telepractices and ASHA: Report of the Telepractices Team*. Retrieved from www.asha.org/policy

American Speech-Language-Hearing Association. (2004a). *Evaluation and treatment for tracheoesophageal puncture and prosthesis: Technical report*. [Technical Report]. Retrieved from www.asha.org/policy

American Speech-Language-Hearing Association. (2004b). *Knowledge and skills for speech-language pathologists with respect to vocal tract visualization and imaging* [Knowledge and Skills]. Retrieved from www.asha.org/policy

American Speech-Language-Hearing Association. (2004c). *Preferred practice patterns for the profession of speech-language pathology* [Preferred Practice Patterns]. Retrieved from www.asha.org/policy

American Speech-Language-Hearing Association. (2004d). *Vocal tract visualization and imaging* [Position Statement]. Retrieved from www.asha.org/policy

American Speech-Language-Hearing Association. (2004e). *Vocal tract visualization and imaging: Technical report* [Technical Report]. Retrieved from www.asha.org/policy

American Speech-Language-Hearing Association (2005a). *The role of the speech-language pathologist, the teacher of singing, and the speaking voice trainer in voice habilitation: Technical report* [Technical Report]. Retrieved from www.asha.org/policy

American Speech-Language-Hearing Association. (2005b). *Speech-language pathologists providing clinical services via telepractice* [Position Statement]. Retrieved from www.asha.org/policy

American Speech-Language-Hearing Association. (2007). *Scope of practice in speech-language pathology* [Scope of Practice]. Retrieved from www.asha.org/policy

American Speech-Language-Hearing Association. (2010). *Professional issues in telepractice for speech-language pathologists* [Professional Issues Statement]. Retrieved from www.asha.org/policy

Amir, O., Biron-Shental, T., & Shabtai, E. (2006). Birth control pills and nonprofessional voice: Acoustic analyses. *Journal of Speech, Language, and Hearing Research, 49,* 1114–1126.

Andreassen, M. L., Leeper, H. A., MacRae, D. L., & Nicholson, I. R. (1994). Aerodynamic, acoustic, and perceptual changes following adenoidectomy. *Cleft Palate–Craniofacial Journal, 31,* 261–270.

Andreassen, M., Smith, B., & Guyette, T. (1992). Pressure-flow measurements for selected oral and nasal sound segments produced by normal adults. *Cleft Palate Journal, 29,* 1–9.

Andrews, M. L. (2006). *Manual of voice treatment: Pediatrics through geriatrics* (3rd ed.). San Diego, CA: Singular.

Andrews, M. L., & Summers, A. C. (2002). *Voice treatment for children and adolescents*. San Diego, CA: Singular.

Andrus, J., & Shapshay, S. (2006). Contemporary management of laryngeal papilloma in adults and children. *Otolaryngologic Clinics of North America, 39,* 135–158.

Angelillo, N., Di Costanzo, B., Angelillo, M., Costa, G., Barillari, M. R., & Barillari, U. (2008). Epidemiological study on vocal disorders in paediatric age. *Journal of Preventive Medicine and Hygiene, 49,* 1–5.

Anvari, M., & Allen, C. (2003). Surgical outcome in gastroesophageal reflux disease patients with inadequate response to proton pump inhibitors. *Surgical Endoscopy, 17,* 1029–1035.

Ardito, G., Revelli, L., D'Alatri, L., Lerro, V., Guidi, M. L., & Ardito, F. (2004). Revisited anatomy of the recurrent laryngeal nerves. *The American Journal of Surgery, 187,* 249–253.

Arndt, W. B., Shelton, R. L., & Bradford, L. J. (1965). Articulation, voice, and obturation in persons with acquired and congenital palate defects. *Cleft Palate Journal, 2,* 377–383.

Arnold, G. E., & Pinto, S. (1960). Ventricular dysphonia: New interpretation of an old observation. *Laryngoscope, 70,* 1608–1627.

Aronson, A. E. (1990). *Clinical voice disorders: An interdisciplinary approach* (3rd ed.). New York: Thieme-Stratton.

Aronson, A. E., & DeSanto, L. W. (1983). Adductor spastic dysphonia: Three years after recurrent laryngeal nerve resection. *Annals of Otolaryngology, Rhinology, and Laryngology, 93,* 1–8.

Arvedson, J. C. (2002). Gastroesophageal/extra-esophageal reflux and voice disorders in children. *ASHA Special Interest Group 3: Perspectives on Voice and Voice Disorders, 12*(1), 17–19.

Arviso, L. C., Klein, A. M., & Johns, M. M. (2012). The management of post-intubation phonatory insufficiency. *Journal of Voice, 26,* 530–533.

Asnaashari, A. M., Rezaei, S., Babaeian, M., Taiarani, M., Shakeri, M. T., Fatemi, S. S., & Darban, A. A. (2012). The effect of asthma on phonation: A controlled study of 34 patients. *Ear Nose Throat Journal, 91,*168–171.

Awan, S. N. (1991). Phonetographic profiles and Fo-SLP characteristics of untrained versus trained vocal groups. *Journal of Voice, 5,* 41–50.

Awan, S. N. (2001). *The voice diagnostic protocol: A practical guide to the diagnosis of voice disorders.* Gaithersburg, MD: Aspen.

Awan, S. N., & Frenkel, M. L. (1994). Improvements in estimating the harmonics-to-noise ratio of the voice. *Journal of Voice, 8,* 255–262.

Awan, S. N., & Lawson, L. L. (2009). The effect of anchor modality on the reliability of vocal severity ratings. *Journal of Voice, 23,* 341–352.

Awan, S. N., Roy, N., Jetté, M. E., Meltzner, G. S., & Hillman, R. E. (2010). Quantifying dysphonia severity using a spectral/cepstral-based acoustic index: Comparisons with auditory-perceptual judgements from the CAPE-V. *Clinical Linguistics and Phonetics, 24,* 742–758.

Baiguera, S., Gonfiotti, A., Jaus, M., Comin, C. E., Paglierani, M., Del Gaudio, C., Bianco, A., Ribatti, D., & Macchiarini, P. (2011). Development of bioengineered human larynx. *Biomaterials, 32,* 4433–4442.

Baken, R. J. (1996). *Clinical measurement of speech and voice.* Boston, MA: College Hill Press.

Baken, R. J. (2005). The aged voice: A new hypothesis. *Journal of Voice, 19,* 317–325.

Baken, R. J., & Orlikoff, R. F. (1988). Changes in vocal fundamental frequency at the segmental level. *Journal of Speech and Hearing Research, 31,* 207–211.

Baker, J., Ben-Tovim, D. I., Butcher, A., Esterman, A., & McLaughlin, K. (2007). Development of a modified diagnostic classification system for voice disorders with inter-rater reliability study. *Logopedics, Phoniatrics, and Vocology, 32,* 99–112.

Baker, S., Sapienza, C. M., & Collins, S. (2003). Inspiratory pressure threshold training in a case of congenital bilateral abductor vocal fold paralysis. *International Journal of Pediatric Otorhinolaryngology, 67,* 414–416.

Baldo, J. V., Wilkins, D. P., Ogar, J., Willock, S., & Dronkers, N. F. (2010). Role of the precentral gyrus of the insula in complex articulation. *Cortex, 47,* 800–807.

Bandura, A. (1997). *Self-efficacy: The exercise of control.* New York: Freeman.

Barkmeier, J. M., & Case, J. L. (2000). Differential diagnosis of adductor-type spasmodic dysphonia, vocal tremor, and muscle tension dysphonia. *Current Opinion in Otolaryngology & Head and Neck Surgery, 8,* 174–179.

Barkmeier, J. M., Case, J. L., & Ludlow, C. L. (2001). Identification of symptoms for spasmodic dysphonia and vocal tremor: A comparison of expert and non-expert judges. *Journal of Communication Disorders, 34,* 21–37.

Barry, H. C., & Eathorne, S. W. (1994). Exercise and aging: Issues for the practitioner. *Medical Clinics of North America, 78,* 357–376.

Bartlett, R. S., Thibeault, S. L., & Prestwich, G. D. (2012). Therapeutic potential of gel-based injectables for vocal fold regeneration. *Biomedical Materials* [epub ahead of print]. doi:10.1088/1748-6041/7/2/024103

Bassich, C. J., & Ludlow, C. L. (1986). The use of perceptual methods by new clinicians for assessing voice quality. *Journal of Speech and Hearing Disorders, 51,* 125–133.

Baylor, C., Burns, M., Eadie, T., Britton, D., & Yorkston, K. (2011). A qualitative study of interference with communicative participation across communication disorders in adults. *American Journal of Speech Language Pathology, 20,* 269–287.

Baylor, C., Yorkston, K., Bamer, A., Britton, D., & Antmann, D. (2010). Variable associated with communicative participation in people with multiple sclerosis: A regression analysis. *American Journal of Speech Language Pathology, 19,* 143–153.

Beaver, M. E., Stasney, C. R., Weitzel, E., Stewert, M. G., Donovan, D. T., Parke, R. B., et al. (2003).

Diagnosis of laryngopharyngeal reflux disease with digital imaging. *Otolaryngology—Head and Neck Surgery, 128,* 103–108.

Bedwell, J., & Zalza, G. (2011). Surgical treatment of laryngomalacia. *Current Pediatric Reviews, 7,* 33–41.

Behlau, M., Zambon, F., Guerrieri, A. C., & Roy, N. (2012). Epidemiology of voice disorders in teachers and nonteachers in Brazil: Prevalence and adverse effects. *Journal of Voice* [epub ahead of print]. doi:10.1016/j.jvoice.2011.09.010

Behrman, A. (2005). Common practices of voice therapists in the evaluation of patients. *Journal of Voice, 19,* 454–469.

Behrman, A. (2006). Facilitating behavioral change in voice therapy: The relevance of motivational interviewing. *American Journal of Speech-Language Pathology, 15,* 215–225.

Behrman, A. (2007). *Speech and voice science.* San Diego, CA: Plural.

Behrman, A., Dahl, L. D., Abramson, A. L., & Schutte, H. K. (2003). Anterior-posterior and medial compression of the supraglottis: Signs of nonorganic dysphonia or normal postures? *Journal of Voice, 17,* 403–410.

Behrman, A., Rutledge, J., Hembree, A., & Sheridan, S. (2008). Vocal hygiene education, voice production therapy, and the role of patient adherence: A treatment effectiveness study in women with phonotrauma. *Journal of Speech, Language and Hearing Research, 51,* 350–366.

Belafsky, P. C. (2011). Bilateral vocal fold immobility. *Current Opinion in Otolaryngology & Head and Neck Surgery, 19,* 415.

Belafsky, P. C., Postma, G. N., Amin, M. R., & Koufman, J. A. (2002). Symptoms and findings of laryngopharyngeal reflux. *Ear, Nose, & Throat Journal, 81*(9 Suppl 2), 10–13.

Belafsky, P. C., Postma, G. N., & Koufman, J. A. (2001). The validity and reliability of the Reflux Finding Score (RFS). *Laryngoscope, 111*(8), 1313–1317.

Belafsky, P. C., Postma, G. N., & Koufman, J. A. (2002a). The association between laryngeal pseudosulcus and laryngopharyngeal reflux. *Journal of Otolaryngology—Head and Neck Surgery, 126*(6), 649–652.

Belafsky, P. C., Postma, G. N., & Koufman, J. A. (2002b). Validity and reliability of the Reflux Symptom Index (RSI). *Journal of Voice, 16,* 274–277.

Bele, I. V. (2005). Reliability in perceptual analysis of voice quality. *Journal of Voice, 19,* 555–573.

Benito-Leon, J., Bermejo-Pareja, F., & Louis, E. D. (2005). Incidence of essential tremor in three elderly populations of central Spain. *Neurology, 64*(10), 1721–1725.

Benninger, M. S. (2000). Microdissection or microspot CO_2 laser for limited vocal fold benign lesions: A predictive randomized trial. *Laryngoscope, 110,* 1–17.

Benninger, M. S., & Jacobson, B. (1995). Vocal nodules, microwebs, and surgery. *Journal of Voice, 9*(3), 326–331.

Berg, E., Hapner, E., Klein, A., & Johns, M. (2008). Voice therapy improves quality of life in age-related dysphonia: A case-control study. *Journal of Voice, 22,* 70–74.

Berke, G. S., Blackwell, K. E., Gerratt, B. R., Verneil, A., Jackson, K. S., & Sercarz, J. A. (1999). Selective laryngeal adductor denervation-renervation: A new surgical treatment for adductor spasmodic dysphonia. *Annals of Otology, Rhinology, and Laryngology, 108,* 227–232.

Berkow, R., Beers, M. H., & Fletcher, A. J. (1997). *Merck manual.* West Point, PA: Merck & Co.

Best, S. R., & Fakhry, C. (2011). The prevalence, diagnosis, and management of voice disorders in a National Ambulatory Medical Care Survey (NAMCS) cohort. *Laryngoscope, 121,* 150–157.

Bhattacharyya, N., Kotz, T., & Shapiro, J. (2002). Dysphagia and aspiration with unilateral vocal cord immobility: Incidence, characterization, and response with surgical treatment. *Annals of Otolaryngology, Rhinology, and Laryngology, 111*(8), 672–679.

Bhuta, T. Patrick, L., & Garnett, J. D. (2004). Perceptual evaluation of voice quality and its correlation with acoustic measurements. *Journal of Voice, 18,* 299–304.

Bickley, C. A., & Stevens, K. N. (1987). Effects of vocal tract constriction of the glottal source: Data from voiced consonants. In T. Baer, C. Sasaki, & K. Harris (Eds.), *Laryngeal functioning phonation and respiration.* Boston, MA: Little, Brown.

Birkent, H., Maronian, N., Waugh, P., Merati, A. L., Perkel, D., & Hillel, A. D. (2009). Dosage changes in patients with long-term botulinum toxin use for laryngeal dystonia. *Otolaryngology—Head and Neck Surgery, 140,* 43–47.

Blager, F. B. (1995). Treatment of paradoxical vocal cord dysfunction. *Voice and Voice Disorders, 5,* 8–11.

Blakiston, J. (1985). *Blakiston's Gould medical dictionary.* New York: McGraw-Hill.

Bless, D. M. (1988). Voice disorders in the adult: Assessment. In D. E. Yoder & R. Kent (Eds), *Decision making in speech-language pathology* (pp. 136–139). Philadelphia, PA: BC Decker.

Blitzer, A. (2010). Spasmodic dysphonia and botulinum toxin: Experience from the largest treatment series. *European Journal of Neurology, 17*(Suppl. 1), 28–30.

Bloch, I., & Behrman, A. (2001). Quantitative analysis of videostroboscopic images in presbylarynges. *Laryngoscope, 111,* 2022–2027.

Block, B. B., & Brodsky, L. (2007). Hoarseness in children: The role of laryngopharyngeal reflux. *International Journal of Pediatric Otorhinolaryngology, 71,* 1361–1369.

Blom, E. D. (1995). Tracheoesophageal speech. *Seminars in Speech & Language, 12,* 191–204.

Blom, E. D., & Singer, M. I. (1979). Surgical prosthetic approaches for postlaryngectomy voice restoration. In R. L. Keith & F. L. Darley (Eds.), *Laryngectomee rehabilitation.* Houston, TX: College Hill Press.

Blom, E. D., Singer, M. I., & Hamaker, R. D. (1998). *Tracheoesophageal voice restoration following total laryngectomy.* San Diego, CA: Singular.

Blomgren, M., Chen, Y., Ng, M. L., & Gilbert, H. R. (1998). Acoustic, aerodynamic, physiological and perceptual properties of modal and vocal fry registers. *Journal of the Acoustical Society of America, 103*(5), 2649–2657.

Blonigen, J. (1994). *Remediation of vocal hoarseness.* Austin, TX: Pro-Ed.

Bogaardt, H. C., Hakkesteegt, M. M., Grolman, W., & Lindeboom, R. (2007). Validation of the Voice Handicap Index using Rasch analysis. *Journal of Voice, 21,* 337–344.

Bogardus, S. T., Yueh, B., & Shekelle, P. G. (2003). Screening and management of adult hearing loss in primary care: Clinical applications. *Journal of the American Medical Association, 289*(15), 1986–1990.

Bonilha, H. S., White, L., Kuckhahn, K., Gerlach, T. T., & Deliyski, D. D. (2012). Vocal fold mucus aggregation in persons with voice disorders. *Journal of Communication Disorders, 45,* 304–311.

Boominathan, P., Mahalingam, S., Samuel, J., Babu, M., & Nallamuthu, A. (2012). Voice characteristics of elderly college teachers: A pilot study. *Laryngology and Voice, 2,* 21–25.

Boone, D. R. (1966a). Modification of the voices of deaf children. *Volta Review, 68,* 686–692.

Boone, D. R. (1966b). Treatment of functional aphonia in a child and an adult. *Journal of Speech and Hearing Disorders, 31,* 69–74.

Boone, D. R. (1971). *The voice and voice therapy.* Englewood Cliffs, NJ: Prentice Hall.

Boone, D. R. (1974). Dismissal criteria in voice therapy. *Journal of Speech and Hearing Disorders, 39,* 133–139.

Boone, D. R. (1982). *The Boone voice program for adults.* Austin, TX: Pro-Ed.

Boone, D. R. (1983). *The voice and voice therapy* (3rd ed.). Englewood Cliffs, NJ: Prentice Hall.

Boone, D. R. (1993). *The Boone voice program for children* (2nd ed.). Austin, TX: Pro-Ed.

Boone, D. R. (1997). *Is your voice telling on you?* (2nd ed.). San Diego, CA: Singular.

Boone, D. R. (1998). *Facilitator application manual.* Lincoln Park, NJ: Kay Elemetrics.

Boone, D. R., & McFarlane, S. C. (1993). A critical study of the yawn-sigh technique. *Journal of Voice, 7,* 75–80.

Boone, D. R., & McFarlane, S. C. (1994). *The voice and voice therapy* (5th ed.). Englewood Cliffs, NJ: Prentice Hall.

Boone, D. R., McFarlane, S. C., Von Berg, S. L., & Zraick, R. I. (2009). *The voice and voice therapy* (8th ed.). Boston, MA: Pearson.

Boone, D. R., & Plante, E. (1993). *Human communication and its disorders* (2nd ed.). Englewood Cliffs, NJ: Prentice Hall.

Boone, D. R., & Wiley, K. D. (2000). *The Boone voice program for adults* (2nd ed.). Austin, TX: Pro-Ed.

Boonin, J. (2006). Rate and volume. In R. K. Adler, S. Hirsch, & M. Mordaunt (Eds.), *Voice and communication therapy for the transgender/transsexual client*. San Diego, CA: Plural.

Borden, G. J., Harris, K. S., & Raphael, L. J. (1994). *Speech science primer: Physiology, acoustics, and perception of speech* (4th ed.). Baltimore, MD: Lippincott.

Boscolo-Rizzo, P., Maronato, F., Marchiori, C., Gava, A., & Da Mosto, M. C. (2008). Long-term quality of life after total laryngectomy and postoperative radiotherapy versus concurrent chemoradiotherapy for laryngeal preservation. *Laryngoscope, 118*, 300–306.

Boseley, M. E., Cunningham, M. J., Volk, M. S., & Hartnick, C. J. (2006). Validation of the pediatric voice-related quality-of-life survey. *Archives of Otolaryngology—Head and Neck Surgery, 132*, 717–720.

Bouchayer, M., & Cornut, G. (1991). Instrumental microscopy of benign lesions of the vocal folds. In C. N. Ford & D. M. Bless (Eds.), *Phonosurgery: Assessment and surgical management of voice disorders* (pp. 143–165). New York: Raven Press.

Bovo, R., Galceran, M., Petruccelli, J., & Hatzopoulos, S. (2007). Vocal problems among teachers: Evaluation of a preventive voice program. *Journal of Voice, 21*, 705–722.

Bowers, M., Adler, R. K., Hirsch, S., & Mordaunt, M. (2006). Endocrinology: Questions and answers. In R. K. Adler, S. Hirsch, & M. Mordaunt (Eds.), *Voice and communication therapy for the transgender/ transsexual client* (pp. 91–100). San Diego, CA: Plural.

Boyle, B. (2000). Voice disorders in school children. *Support for Learning, 15*, 71–75.

Boyle, P., & Levin, B. (2008). *World Cancer Report, 2008*. Geneva, Switzerland: World Health Organization.

Bradford, L. I., Brooks, A. R., & Shelton, R. L. (1964). Clinical judgment of hypernasality in cleft palate children. *Cleft Palate Journal, 1*, 329–335.

Branski, R. C., Cukier-Blaj, S., Pusic, A., Cano, S. J., Klassen, A., Mener, D., et al. (2010). Measuring quality of life in dysphonic patients: A systematic review of content development in patient-reported outcomes measures. *Journal of Voice, 24*, 193–198.

Branski, R. C., Verdolini, K., Sandulache, V., Rosen, C. A., & Hebda, P. A. (2006). Vocal fold wound healing: A review for clinicians. *Journal of Voice, 20*, 432–442.

Brewer, D. W., & McCall, G. (1974). Visible laryngeal changes during voice therapy: Fiber-optic study. *Annals of Otology, Rhinology, Laryngology, 83*(4), 423–427.

Brockmann, M., Drinnan, M. J., Storck, C., & Carding, P. N. (2011). Reliable jitter and shimmer measurements in voice clinics: The relevance of vowel, gender, vocal intensity, and fundamental frequency effects in a typical clinical task. *Journal of Voice, 25*, 44–53.

Brockmann-Bauser, M., & Drinnan, M. J. (2011). Routine acoustic voice analysis: Time to think again? *Current Opinion in Otolaryngology, Head and Neck Surgery, 19*, 165–170.

Brodnitz, F. S., & Froeschels, E. (1954). Treatment of nodules of vocal cords by the chewing method. *Archives of Otolaryngology, 59*, 560–566.

Brookshire, R. H. (2007). *Introduction to neurogenic communication disorders* (7th ed.). St. Louis, MO: Mosby.

Broomfield, J., & Dodd, B. (2004). Children with speech and language disability: Caseload characteristics. *International Journal of Language and Communication Disorders, 39*, 303–325.

Brown, O. L. (1996). *Discover your voice*. San Diego, CA: Singular.

Brown, S., Ngan, E., & Liotti, M. (2008). A larynx area in the human motor cortex. *Cerebral Cortex, 18*, 837–845.

Brown, W. S., Vinson, B. P., & Crary, M. A. (1996). *Organic voice disorders: Assessment and treatment*. San Diego, CA: Singular.

Burns, J. A., Zeitels, S. M., Akst, L. M., Broadhurst, M. S., Hillman, R. E., & Anderson, R. (2007). 532 nm pulsed potassium-titanyl-phosphate laser treatment of laryngeal papillomatosis under general anesthesia. *Laryngoscope, 117*(8), 1500–1504.

Butler, C., & Darrah, J. (2001). Effects of a neuro-development treatment (NDT) for cerebral palsy: An AACPDM evidence report. *Developmental Medicine and Child Neurology, 43*, 778–790.

Bzoch, K. R. (1989). *Communicative disorders related to cleft lip and palate* (3rd ed.). Austin, TX: Pro-Ed.

Callan, D. E., Kent, R. D., Guenther, F. H., & Varperian, H. K. (2000). An auditory-feedback-based neural network model of speech production that is robust to developmental changes in the size and shape of the articulatory system. *Journal of Speech, Language and Hearing Research, 43,* 721–736.

Campisi, P., Low, A., Papsin, B., Mount, R., Cohen-Kerem, R., & Harrison, R. (2005). Acoustic analysis of the voice in pediatric cochlear implant recipients: A longitudinal study. *Laryngoscope, 115,* 1046–1050.

Carding, P., Carlson, E., Epstein, R., Mathieson, L., & Shewell, C. (2000). Formal perceptual evaluation of voice quality in the United Kingdom. *Logopedics Phoniatrics Vocology, 25,* 133–138.

Carding, P. N., Horsley, I. A., & Docherty, G. J. (1999). A study of the effectiveness of voice therapy in the treatment of 45 patients with nonorganic dysphonia. *Journal of Voice, 13,* 72–104.

Carding, P. N., Roulstone, S., Northstone, K., & ALSPAC Study Team. (2006). The prevalence of childhood dysphonia: A cross-sectional study. *Journal of Voice, 20,* 623–630.

Carroll, T. L., & Rosen, C. A., (2011). Long-term results of calcium hydroxylapatite for vocal fold augmentation. *Laryngoscope, 121,* 313–319.

Caruso, A. J., & Mueller, P. B. (1997). Age-related changes in speech, voice and swallowing. In B. B. Shaden & M. A. Toner (Eds.), *Aging and communication: For clinicians, by clinicians* (pp. 117–134). Austin, TX: Pro-Ed.

Case, J. L. (2002). *Clinical management of voice disorders* (4th ed.). Austin, TX: Pro-Ed.

Casper, J. (2000). Confidential voice. In J. C. Stemple (Ed.), *Voice therapy: Clinical studies* (2nd ed.). San Diego, CA: Singular.

Chan, K. M. K., & Yiu, E. M. L. (2002). The effect of anchors and training on the reliability of perceptual voice evaluation. *Journal of Speech, Language, and Hearing Research, 45,* 111–126.

Chan, K. M. K., & Yiu, E. M. L. (2006). A comparison of two perceptual voice evaluation training programs for naive listeners. *Journal of Voice, 20,* 229–241.

Chang, C. Y., Chabot, P., & Walz, C. M. (2009). A survey of current practices of physicians who treat adductor spasmodic dysphonia in the U.S. *ENT: Ear, Nose & Throat Journal, 88,* E. 18.

Chaturvedi, A. K., Engels, E. A., & Pfeiffer, R. M. (2011). Human papillomavirus and rising oropharyngeal cancer incidence in the United States. *Journal of Clinical Oncology, 29*(32), 4294–4301.

Chen, S. H., Hsiao, T. Y., Hsiao, L. C., Chung, Y. M., & Chiang, S. C. (2007). Outcome of resonant voice therapy for female teachers with voice disorders: Perceptual, physiological, acoustic, aerodynamic, and functional measurements, *Journal of Voice, 21,* 415–425.

Chen, Y., Robb, M. P., & Gilbert, H. R. (2002). Electroglottographic evaluation of gender and vowel effects during modal and vocal fry phonation. *Journal of Speech, Language, and Hearing Research, 45,* 821–829.

Cheyne, H. A., Hanson, H. M., Genereaux, R. P., Stevens, K. N., & Hillman, R. E. (2003). Development and testing of a portable vocal accumulator. *Journal of Speech, Language, and Hearing Research, 46,* 1457–1467.

Chiou, E., Rosen, R., & Nurko, S. (2011). Effect of different pH criteria on dual-sensor pH monitoring in the evaluation of supraesophageal gastric reflux in children. *Journal of Pediatric Gastroenterology and Nutrition, 52,* 399–403.

Chodzko-Zajko, W. J. (1997). Normal aging and human physiology. *Seminars in Speech and Language, 18*(2), 95–106.

Chone, C. T., Gripp, F. M., Spina, A. L., & Crespo, A. N. (2005). Primary versus secondary tracheoesophageal puncture for speech rehabilitation in total laryngectomy: Long-term results with indwelling voice prosthesis. *Otolaryngology—Head and Neck Surgery, 133,* 89–93.

Clements, K. S., Rassekh, C. H., Seikaly, H., Hokanson, J. A., & Calhoun, K. H. (1997). Communication after laryngectomy: An assessment of patient satisfaction. *Archives of Otolaryngology Head and Neck Surgery, 123*(5), 493–496.

Cleveland, T. F. (1994). A clearer view of singing voice production: 25 years of progress. *Journal of Voice, 8,* 18–23.

Coffin, B. (1981). *Overtones of Bel Canto.* Metuchen, NJ: Scarecrow.

Cohen, S. M. (2010). Self-reported impact of dysphonia in a primary care population: An epidemiologic study. *Laryngoscope, 120,* 2022–2032.

Cohen, S. M., Dupont, W. D., & Courey, M. S. (2006). Quality of life impact of non-neoplastic voice disorders: A meta-analysis. *Annals of Otology, Rhinology, and Laryngology, 115,* 128–134.

Cohen, S. M., & Garrett, C. G. (2007). Utility in voice therapy management of vocal fold polyps and cysts. *Otolarynology Head and Neck Surgery, 136,* 742–746.

Cohen, S. M., Jacobson, B. H., Garrett, C. G., Nordzij, J. P., Stewart, M. G., Attia, A., et al. (2007). Creation and validation of the Singing Voice Handicap Index. *Annals of Otology, Rhinology & Laryngology 116,* 402–406.

Cohen, S. M., Kim, J., Roy, N., Asche, C., & Courey, M. (2012a). Direct health care costs of laryngeal diseases and disorders. *Laryngoscope, 122,* 1582–1588.

Cohen, S. M., Kim, J., Roy, N., Asche, C., & Courey, M. (2012b). Prevalence and causes of dysphonia in a large treatment-seeking population. *Laryngoscope, 122,* 343–348.

Cohen, S. M., Mehta, D. K., Maguire, R. C., & Simons, J. P. (2011). Injection medialization laryngoplasty in children. *Archives of Otolaryngology, Head and Neck Surgery, 137,* 264–268.

Cohen, S. M., Pitman, M. J., Noordzij, P., & Courey, M. (2012). Management of dysphonic patients by otolaryngologists. *Otolaryngology—Head and Neck Surgery, 147,* 289–294.

Cohen, S. M., Statham, M., Rosen, C. A., & Zullo, T. (2009). Development and validation of the Singing Voice Handicap–10. *Laryngoscope, 119,* 1864–1869.

Cohen, S. M., & Turley, R. (2009). Coprevalence and impact of dysphonia and hearing loss in the elderly. *Laryngoscope, 119,* 1870–1873.

Cohen-Kettenis, P. T., & Pfafflin, F. (2010). The DSM diagnostic criteria for gender identity disorders in adolescents and adults. *Archives of Sexual Behavior, 39,* 499–513.

Coletti, R. B., Christei, D. L., & Orenstein, S. R. (1995). Indications for pediatric esophageal pH monitoring. *Pediatric Gastroenterology Nutrition, 21,* 253–262.

Colton, J., & Casper, J. (1996) *Understanding voice problems: A physiological perspective for diagnosis and treatment.* Baltimore, MD: Lippincott Williams and Wilkins.

Colton, J., Casper, J., & Leonard, R. (2011) *Understanding voice problems: A physiological perspective for diagnosis and treatment* (4th ed.). Baltimore, MD: Lippincott Williams and Wilkins.

Congdon, N. G., Friedman, D. S., & Lietman, T. (2004). Important causes of visual impairment in the world today. *Journal of the American Medical Association, 290,* 2057–2060.

Connor, N., Cohen, S., Theis, S., Thibeault, S., Heatley, D., & Bless, D. (2008). Attitudes of children with dysphonia. *Journal of Voice, 22,* 197–209.

Cooper, M. (1990). *Winning with your voice.* Hollywood, FL: Fell.

Cornut, G., & Troillet-Cornut, A. (1995). Childhood dysphonia: Clinical and therapeutic considerations. *Voice, 4,* 70–76.

Costa, H. O., & Matias, C. (2005). Vocal impact on quality of life of elderly female subjects. *Revista Brasileira Otorrinolaringologia, 71,* 172–178.

Courey, M. S., Garrett, C. G., & Ossoff, R. H. (1997). Medial microflap for excision of benign vocal fold lesions. *Laryngoscope, 107,* 340–344.

Courey, M. S., Shohet, J. A., Scott, M. A., & Ossoff, R. H. (1996). Immunohistochemical characterization of benign laryngeal lesions. *Annals of Otology, Rhinology, and Laryngology, 105,* 525–531.

Coutinho, S. B., Diaferi, G., Olivera, G., & Belhau, M. (2009). Voice and speech of individuals with Parkinson's diease during amplication, delay and masking situations. *Pro-Fono-Revista de Ataulizaxaxao Clientifica, jul-set, 21*(3), 219–224.

Culton, G. L., & Gerwin, J. M. (1998). Current trends in laryngectomy rehabilitation: A survey of speech-language pathologists. *Journal of Otolaryngology—Head and Neck Surgery, 118*(4), 458–463.

Dacakis, G., Oates, J., & Douglas, J. (2012). Beyond voice: Perceptions of gender in male-to-female transsexuals. *Current Opinion in Otolaryngology & Head & Neck Surgery, 20,* 165–170.

Da Costa, V., Prada, E., Roberts, A., & Cohen, S. M. (2012). Voice disorders in primary school teachers and barriers to care. *Journal of Voice, 26,* 69–76.

Dagli, M., Acar, A., Stone, R. E., & Erythmaz, A. (2008). Mutational falsetto: Intervention outcomes in 45 patients. *Journal of Otolaryngology and Otology, 12,* 277–281.

Dailey, S., Hillman, R. E., & Stemple, J. (2011). New frontiers and emerging technologies in comprehensive voice care. Short course at the annual convention of the American Speech and Hearing Association, San Diego, CA.

Daniloff, R. G. (1985). *Speech science*. San Diego, CA: College Hill Press.

D'Antonio, L. L., Muntz, H. R., Province, M. A., & Marsh, J. L. (1988). Laryngeal/voice findings in persons with velopharyngeal dysfunction. *Laryngoscope, 98*, 432–438.

Darley, F. L., Aronson, A. E., & Brown, J. R. (1975). *Motor speech disorders*. Philadelphia, PA: Saunders.

Davids, T., Klein, A. M., & Johns, M. M. (2012). Current dysphonia trends in patients over the age of 65: Is vocal atrophy becoming more prevalent? *Laryngoscope, 122*, 332–335.

Davis, A., Stephens, D., Rayment, A., & Thomas, K. (1997). Hearing impairments in middle age: The acceptability, benefit and cost of detection (ABCD). *British Journal of Audiology, 26*, 1–14.

Davis, C. N., & Harris, T. B. (1992). Teachers' ability to accurately identify disordered voices. *Language, Speech, and Hearing Services in Schools, 23*, 136–140.

Davis, P. J., Boone, D. R., Carroll, R. L., Darveniza, F., & Harrison, G. A. (1988). Adductor spastic dysphonia: Heterogeneity of physiological and phonatory characteristics. *Archives of Otolaryngology, 97*, 179–185.

Davis, P. J., Zhang, S. P., Winkworth, A., & Bandler, R. (1996). Neural control of vocalization: Respiratory and emotional influences. *Journal of Voice, 10*, 23–38.

Dean, C. M., Ahmarani, C., Bettez, M., & Heuer, R. J. (2001). The adjustable laryngeal implant. *Journal of Voice, 15*, 141–150.

Deary, I. J., Wilson, J. A., Carding, P. N., & MacKenzie, K. (2003). VoiSS: A patient-derived voice symptom scale. *Journal of Psychosomatic Research, 54*, 483–489.

Deary, V., & Miller, T. (2011). Reconsidering the role of psychosocial factors in functional dysphonia. *Current Opinion in Otolaryngology and Head and Neck Surgery, 19*, 150–154.

De Bodt, M. S., Ketelslagers, K., Peeters, T., Wuyts, F., Mertens, F., Pattyn, J., et al. (2007). Evolution of vocal fold nodules from childhood to adolescence. *Journal of Voice, 21*, 151–156.

Dedo, H. H. (1976). Recurrent laryngeal nerve section for spastic dysphonia. *Annals of Otology, Rhinology, and Laryngology, 85*, 451–459.

Dedo, H. H. (1992). Injection and removal of Teflon for unilateral vocal cord paralysis. *Annals of Otology, Rhinology, and Laryngology, 101*, 81–86.

Dedo, H. H., & Izdebski, K. (1983). Intermediate results of 306 recurrent laryngeal nerve sections for spastic dysphonia. *Laryngoscope, 93*, 9–16.

de Jong, F. I. C. R. S., Kooijman, P. G. C., Thomas, G., Huinck, W. J., Graamans, K., & Schutte, H. K. (2006). Epidemiology of voice problems in Dutch teachers. *Folia Phoniatrica Logopaedica, 58*, 186–198.

De Letter, M., Santens, P., De Bodt, M., Van Maele, G., Van Borsel, J., & Boon, P. (2007). The effect of levodopa on respiration and word intelligibility in people with advanced Parkinson's disease. *Clinical Neurology and Neurosurgery, 109*, 495–500.

de Medeiros, A. M., Assunção, A. A., & Barreto, S. M. (2011). Absenteeism due to voice disorders in female teachers: A public health problem. *International Archives of Occupational Environmental Health, 85*, 853–864.

Derkay, C. S. (1995). Task force on recurrent respiratory papillomas: A preliminary report. *Archives of Otolaryngolgy, Head and Neck Surgery, 121*, 1386–1391.

Derkay, C. S. (2001). Recurrent respiratory papillomatosis. *Laryngoscope, 11*, 57–69.

Desai, V., & Mishra, P. (2012). Voice therapy outcome in puberphonia. *Journal of Laryngology and Voice, 2*, 26–29.

de Swart, B. J., Willemse, S. C., Maassen, B. A., & Horstink, M. W. (2003). Improvement in voicing in patients with Parkinson's disease by speech therapy. *Neurology, 60*(3), 498–500.

Deuschl, G., Raethjen, J., Hellriegel, H., & Elble, R. (2011). Treatment of patients with essential tremor. *The Lancet Neurology, 10*, 148–161.

Dickson, D. R. (1962). Acoustic study of nasality. *Journal of Speech and Hearing Research, 5*, 103–111.

Diedrich, W. M., & Youngstrom, K. A. (1966). *Alaryngeal speech*. Springfield, IL: Charles C. Thomas.

Dietrich, M., Verdolini-Abbott, K., Gartner-Schmidt, J., & Rosen, C. A. (2008). The frequency of perceived stress, anxiety, and depression in patients with common pathologies affecting voice. *Journal of Voice, 22*, 472–488.

Djukanović, R., Homeyard, S., Gratziou, C., Madden, J., Walls, A., Montefort, S., et al. (1997). The effect of treatment with oral corticosteroids on asthma symptoms and airway inflammation. *American Journal of Respiratory Critical Care Medicine, 155*, 826–832.

Downie, A., Low, J. M., & Lindsay, D. D. (1981). Speech disorders in Parkinsonism: Usefulness of delayed auditory feedback in selected cases. *British Journal of Disorders of Communication, 16*, 135–139.

Doyle, P. C., Danhauer, J. L., & Reed, C. G. (1988). Listeners' perceptions of consonants produced by esophageal and tracheoesophageal talkers. *Journal of Speech and Hearing Disorders, 53*, 400–407.

Doyle, P. C., & Keith R. L. (2005). *Contemporary considerations in the treatment and rehabilitation of head and neck cancer.* Austin, TX: Pro-Ed.

Dromey, C., Nissen, S. L., Roy, N., & Merrill, R. M. (2008). Articulatory changes following treatment of muscle tension dysphonia: Preliminary acoustic evidence. *Journal of Speech, Language, and Hearing Research, 51*, 196–208.

Dronkers, N. F. (1996). A new brain region for coordinating speech articulation. *Nature, 384*, 159–161.

Duff, M. C., Proctor, A., & Yairi, E. (2004). Prevalence of voice disorders in African American and European American preschoolers. *Journal of Voice, 18*, 348–353.

Duffy, J. R. (2005). *Motor speech disorders: Substrates, differential diagnosis and management.* St. Louis, MO: Elsevier Mosby.

Duffy, O. M., & Hazlett, D. E. (2004). The impact of preventive voice care programs for training teachers. *Journal of Voice, 18*, 63–70.

Dursun, G., Boynukalin, S., Bagis Ozgursoy, O., & Coruh, I. (2008). Long-term results of different treatment modalities for glottic insufficiency. *American Journal of Otolaryngology, 29*(1), 7–12.

Dursun, G., Ozgursoy, O. B., Kemal, O., & Coruh, I. (2007). One-year follow-up results of combined use of CO_2 laser and cold instrumentation for Reinke's edema surgery in professional voice users. *European Archives of Otorhinolaryngology, 264*, 1027–1032.

Dworkin, J. P. (2008). Laryngitis: Types, causes, and treatments. *Otolaryngologic Clinics of North America, 41*, 419–436.

Dworkin, J. P., Marunick, M. T., & Krouse, J. H. (2004). Velopharyngeal dysfunction: Speech characteristics, variable etiologies, evaluation techniques and differential treatments. *Language, Speech, and Hearing in Schools, 35*, 333–352.

Dworkin, J. P., Meleca, R. J., & Abkarian, G. G. (2000). Muscle tension dysphonia. *Current Opinion in Otolaryngology & Head and Neck Surgery, 8*, 169–173.

Dworkin, J. P., & Treadway, C. (2009). Idiopathic vocal fold paralysis: Clinical course and outcomes. *Journal of the Neurological Sciences, 284*, 56–62.

Eadie, T. L., & Baylor, C. R. (2006). The effect of perceptual training on inexperienced listeners' judgments of dysphonic voice. *Journal of Voice, 20*, 527–544.

Eadie, T. L., & Doyle, B. C. (2005). Classification of dysphonic voice: Acoustic and auditory-perceptual measures. *Journal of Voice, 19*, 1–14.

Eadie, T. L., Van Boven, L., Stubbs, K., & Giannini, E. (2010). The effect of musical background on judgments of dysphonia. *Journal of Voice, 24*, 93–101.

Eckel, F. C., & Boone, D. R. (1981). The s/z ratio as an indicator of laryngeal pathology. *Journal of Speech and Hearing Disorders, 46*, 147–150.

El Hakim, H., Waddell, A. N., & Crysdale, W. S. (2002). Observations on the early results of treatment of recurrent respiratory papillomatosis using cidfovir. *Journal of Otolaryngology, 31*(6), 333–335.

Eliot, R. S. (1994). *From stress to strength: How to lighten your load.* New York: Chelsea House.

Ellis, P. D. M., & Bennett, J. (1977). Laryngeal trauma after prolonged endotracheal intubation. *Journal of Laryngology, 91*, 69–76.

Elluru, R. G. (2006). Reconstruction techniques for the treatment of anatomical upper respiratory tract anomalies in children. *ASHA Special Interest Group 3: Perspectives on Voice and Voice Disorders, 15*(3), 3–11.

Emami, A., Morrison, L., Rammage, L., & Bosch, D. (1999). Treatment of laryngeal contact ulcers and granulomas: A 12-year retrospective analysis. *Journal of Voice, 13,* 612–617.

Epstein, R., Hirani, S. P., Stygall, J., & Newman, S. P. (2009). How do individuals cope with voice disorders? Introducing the Voice Disability Coping Questionnaire. *Journal of Voice, 23,* 209–217.

Erkan, A., Yavuz, H., Bolat, F., & Yilmaz, I. (2007). Hemangioma of the vocal cords: Review of two cases. *Journal of Otolaryngology, 36,* E48–E50.

Fahr, S., Elton, R. I., & UPDRS Development Committee. (1987). Unified Parkinson's disease rating scale. In S. Fahr, C. D. Marsden, D. B. Calne, & M. Goldstein (Eds.), *Recent developments in Parkinson's disease* (pp. 153–304). New York: Macmillan.

Farwell, D. G. (2012). Personal communication. Associate Professor, Department of Otolaryngology—Head and Neck Surgery, University of California, Davis.

Fattaha, H. A., Gaafara, A. H., & Mandoura, Z. M. (2011). Laryngomalacia: Diagnosis and management. *Egyptian Journal of Ear, Nose, Throat, and Allied Sciences, 12,* 149–153.

Faust, R. A. (2003). Childhood voice disorders: Ambulatory evaluation and operative diagnosis. *Clinical Pediatrics, 42,* 1–9.

Feigin, V. L., Lawes, C. M. M., Bennett, D. A., Anderson, C. S. (2003). Stroke epidemiology: A review of population-based studies of incidence, prevalence, and case fatality in the later 20th century. *Lancet Neurology, 2,* 43–53.

Feldman, R. S. (1992). *Understanding stress.* New York: Venture.

Fendler, M., & Shearer, W. M. (1988). Reliability of s/z ratio in normal children's voices. *Language, Speech and Hearing Services in the Schools, 19,* 2–4.

Ferrand, C. T. (2000). Harmonics-to-noise ratios in normally speaking prepubescent girls and boys. *Journal of Voice, 14,* 17–21.

Ferrand, C. T. (2002). Harmonics-to-noise ratio: An index of vocal aging. *Journal of Voice, 16,* 480–487.

Ferrand, C. T. (2006). Relationship between masking levels and phonatory stability in normal-speaking women. *Journal of Voice, 20,* 223–228.

Ferrand, C. T. (2007). *Speech science: An integrated approach to theory and clinical practice* (2nd ed.). Boston, MA: Allyn and Bacon.

Ferrand, C. T. (2012). *Voice disorders, scope of theory and practice.* Boston, MA: Pearson.

Filter, M. D., & Urioste, K. (1981). Pitch imitation abilities of college women with normal voices. *Journal of Speech and Hearing Association, 22,* 20–26.

Finitzo, T., & Freeman, F. (1989). Spasmodic dysphonia, whether and where: Results of seven years of research. *Journal of Speech and Hearing Research, 32,* 541–555.

Finnegan, D. E. (1984). Maximum phonation time for children with normal voices. *Journal of Communicative Disorders, 17,* 309–317.

Fisher, H. B. (1975). *Improving voice and articulation* (2nd ed.). New York: Houghton Mifflin.

Fitzsimmons, M., Sheahan, N., & Staunton, H. (2001). Gender and the integration of acoustic dimensions of prosody. *Brain and Language, 78,* 84–108.

Fletcher, S. (1973). *Manual for measurement and modification of nasality with TONAR II.* Birmingham: University of Alabama Press.

Fletcher, S. G. (1972). Contingencies for bioelectronic modification of nasality. *Journal of Speech and Hearing Disorders, 37,* 329–346.

Fletcher, S. G. (1978). *Diagnosing speech disorder for cleft palate.* New York: Grune & Stratton.

Fletcher, S. G., Adams, L. E., & McCutcheon, M. J. (1989). Cleft palate speech assessment through oral-nasal acoustic measures. In K. R. Bzoch (Ed.), *Communicative disorders related to cleft lip and palate* (3rd ed.). Boston, MA: College Hill Press.

Ford, C. N. (2005). Evaluation and management of laryngopharyngeal reflux. *JAMA, 294,* 1534–1540.

Ford, C. N., Inagi, K., Bless, D. M., Khidr, A., & Gilchrist, K. W. (1996). Sulcus vocalis: A rational analytical approach to diagnosis and management. *Annals of Otolaryngology, Rhinology and Laryngology, 105,* 189–200.

Forrest, L. A., Husein, T., & Husein, O. (2012). Paradoxical vocal cord motion: Classification and treatment. *Laryngoscope, 122,* 844–853.

Franic, D. M., Bramlett, R. E., & Bothe, A. C. (2004). Psychometric evaluation of disease specific quality of life instruments in voice disorders. *Journal of Voice, 19,* 300–315.

Friederici, A. (2011). The brain basis of language processing: From structure to function. *Physiological Reviews, 91,* 1357–1392.

Friedrich, G., Kiesler, K., & Gugatschka, M. (2010). Treatment of functional ventricular fold phonation by temporary suture lateralization. *Journal of Voice, 24,* 606–609.

Fujimoto, F. A., Madison, C. L., & Larrigan, L. B. (1991). The effects of a tracheostoma valve on the intelligibility and quality of tracheoesophageal speech. *Journal of Speech and Hearing Research, 34,* 33–36.

Gallivan, G. J., Hoffman, L., & Gallivan, K. H. (1996). Episodic paroxysmal laryngospasm: Voice and pulmonary function assessment and management. *Journal of Voice, 10,* 93–105.

Gandini, S., Botteri, E., & Iodice, S. (2008). Tobacco smoking and cancer: A meta-analysis. *International Journal of Cancer, 122*(1), 155–164.

Garcia, I., Krishna, P., & Rosen, C. A. (2006). Severe laryngeal hyperkeratosis secondary to laryngopharyngeal reflux. *Ear, Nose and Throat Journal, 85*(7), 417.

Gelfer, M. P., & Pazera, J. F. (2006). Maximum duration of sustained /s/ and /z/ and the s/z ratio with controlled intensity. *Journal of Voice, 20,* 369–379.

Gelfer, M. P., & Schofield, K. J. (2000). Comparison of acoustic and perceptual measures of voice in male-to-female transsexuals. *Journal of Voice, 14,* 22–33.

Gerritsma, E. J. (1991). An investigation into some personality characteristics of patients with psychogenic aphonia and dysphonia. *Folia Phoniatrica et Logopaedica, 42*(1), 13–20.

Ghandi, S., & Jacobs, R. (2012). Remission in juvenile-onset recurrent respiratory papillomatosis. *Journal of Laryngology and Voice, 2,* 30–34.

Gilger, M. A. (2003). Pediatric otolaryngologic manifestations of gastroesophageal reflux disease. *Current Gastroenterology Reports, 5*(3), 247–252.

Gillivan-Murphy, P., & Miller, N. (2011). Voice tremor: What we know and what we do not know. *Current Opinion in Otolaryngology & Head & Neck Surgery, 19,* 155–159.

Giovanni, A., Chanteret, C., & Lagier, A. (2007). Sulcus vocalis: A review. *European Archives of Otorhinolaryngology, 264*(4), 337–344.

Glaze, L. E. (1996). Treatment of voice hyperfunction in the pre-adolescent. *Language, Speech and Hearing in Schools, 27,* 244–250.

Glicklich, R. E., Glovsky, R. M., & Montgomery, W. W. (1999). Validation of a voice outcome survey for unilateral vocal cord paralysis. *Journal of Otolaryngology—Head & Neck Surgery, 120,* 153–158.

Golding-Kushner, K. J. (2001). *Therapy techniques for cleft palate speech and related disorders.* San Diego, CA: Singular.

Goldman-Eisler, F. (1968). *Psycholinguistics: Experiments in spontaneous speech.* New York: Academic Press.

Golub, J. S., Chen, P., Otto, K. J., Hapner, E., & Johns, M. M. (2006). Prevalence of perceived dysphonia in a geriatric population. *Journal of the American Geriatric Society, 54,* 1736–1739.

Goon, P., Sonnex, C., Jani, P., Stanley, M., & Sudho, H. (2008). Recurrent respiratory papillomatosis: An overview of current thinking and treatment. *European Archives of Otorhinolaryngology, 265,* 147–151.

Gorham-Rowan, M. M., & Laures-Gore, J. (2006). Acoustic-perceptual correlates of voice quality in elderly men and women. *Journal of Communication Disorders, 39,* 171–184.

Gottliebson, R. O., Lee, L., Weinrich, B., & Sanders, J. (2007). Voice problems of future speech-language pathologists. *Journal of Voice, 21,* 699–704.

Grace, S. G. (1984). Speech pathology: Views from medicine and dentistry. In S. C. McFarlane (Ed.), *Coping with communicative handicaps.* San Diego, CA: College Hill Press.

Green, G. (1989). Psycho-behavioral characteristics of children with vocal nodules: WPBIC ratings. *Journal of Speech and Hearing Disorders, 54,* 306–312.

Greene, M. C. L. (1980). *The voice and its disorders* (4th ed.). Philadelphia, PA: J. B. Lippincott.

Gregory, N. D., Chandran, S., Lurie, D., & Sataloff, R. T. (2012). Voice disorders in the elderly. *Journal of Voice, 26,* 254–258.

Grillo, E. U., & Fugowski, J. (2011). Voice characteristics of female education student teachers. *Journal of Voice, 25,* 149–157.

Grover, N., & Bhattacharyya, A. (2012). Unilateral pediatric vocal fold paralysis: Evolving trends. *Journal of Laryngology and Voice, 2,* 5–9.

Gupta, R., & Sataloff, R. T. (2009). Laryngopharyngeal reflux: Current concepts and questions. *Current Opinion in Otolaryngology & Head and Neck Surgery, 17*(3), 143–148.

Guss, J., & Mirza, N. (2006). Methacholine challenge testing in the diagnosis of paradoxical vocal fold motion. *Laryngoscope, 116*(9), 1558–1561.

Guttman, M. R. (1932) Rehabilitation of the voice in laryngectomized patients. *Archives of Otolaryngology, 15,* 478–488.

Guyette, T., Polley, J., Botts, J., Figueroa, A., & Smith, B. (2001). Changes in speech following mandibular distraction osteogenesis. *The Cleft Palate–Craniofacial Journal, 38,* 179–184.

Guyette, T., Polley, J., Figueroa, A., & Smith, B. (2001). Changes in speech following maxillary distraction osteogenesis. *The Cleft Palate–Craniofacial Journal, 38,* 199–205.

Habermann, W., Schmid, C., Neumann, K., DeVaney, T., & Hammer, H. F. (2012). Reflux Symptom Index and Reflux Finding Score in otolaryngologic practice. *Journal of Voice, 26,* e123–e127.

Hacki, T., & Heitmuller, S. (1999). Development of the child's voice: Premutation, mutation. *International Journal of Pediatric Otorhinolaryngology, 49,* 141–144.

Haigentz, M., Silver, C. E., Hartl, D. M., Takes, R. P., Rodrigo, J. P., Robbins, K. T., et al. (2010). Chemotherapy regimens and treatment protocols for laryngeal cancer. *Expert Opinion on Pharmacotherapy, 11*(8), 1305–1316.

Hamaker, R. C., & Hamaker, R. A. (1995). Surgical treatment of laryngeal cancer. *Seminars in Speech and Language, 12,* 221–232.

Hamdan, A. L., Al Barazi, R., Kanaan, A., Sinno, S., & Soubra, A. (2011). Vocal symptoms in women undergoing in vitro fertilization. *American Journal of Otolaryngology—Head and Neck Medicine and Surgery, 33,* 239–243.

Hamdan, A. L., Sharara, A. I., Younes, A., & Fuleihan, N. (2001). Effect of aggressive therapy on laryngeal symptoms and voice characteristics in patients with gastroesophageal reflux. *Acta Otolaryngology, 121,* 868–872.

Hamel, W., Fietzek, U., Morsnowski, A., Schrader, B., Herzog, J., Weinert, D., et al. (2003). Deep brain stimulation of the subthalamic nucleus in Parkinson's disease: Evaluation of active electrode contacts. *Journal of Neurology, Neurosurgery and Psychiatry, 74*(8), 1036–1046.

Hamilton, S., Husein, M., & Dworschak-Stokan, A. (2008). Velopharyngeal insufficiency clinic: The first 18 months. *Journal of Otolaryngology—Head & Neck Surgery, 37,* 586–590.

Hancock, A. B., Krissinger, J., & Owen, K. (2011) Voice perception and quality of life for transgender people. *Journal of Voice, 25,* 553–558.

Hanson, W., & Metter, E. (1983). DAF speech rate modification in Parkinson's disease: A report of two cases. In W. Berry (Ed.), *Clinical dysarthria.* Austin, TX: Pro-Ed.

Hapner, E. R., & Johns, M. M. (2004). *The use of virtual reality in voice therapy.* Paper presented at the ASHA, Philadelphia, PA.

Haque, R., Usmani, O., & Barnes, P. (2005). Chronic idiopathic cough: A discrete clinical entity? *Chest, 127,* 1710–1713.

Harris, A. T., Atkinson, H., Vaughan, C., Knight, L. C. (2012). Presentation of laryngeal papilloma in childhood: The Leeds experience. *The International Journal of Clinical Practice, 66*(2), 183–184.

Harrison, G. A., Davis, P. J., Troughear, R. H., & Winkworth, A. L. (1992). Inspiratory speech as a management option for spastic dysphonia. *Annals of Otology, Rhinology, and Laryngology, 101,* 375–382.

Hartnick, C. J. (2002). Validation of a pediatric voice quality-of-life instrument: The Pediatric Voice Outcome Survey. *Archives of Otolaryngology—Head and Neck Surgery, 128,* 919–922.

Harvey-Woodnorth, G. (2004). Assessing and managing medically fragile children: Tracheostomy and ventilatory support. *Language, Speech, and Hearing Services in Schools, 35*(4), 363–373.

Hazlett, D. E., Duffy, O. M., & Moorhead, S. A. (2011). Review of the impact of voice training on the vocal quality of professional voice users: Implications for vocal health and recommendations for further research. *Journal of Voice, 25,* 181–191.

Heatley, D. G., & Swift, E. (1996). Paradoxical vocal cord dysfunction in an infant with stridor and gastroesophageal reflux. *International Journal of Pediatric Otorhinolaryngology, 34,* 149–151.

Helou, L. B., Solomon, N. P., Henry, L. R., Coppit, G. L., Howard, R. S., & Stojadinovic, A. (2010). The role of listener experience on Consensus Auditory-Perceptual Evaluation of Voice (CAPE-V) ratings of postthyroidectomy voice. *American Journal of Speech-Language Pathology, 19,* 248–258.

Heman-Ackah, Y. D., Joglekar, S. S., Caroline, M., Becker, C., Kim, E-J., Gupta, R., et al. (2011). The prevalence of undiagnosed thyroid disease in patients with symptomatic vocal fold paresis. *Journal of Voice, 25,* 496–500.

Herrington-Hall, B., Lee, L., Stemple, J. C., Niemi, K. R., & McHone, M. M. (1988). Description of laryngeal pathologies by age, sex, and occupation in a treatment-seeking sample. *Journal of Speech and Hearing Disorders, 53,* 57–64.

Heylen, D., Wuyts, F., Mertens, F., De Bodt, M., Pattyn, J., Croux, C., et al. (1998). Evaluation of the vocal performance of children using a voice range profile index. *Journal of Speech, Language, and Hearing Research, 41,* 232–238.

Heylen, L., Wuyts, F. L., Mertens, F., DeBodt, M., & Van De Heyning, P. (2002). Normative voice range profiles of male and female professional voice users. *Journal of Voice, 16,* 1–7.

Higgins, M. B., McCleary, E. A., Ide-Helvie, D. L., & Carney, A. E. (2005). Speech and voice physiology of children who are hard of hearing. *Ear and Hearing, 26,* 546–558.

Hillman, R. E., & Mehta, D. D. (2011). Ambulatory monitoring of daily voice use. *ASHA Special Interest Group 3: Perspectives on Voice and Voice Disorders, 21,* 56–61.

Hillman, R. E., & Verdolini, K. (1999). *Management of hyperfunctional voice disorders: Unifying concepts and strategies.* ASHA and RTN HealthCare Group, 99S05.

Hillman, R. E., Walsh, M. J., Wolf, G. T., Fisher, S. G., & Hong, W. K. (1998). Functional outcomes following treatment of advanced laryngeal cancer. *Annals of Otolaryngology, Rhinology, and Laryngology, 172,* 1–27.

Hirano, M. (1981). *Clinical examination of the voice.* New York: Springer-Verlag.

Hirano, M., & Bless, D. M. (1993). *Videostroboscopic examination of the larynx.* San Diego, CA: Singular.

Hirano, M., Kurita, S., & Nakashima, T. (1983). Growth, development and aging of human vocal folds. In D. Bless (Ed.), *Vocal fold physiology: Contemporary research and clinical issues* (pp. 22–43). San Diego, CA: College Hill Press.

Hirano, S., Kojima, H., Tateya, I., & Ito, J. (2002). Fiberoptic laryngeal surgery for vocal process granuloma. *Annals of Otology, Rhinology, and Laryngology, 111*(9), 789–793.

Hirano, S., Yamashita, M., Ohno, T., Kitamura, M., Kanemaru, S., & Ito, J. (2008). Phonomicrosurgery for posterior glottic lesions using triangular laryngoscope. *European Archives of Otorhinolaryngology, 265,* 435–440.

Hirano, M., Yoshida, T., Tanaka, S., & Hibi, S. (1990). Sulcus vocalis: Functional aspects. *Annals of Otology, Rhinology, and Laryngology, 99,* 679–683.

Hirsch, S., & Van Borsel, J. (2006). Nonverbal communication: A multicultural view. In R. K. Adler, S. Hirsch, & M. Mordaunt (Eds.), *Voice and communication therapy for the transgender/transsexual client.* San Diego, CA: Plural.

Hixon, T. J., & Abbs, J. H. (1980). Normal speech production. In T. J. Hixon, L. D. Shriberg, & J. H. Saxman (Eds.), *Introduction to Communication Disorders.* Upper Saddle River, NJ: Prentice Hall.

Hixon, T. J., Hawley, J. L., & Wilson, K. J. (1982). An around-the-house device for the clinical determination of respiratory driving pressure: A note on making the simple even simpler. *Journal of Speech and Hearing Disorders, 47,* 413–415.

Hixon, T. J., & Hoit, J. D. (1998). Physical examination of the diaphragm by the speech-language pathologist. *American Journal of Speech-Language Pathology, 7,* 37–45.

Hixon, T. J., & Hoit, J. D. (1999). Physical examination of the abdominal wall by the speech-language pathologist. *American Journal of Speech-Language Pathology, 8,* 35–46.

Hixon, T. J., & Hoit, J. D. (2000). Physical examination of the rib cage by the speech-language pathologist. *American Journal of Speech-Language Pathology, 9,* 179–196.

Hixon, T. J., & Hoit, J. D. (2005). *Evaluation and management of speech breathing disorders: Principles and methods.* Tucson, AZ: Reddington Brown.

Hixon, T. J., Weismer, G., & Hoit, J. D. (2008). *Preclinical Speech Science: Anatomy, Physiology, Acoustics, Perception.* San Diego, CA: Plural.

Hobbs, F., & Stoops, N. (2002). *Demographic trends in the 20th century.* U.S. Census Bureau, Census 2000 Special Reports, Series CENSR-4. Washington, DC: U.S. Government Printing Office.

Hochman, I. I., & Zeitels, S. M. (2000). Phonomicrosurgical management of vocal fold polyps: The subepithelial microflap resection technique. *Journal of Voice, 14,* 112–118.

Hoffman, L., Bolton, J., & Ferry, S. (2008). Passy-Muir speaking valve use in a children's hospital: An interdisciplinary approach. *ASHA Special Interest Group 3: Perspectives on Voice and Voice Disorders, 18,* 2.

Hogikyan, N. D., & Sethuraman, G. (1999). Validation of an instrument to measure voice-related quality of life (V-RQOL). *Journal of Voice, 13,* 557–569.

Hoit, J. D., & Hixon, T. J. (1987). Age and speech breathing. *Journal of Speech and Hearing Research, 30,* 351–366.

Hoit, J. D., Hixon, T. J., Altman, M. E., & Morgan, W. J. (1989). Speech breathing in women. *Journal of Speech and Hearing Research, 32,* 353–365.

Hoit, J. D., Hixon, T. J., Watson, P. J., & Morgan, W. J. (1990). Speech breathing in children and adolescents. *Journal of Speech and Hearing Research, 33,* 51–69.

Holinger, L. D. (1997). Congenital laryngeal anomalies. In L. D. Holinger, R. P. Lusk, & C. G. Green (Eds.), *Pediatric laryngology and bronchoesophagology* (pp. 139–142). Philadelphia, PA: Lippincott-Raven.

Holler, T., Campisi, P., Allegro, J., Chadha, N. K., Harrison, R. V., Papsin, B., et al. (2010). Abnormal voicing in children using cochlear implants. *Archives of Otolaryngology, Head and Neck Surgery, 136,* 17–22.

Hollien, H. (1974). On vocal registers. *Journal of Phonetics, 2,* 125–143.

Hollien, H. (1987). Old voices: What do we really know about them? *Journal of Voice, 1,* 2–17.

Hollien, H., Dew, D., & Philips, P. (1971). Data on adult phonational ranges. *Journal of Speech and Hearing Research, 14,* 755–760.

Holmberg, E. B., Hillman, R. E., Hammarberg, B., Södersten, M., & Doyle, P. (2001). Efficacy of a behavioral based voice therapy protocol for vocal nodules. *Journal of Voice, 15,* 395–412.

Holmberg, E. B., Ihre, E., & Södersten, M. (2007). Phonetograms as a tool in the voice clinic: Changes across voice therapy for patients with vocal fatigue. *Logopedics Phoniatrics Vocology, 32*(3), 113–127.

Holt, C., & Dowell, R. C. (2011). Actor vocal training for the habilitation of speech in adolescent users of cochlear implants. *Journal of Deaf Studies and Deaf Education, 16,* 140–151.

Hooper, C. R. (2006). Language: Syntax and semantics. In R. K. Adler, S. Hirsch, & M. Mordaunt (Eds.), *Voice and communication therapy for the transgender/transsexual client.* San Diego, CA: Plural.

Horga, D., & Liker, M. (2006). Voice and pronunciation of cochlear implant speakers. *Clinical Linguistics and Phonetics, 20,* 211–217.

Horii, Y., & Fuller, B. (1990). Selected acoustic characteristics of voices before intubation and after extubation. *Journal of Speech and Hearing Research, 33,* 505–510.

House, A., & Andrews, H. B. (1987). The psychiatric and social characteristics of patients with functional dysphonia. *Journal of Psychosomatic Research, 31,* 483–490.

Hudgins, C. V., & Stetson, R. H. (1937). Relative speed of articulatory movements. Amsterdam: Archives Neérlandaises de Phonétique Experimentale.

Hufnagle, J., & Hufnagle, K. K. (1988). s/z ratio in dysphonic children with and without vocal cord nodules. *Language, Speech and Hearing Services in the Schools, 19,* 418–422.

Hughes, C. A., Troost, S., Miller, S., & Troost, T. (2000). Unilateral true vocal fold paralysis: Cause of right-sided lesions. *Journal of Otolaryngology—Head and Neck Surgery, 122*(5), 678–680.

Hummert, M. L., Mazloff, D., & Henry, C. (1999). Vocal characteristics of older adults and stereotyping. *Journal of Nonverbal Behavior, 23,* 111–132.

Huntley, R., Hollien, H., & Shipp, T. (1980). Influences of listener characteristics on perceived age estimations. *Journal of Voice, 1,* 49–52.

Hutchinson, J., Robinson, K., & Nerbonne, M. (1978). Patterns of nasalance in a sample of normal gerontologic subjects. *Journal of Communication Disorders, 11,* 469–481.

Ik, L., Ep, M., & Em, Y. (2009). Speech intelligibility, acceptability, and communication-related quality of life in Chinease alaryngeal speakers. *Archives of Otolaryngology, Head and Neck Surgery, 135*(7), 704–711.

Isenberg, J. S., Crozier, D. L., & Dailey, S. H. (2008). Institutional and comprehensive review of laryngeal leukoplakia. *Annals of Otology, Rhinology and Laryngology, 117*(1), 74–79.

Ishi, C., Ishiguro, H., & Hagita, N. (2006). Acoustic analysis of pressed voice. *The Journal of the Acoustical Society of America, 120,* 3374.

Isshiki, N., Okamura, H., & Ishiwaka, T. (1975). Thyroplasty type I (lateral compression) for dysphonia due to vocal cord paralysis or atrophy. *Acta Otolaryngologica (Stockholm), 80,* 465–473.

Isshiki, N., Shoji, K., Kojima, H., & Hirano, S. (1996). Vocal fold atrophy and its surgical treatment. *Annals of Otology, Rhinology and Laryngology, 105,* 182–188.

Isshiki, N., Taira, T., & Tanabe, M. (1983). Surgical alteration of the vocal pitch. *Journal of Otolaryngology, 12,* 335–340.

Izdebski, K., Dedo, H. H., & Boles, L. (1984). Spastic dysphonia: A patient profile of 200 cases. *American Journal of Otolaryngology, 5,* 7–14.

Jacobson, B. H., Johnson, A., Grywalski, C., Silbergleit, A., Jacobson, G., & Benninger, M. S. (1997). The Voice Handicap Index (VHI): Development and validation. *American Journal of Speech-Language Pathology, 6,* 66–70.

Jacobson, B. H., & Zraick, R. I. (2011). Voice-related quality of life in persons with dysphonia. In E. Ma & E. Yiu (Eds.), *Handbook of voice assessments.* San Diego, CA: Plural.

Jamison, W. (1996). Some practical considerations when evaluating the exceptional adolescent singing voice. *Language, Speech, and Hearing Services in Schools, 27,* 292–300.

Jankovic, J. (1986). Cranial-cervical dyskinesias. In S. H. Appel (Ed.), *Current neurology* (p. 6). Chicago, IL: Mosby-Year Book.

Jemal, A., Siegel, R., Xu, J., & Ward, E. (2010). Cancer statistics, 2008. *CA: A Cancer Journal for Clinicians, 60*(5), 277–300.

Johns, M. M., Arviso, L. C., & Ramadan, F. (2011). Challenges and opportunities in the management of the aging voice. *Journal of Otolaryngology—Head and Neck Surgery, 145,* 1–6.

Ju, S., Raghunathan, A., Cheung, S-C. S., & Patel, R. (2011). *Automatic content generation for video self modelling.* Paper presented at the IEEE International conference, University of Kentucky, United States.

Kahane, J. (1981). Anatomic and physiologic changes in the aging peripheral speech mechanism. In D. S. Beasley & G. A. Davis (Eds.), *Aging communication processes and disorders* (pp. 21–45). New York: Grunne and Stratton.

Kahane, J., & Beckford, N. (1991). The aging larynx and voice. In D. Ripich (Ed.), *Handbook of geriatric communication disorders* (pp. 165–186). Austin, TX: Pro-Ed.

Kahane, J., & Mayo, R. (1989). The need for aggressive pursuit of healthy childhood voices. *Language, Speech, and Hearing Services in Schools, 20,* 102–107.

Kamargiannis, N., Gouveris, H., Katsinelos, P., Katotomichelakis, M., Riga, M., Beltsis, A., et al. (2011). Chronic pharyngitis is associated with severe acidic laryngopharyngeal reflux in patients with Reinke's edema. *Annals of Otology Rhinology and Laryngology, 120,* 722–726.

Kaptein, A. A., Hughes, B. M., Scharloo, M., Hondebrink, N., & Langeveld, T. P. M. (2010). Psychological aspects of adductor spasmodic dysphonia: A prospective population controlled questionnaire study. *Clinical Otolaryngology, 35,* 31–38.

Karkos, P. D., Leong, S. C., Apostolidou, M. T., & Apostolidis, T. (2006). Laryngeal manifestations and pediatric laryngopharyngeal reflux. *American Journal of Otolaryngology—Head and Neck Medicine and Surgery, 27*(Suppl. 1), 200–203.

Kazandijian, M., & Dikeman, K. (2008). Communication options for tracheostomy and ventilator-dependent patients. In E. N. Myers & J. T. Jonas (Eds.), *Tracheostomy: Airway management, communication and swallowing* (pp. 187–214). San Diego, CA: Plural.

Keith, R. L., & Darley, F. L. (1994). *Laryngectomee rehabilitation* (3rd ed.). Austin, TX: Pro-Ed.

Kelchner, L. N., Brehm, S. B., de Alarcon, A., & Weinrich, B. (2012). Update on pediatric voice and airway disorders: Assessment and care. *Current Opinion in Otolaryngology & Head & Neck Surgery, 20,* 160–164.

Kelchner, L. N., Brehm, S. B., Weinrich, B., Middendorf, J., de Alarcan, A., Levin, L., et al. (2010). Perceptual evaluation of severe pediatric voice disorders: Rater reliability using the Consensus Auditory Perceptual Evaluation of Voice. *Journal of Voice, 24,* 441–449.

Kelly-Campbell, R. J., & Robinson, G. C. (2011). Disclosure of membership in the lesbian, gay, bisexual, and transgender community by individuals with communication impairments: A preliminary web-based survey. *American Journal of Speech-Language Pathology, 20,* 86–94.

Kempster, G. B., Gerratt, B. R., Verdolini Abbott, K., Barkmeier-Kraemer, J., & Hillman, R. E. (2009). Consensus auditory-perceptual evaluation of voice: Development of a standardized clinical protocol. *American Journal of Speech-Language Pathology, 18*(2), 124–132.

Kendall, K. (2007). Presbyphonia: A review. *Current Opinion in Otolaryngology & Head and Neck Surgery, 15,* 137–140.

Kendall, K. A. (2009). High-speed laryngeal imaging compared with videostroboscopy in healthy subjects. *Archives of Otolaryngology, Head and Neck Surgery, 135,* 274–281.

Kendall, K. A., Browning, M. M., & Skovlund, S. M. (2005). Introduction to high-speed imaging of the larynx. *Current Opinion in Otolaryngology & Head and Neck Surgery, 13,* 135–137.

Kendall, K. A., & Leonard, R. J. (1997). Treatment of ventricular dysphonia with botulinum toxin. *Laryngoscope, 107,* 948–953.

Kendall, K. A., & Leonard, R. J. (2011). Interarytenoid muscle Botox injection for treatment of adductor spasmodic dysphonia with vocal tremor. *Journal of Voice, 25,* 114–119.

Kendall, K. A., & Leonard, R. J. (2012). *Laryngeal evaluation: Indirect laryngoscopy to high-speech digital imaging.* New York: Thieme.

Kent, R. D. (1994). *Reference manual for communicative sciences and disorders: Speech and language.* Austin, TX: Pro-Ed.

Kent, R. D. (1996). Hearing and believing: Some limits to the auditory-perceptual assessment of speech and voice. *American Journal of Speech-Language Pathology, 5,* 7–23.

Kent, A., & Graubard, B. (2010). Contributors of water intake in US children and adolescents: Associations with dietary and meal characteristics—National Health and Nutrition Examination Survey 2005–2006. *American Journal of Clinical Nutrition, 92,* 887–896.

Kent, R. D., Kent, J. F., & Rosenbek, J. C. (1987). Maximum performance tests of speech production. *Journal of Speech and Hearing Disorders, 52,* 367–387.

Kent, R. D., & Read, C. (2002). *The acoustic analysis of speech.* Albany, NY: Thomson Learning.

Khan, K., Krosch, T. C., Eickoff, J. C., Sabati, A. A., Brudney, J., Rivard, A. L., et al. (2009). Achievement of feeding milestones after primary repair of long-gap esophageal atresia. *Early Human Development, 85,* 387–392.

King, S. N., Davis, L., Lehman, J. J., & Hoffman-Ruddy, B. (2011). A model for treating voice disorders in school-age children within a video gaming environment. *Journal of Voice, 26,* 656–663.

Kishimoto, Y., Hirano, S., Kojima, T., Kanemaru, S., & Ito, J. (2009). Implantation of an atelocollagen sheet for the treatment of vocal fold scarring and sulcus vocalis. *Annals of Otology, Rhinology, & Laryngology, 119,* 613–620.

Klein, A. M., Lehmann, M., Hapner, E. R., & Johns, M. M. (2009). Spontaneous resolution of hemorrhagic polyps of the true vocal fold. *Journal of Voice, 23,* 132–135.

Klein, S., Piccirillo, J. F., & Painter, C. (2000). Comparative contrast of voice measurements. *Journal of Otolaryngology—Head and Neck Surgery, 123,* 164–169.

Kleinsasser, O. (1979). *Microlaryngoscopy and endolaryngeal microsurgery: Technique and typical findings*. Baltimore, MD: University Park.

Kleinsasser, O. (1982). Pathogenesis of vocal cord polyps. *Annals of Otology, Rhinology and Laryngology, 91*, 378–381.

Klostermann, F., Ehlen, F., Vesper, J., Nubel, K., Gross, M., Marzinzik, F., et al. (2008). Effects of subthalamic deep brain stimulation on dysarthrophonia in Parkinson's disease. *Journal of Neurology, Neurosurgery and Psychiatry with Practical Neurology, 79*, 522–529.

Knott, P., Hicks, D., Braun, W., & Strome, M. (2011). A 12-year perspective on the world's first total laryngeal transplant. *Transplantation, 91*(7), 804–805.

Koike, M., Kobayashi, N., Hirose, H., & Hara, Y. (2002). Speech rehabilitation after total laryngectomy. *Acta Otolaryngology Supplement, 547*, 107–112.

Kollbrunner, J., Menet, A. D., & Seifert, E. (2010). Psychogenic aphonia: No fixation even after a lengthy period of aphonia. *Swiss Medical Weekly, 140*, 12–17.

Konst, E. M., Rietveld, T., Peters, H. F., & Prahl-Andersen, B. (2003). Phonological development of toddlers with unilateral cleft lip and palate who were treated with and without infant orthopedics: A randomized clinical trial. *Cleft Palate–Craniofacial Journal, 40*(1), 32–39.

Kooijman, P. G., de Jong, F. I., Oudes, M. J., Huinck, W., van Acht, H., & Graamans, K. (2005). Muscular tension and body posture in relation to voice handicap and voice quality in teachers with persistent voice complaints. *Folia Phoniatrica et Logopaedica, 57*(3), 134–147.

Kotby, M., El-Sady, S., Baslouny, S., Abou-Rass, Y., & Hegazi, M. (1991). Efficacy of the accent method of voice therapy. *Journal of Voice, 5*, 316–320.

Kotsis, G. P., Nikolopoulos, T. P., Yiotakis, I. E., Papacharalampous, G. X., & Kandiloros, D. C. (2009). Recurrent acute otitis media and gastroesophageal reflux disease in children: Is there an association? *Journal of Pediatric Otorhinolaryngology, 73*, 1373–1380.

Koufman, J. A. (1991). The otolaryngologic manifestations of gastroesophageal reflux disease (GERD). *Laryngoscope, 101*(4 Pt 2 Suppl 53), 1–78.

Koufman, J. A., & Belafsky, P. C. (2001). Unilateral or localized Reinke's edema (pseudocyst) as a manifestation of vocal fold paresis: The paresis podule. *Laryngoscope, 111*(4), 576–580.

Koufman, J. A., Radomski, T. A., Joharji, G. M., Russell, G. B., & Pillsbury, D. C. (1996). Laryngeal biomechanics of the singing voice. *Journal of Otolaryngology—Head and Neck Surgery, 115*, 527–537.

Krauss, R. M., Freyberg, R., & Morsella, E. (2002). Inferring speakers' physical attributes from their voices. *Journal of Experimental Social Psychology, 38*, 618–625.

Kreiman, J., & Gerratt, B. R. (2005). Perception of aperiodicity in pathological voice. *Journal of the Acoustical Society of America, 117*, 2201–2211.

Kreiman, J., Gerratt, B. R., Kempster, G. B., Erman, A., & Berke, G. S. (1993). Perceptual evaluation of voice quality: Review, tutorial, and a framework for future research. *Journal of Speech and Hearing Research, 36*, 21–40.

Kuehn, D. P. (1997). The development of a new technique for treating hypernasality: CPAP. *American Journal of Speech-Language Pathology, 6*, 5–8.

Kummer, A. W. (2011). Perceptual assessment of resonance and velopharyngeal function. *Seminars in Speech and Language, 32*, 159–167.

Kummer, A. W., & Lee, L. (1996). Evaluation and treatment of resonance disorders. *Language, Speech, and Hearing Services in Schools, 27*, 271–281.

La, F. M., Ledger, W. L., Davidson, J. W., Howard, D. M., & Jones, G. L. (2007). The effects of a third-generation combined oral contraceptive pill on the classical singing voice. *Journal of Voice, 21*(6), 754–761.

La, F. M. B., & Sundberg, J. (2012). Pregnancy and the singing voice: Reports from a case study. *Journal of Voice, 26*, 431–439.

Lakhani, R., Fishman, J. M., Bleach, N., & Costello, D. (2011). Injectable materials for vocal fold medialisation in unilateral vocal fold paralysis (Protocol). *Cochrane Database of Systematic Reviews, 7*, Art. No.: CD009239. doi:10.1002/14651858.CD009239

Larson, G. W., Mueller, P. B., & Summers, P. A. (1990). Effects of procedural variations in determining the s/z ratio of young children. *Journal of the British College of Speech Therapists, 863*, 7–8.

Lau, P. (2008). *The Lombard effect as a communicative phenomenon*. UC Berkeley Phonology Lab Annual Report.

Lauder, E. (2001). *Self-help for the laryngectomee*. Carpinteria, CA: Author.

Laver, J. (1980). *The phonetic description of voice quality*. Cambridge, UK: Cambridge University Press.

Lavorato, A. S., & McFarlane, S. C. (1983). Treatment of the professional voice. In W. H. Perkins (Ed.), *Current therapy of communication disorders: Voice disorders*. New York: Thieme-Stratton.

Law, T., Kim, J. H., Lee, K. Y., Tang, E. C., Lam, J. H., van Hasselt, A. C., et al. (2012). Comparison of rater's reliability on perceptual evaluation of different types of voice sample. *Journal of Voice* [epub ahead of print]. doi:10.1016/j.jvoice.2011.08.003

Le, C. T., & Boen, J. R. (1995). Health and numbers: Basic biostatistical methods. New York: Wiley-Liss.

Lederele, A., Barkmeier-Kraemer, J., & Finnegan, E. (2012). Perception of vocal tremor during sustained phonation compared with sentence context. *Journal of Voice* [epub ahead of print]. doi:10.1016/j.jvoice.2011.11.001

Lee, G. S., Hsiao, T. Y., Yang, C. C. H., & Kuo, T. B. J. (2007). Effects of speech noise on vocal fundamental frequency using power spectral analysis. *Ear and Hearing, 28,* 343–350.

Lee, E-K., & Son, Y-I. (2005). Muscle tension dysphonia in children: Voice characteristics and outcome of voice therapy. *International Journal of Pediatric Otorhinolaryngology, 69,* 911–917.

Lee, L., Stemple, J. C., & Glaze, L. (2005). *Quick screen for voice*. San Diego, CA: Plural.

Lee, L., Stemple, J. C., Glaze, L., & Kelchner, L. N. (2004). Quick screen for voice and supplementary documents for identifying pediatric voice disorders. *Language, Speech, and Hearing Services in Schools, 35*(4), 308–320.

Lee, S-H., Yeo, J-O., Choi, J-I., Jin, H-J., Kim, J-P., Woo, S-H., & Jin, S-M. (2011). Local steroid injection via the cricothyroid membrane in patients with a vocal nodule. *Archives of Otolaryngology—Head Neck Surgery, 137,* 1011–1016.

Leeper, H. A., Tissington, M. L., & Munhall, K. G. (1998). Temporal characteristics of velopharyngeal function in children. *Cleft Palate Journal, 35,* 215–221.

Lehmann, Q. H. (1965). Reverse phonation: A new maneuver for eliminating the larynx. *Radiology, 84,* 215–222.

Leonard, R. (2009). Voice therapy and vocal nodules in adults. *Current Opinion in Otolaryngology, Head and Neck Surgery, 17,* 453–457.

Leonard, R., & Kendall, K. (1997). *Dysphagia assessment and treatment planning: A team approach*. San Diego, CA: Singular.

Leonard, R., & Kendall, K. (1999). Differentiation of spasmodic and psychogenic dysphonias with phonoscopic evaluation. *Laryngoscope, 109,* 295–300.

Levitzky, M. G. (2007). *Pulmonary Physiology* (7th ed.). New York: McGraw-Hill.

Lewin, J. S., Lemon, J., Bishop-Leone, J. K., Leyk, S., Martin, J. W., & Gillenwater, A. M. (2000). Experience with Barton button and peristomal breathing valve attachments for hands-free tracheoesophageal speech. *Head and Neck, 22*(2), 142–148.

Lewis, J. R., Andreassen, M. L., Leeper, H. A., MacRae, D. L., & Thomas, J. (1998). Vocal characteristics of children with cleft lip and palate and associated velopharyngeal incompetence. *Journal of Otolaryngology, 22,* 113–117.

Leydon, C., Sivasankar, M., Lodewyck, D. L., Atkins, C., & Fisher, K. V. (2009). Vocal fold surface hydration: A review. *Journal of Voice, 23,* 658–665.

Lindestadt, P., Hertegard, S., & Bjorck, G. (2004). Laryngeal adduction asymmetries in normal speaking. *Logopedics, Phoniatrics, and Vocology, 29,* 128–134.

Linville, S. E., & Fisher, H. B. (1985). Acoustic characteristics of women's voices with advancing age. *Journal of Gerontology, 40,* 324–330.

Linville, S. E., & Rens, J. (2001). Vocal tract resonance analysis of aging voice using long-term average spectra. *Journal of Voice, 15,* 323–330.

Liss, J. M., Weismer, G., & Rosenbek, J. C. (1990). Selected acoustic characteristics of speech production in very old males. *Journal of Gerontology, 45,* 35–45.

Liu, X. Z., & Yan, D. (2007). Ageing and hearing loss. *Journal of Pathology, 211,* 188–197.

Logemann, J. A. (1998). *Evaluation and treatment of swallowing disorders* (2nd ed.). Austin, TX: Pro-Ed.

Loucks, T. M. J., Poletto, C. J., Simonyan, K., Reynolds, C. L., & Ludlow, C. L. (2007). Human brain activation during phonation and exhalation: Common volitional control for two upper airway functions. *NeuroImage, 36*, 131–143.

Loughran, S., Alves, C., & MacGregor, F. B. (2002). Current aetiology of unilateral vocal fold paralysis in a teaching hospital in the West of Scotland. *Journal of Laryngology and Otology, 116*, 907–910.

Lowell, S. Y., Colton, R. H., Kelley, R. T., & Hahn, Y. C. (2011). Spectral- and cepstral-based measures during continuous speech: Capacity to distinguish dysphonia and consistency within a speaker. *Journal of Voice, 25*, e223–e232.

Lowell, S. Y., Kelley, R. T., Colton, R. H., Smith, P. B., & Portnoy, J. E. (2012). Position of the hyoid and larynx in people with muscle tension dysphonia. *Laryngoscope, 122*, 370–372.

Luchsinger, R., & Arnold, G. E. (1965). *Voice-speech-language clinical communicology: Its physiology and pathology*. Belmont, CA: Wadsworth.

Lundström, E., Hammarberg, B., Munck-Wikland, E., & Edsborg, N. (2008). The pharyngoesophageal segment in laryngectomees—videoradiographic, acoustic, and voice quality perceptual data. *Logopedics, Phoniatrics, and Vocology, 33*, 115–125.

Lyden, D., Welch, D. R., & Psaila, B. (2011). *Cancer metastasis: Biologic basis and therapeutics* (pp. 296–298). Cambridge, England: Cambridge University Press.

Ma, E., Robertson, J., Radford, C., Vagne, S., El-Halabi, R., & Yiu, E. (2007). Reliability of speaking and maximum voice range measures in screening for dysphonia. *Journal of Voice, 21*, 397–406.

Ma, E., & Yiu, E. (2001). Voice activity and participation profile: Assessing the impact of voice disorders on daily activities. *Journal of Speech, Language, and Hearing Research, 44*, 511–524.

Ma, E., & Yiu, E. (2006). Multiparametric evaluation of dysphonic severity. *Journal of Voice, 20*, 380–390.

Ma, E., & Yiu, C. (2009). *Teachers' attitudes towards children with voice problems*. Presented at the 8th Pan European Voice Conference, August 26, 2009; Dresden, Germany.

Ma, W., Yu, L., Wang, Y., Li, X., Lu, H., & Qiu, Z. (2009). Changes in health related quality of life and clinical implications in Chinese patients with chronic cough. *Cough, 5*, 7.

Maier, W., Lohle, E., & Welte, V. (1994). Pathogenic and therapeutic aspects of contact granuloma. *Laryngorhinootologie, 73*, 488–491.

Makowska, W., Bogacka-Zatorska, E., & Rogozinski, T. (2001). Human papillomavirus in laryngeal leukoplakia. *Otolaryngology Polska, 55*, 395–398.

Marchant, H., Supiot, F., Choufani, G., & Hassid, S. (2003). Bilateral vocal fold palsy caused by chronic axonal neuropathy. *Journal of Laryngology and Otology, 117*, 414–416.

Marcotullio, D., Magliulo, G., & Pezone, T. (2002). Reinke's edema and risk factors: Clinical and histopathologic aspects. *American Journal of Otolaryngology, 23*, 81–84.

Marcum, K. K., Wright, S. C., Kemp, E. S., & Kitse, D. J. (2010). A novel modification of the ansa to recurrent laryngeal nerve procedure for young children. *International Journal of Pediatric Otorhinolaryngology, 74*, 1335–1337.

Marina, M. B., Marie, J. P., Birchall, M. A. (2011). Laryngeal reinnervation for bilateral vocal fold paralysis. *Current Opinion in Otolaryngology and Head & Neck Surgery, 19*, 434–438.

Martins, R. H. C., Defaveri, J., Domingues, M. A. C., Silva, R. D., & Fabio, A. T. (2010). Vocal fold nodules: Morphological and immunohistochemical investigation. *Journal of Voice, 24*, 521–539.

Martins, R. H. C., Fabior, A. T., Domingues, M. A. C., Chi, A. P., & Gregorio, E. O. (2009). Is Reinke's edema a precancerous lesion? Histological and electron microscopic aspects. *Journal of Voice, 23*, 721–725.

Maryn, Y., De Bodt, M. S., & Van Cauwenberge, P. (2003). Ventricular dysphonia: Clinical aspects and therapeutic options. *Laryngoscope, 113*, 859–866.

Mashima, P. A., Birkmire-Peters, D. P., Syms, M. J., Holtel, M. R., Burgess, L. P., & Peters, L. J. (2003). Telehealth: Voice therapy using telecommunications technology [Research Support, U.S. Gov't, Non-P.H.S.]. *American Journal of Speech-Language Pathology, 12*(4), 432–439.

Maslan, J., Leng, X., Rees, C., Blalock, D., & Butler, S. (2011). Maximum phonation time in healthy older adults. *Journal of Voice, 25,* 709–713.

Mason, M. F. (1993). *Speech pathology for tracheostomized and ventilator dependent patients.* Newport Beach, CA: Voicing.

Mason, R. M., & Warren, D. W. (1980). Adenoid involution and developing hypernasality in cleft palate. *Journal of Speech and Hearing Disorders, 45,* 469–480.

Mate, M. A., Cobeta, I., Jimenez-Jimenez, F. J., & Figueiras, R. (2011). Digital voice analysis in patients with advanced Parkinson's disease undergoing deep brain stimulation therapy. *Journal of Voice, 26,* 496–501.

Mathieson, L. (2011). The evidence for laryngeal manual therapies in the treatment of muscle tension dysphonia. *Current Opinion in Otolaryngology and Head and Neck Surgery, 19,* 171–176.

Mattioli, F., Bergmini, G., & Alicandri-Ciufelli, M. R. (2011). The role of early voice therapy in the incidence of motility recovery in unilateral vocal fold paralysis. *Logopedics Phoniatrics Vocology, 36,* 40–47.

Maturo, S., Hill, C., Bunting, G., Baliff, C., Ramakrishna, J., Scirica, C., et al. (2011). Pediatric paradoxical vocal fold motion: Presentation and natural history. *Pediatrics, 128,* e1443–e1449.

Max, L., DeBruyn, W., & Steurs, W. (1997). Intelligibility of oesophageal and tracheooesophageal speech: Preliminary observations. *European Journal of Disorders of Communication, 32,* 429–440.

Mayer, R. M., & Gelfer, M. P. (2008). *Outcomes of voice therapy for male-to-female transgendered individuals.* Seminar at the ASHA Annual Convention, Chicago, IL.

Mazaheri, M. (1979). Prosthodontic care. In H. K. Cooper, R. L. Harding, M. M. Krogman, M. Mazaheri, & R. T. Millard (Eds.), *Cleft palate and cleft lip: A team approach.* Philadelphia, PA: Saunders.

McAllister, A. M., Granqvist, S., Sjölander, P., & Sundberg, J. (2009). Child voice and noise: A pilot study of noise in day cares and the effects on 10 children's voice quality according to perceptual evaluation. *Journal of Voice, 23,* 587–593.

McCabe, D., & Titze, I. R. (2002). Chant therapy for treating vocal fatigue among public school teachers: A preliminary study. *American Journal of Speech-Language Pathology, 11,* 356–369.

McCory, E. (2001). Voice therapy outcomes in vocal fold nodules: A retrospective audit. *International Journal of Language and Communication Disorders, 26*(s1), 19–24.

McFarlane, S. C. (1990). Videolaryngoendoscopy and voice disorders. *Seminars in Speech and Language, 11,* 162–171.

McFarlane, S. C., Fujiki, M., & Brinton, B. (1984). *Coping with communicative handicaps: Resources for the practicing clinician.* San Diego, CA: College Hill Press.

McFarlane, S. C., Holt-Romeo, T. L., Lavorato, A. S., & Warner, L. (1991). Unilateral vocal fold paralysis: Perceived vocal quality following three methods of treatment. *American Journal of Speech-Language Pathology, 1,* 45–48.

McFarlane, S. C., & Lavorato, A. S. (1984). The use of videoendoscopy in the evaluation and treatment of dysphonia. *Communicative Disorders, 9,* 117–126.

McFarlane, S. C., Nelson, W., & Watterson, T. L. (1998). Acoustic, physiologic and aerodynamic effects of tongue protrusion /i/ in dysphonia. *ASHA Leader, 18,* 72.

McFarlane, S. C., & Shipley, K. G. (1979). Spastic dysphonia: Laryngeal stuttering? *ASHA Leader, 21,* 710.

McFarlane, S. C., & Von Berg, S. (1998). Facilitative techniques in intervention for dysphonia. *Current Opinion in Otolaryngology & Head and Neck Surgery, 6,* 161–165.

McFarlane, S. C., & Watterson, T. L. (1990). Vocal nodules: Endoscopic study of their variations and treatment. *Seminars in Speech and Language, 11,* 47–59.

McFarlane, S. C., & Watterson, T. L. (1995a). General principles of working to develop alaryngeal speech. *Seminars in Speech and Language, 12,* 175–180.

McFarlane, S. C., & Watterson, T. L. (1995b). Laryngectomee rehabilitation. *Seminars in Speech and Language, 12,* 175–239.

McFarlane, S. C., Watterson, T. L., & Brophy, J. (1990). Transnasal videoendoscopy of the laryngeal mechanisms. *Seminars in Speech and Language, 11*, 8–16.

McFarlane, S. C., Watterson, T. L., Lewis, K., & Boone, D. R. (1998). Effect of voice therapy facilitation techniques on airflow in unilateral paralysis patients. *Phonoscope, 1*, 187–191.

McFerran, D. J., Abdullah, V., Gallimore, A. P., Pringle, M. B., & Croft, C. B. (1994). Vocal process granulomata. *Journal of Laryngology and Otology, 108*, 216–220.

McKinney, J. C. (1994). *The diagnosis and correction of vocal faults.* San Diego, CA: Singular.

McKinnon, D. H., McLeod, S., & Reilly, S. (2007). The prevalence of stuttering, voice, and speech-sound disorders in primary school students in Australia. *Language, Speech, and Hearing Services in Schools, 38*, 5–15.

McMurray, J. S. (2003). Disorders of phonation in children. *Pediatric Clinics of North America, 50*, 363–380.

McNeil, M. R., (2009). *Clinical management of sensorimotor speech disorders* (2nd ed.). New York: Thieme Medical Publishing.

McNeill, E. J. M., Wilson, J. A., Clark, S., & Deakin, J. (2008). Perception of voice in the transgender client. *Journal of Voice, 22*, 727–733.

McWilliams, B. J., Morris, H. L., & Shelton, R. L. (1990). *Cleft palate speech* (2nd ed.). Philadelphia, PA: B.C. Decker.

Merati, A. L., Keppel, K., Braun, N. M., Blumin, J. H., & Kerschner, J. E. (2008). Pediatric voice-related quality of life: Findings in healthy children and in common laryngeal disorders. *Annals of Otology, Rhinology and Laryngology, 117*, 259–262.

Mersbergen, M. (2011). Voice disorders and personality: Understanding their interactions. *ASHA Special Interest Group 3: Perspectives on Voice and Voice Disorders, 21*, 31–38.

Meurer, E. M., Garcez, V., von Eye Corleta, H., & Capp, E. (2009). Menstrual cycle influences on voice and speech in adolescent females. *Journal of Voice, 23*, 109–113.

Milisen, R. (1957). Methods of evaluation and diagnosis of speech disorders. In L. E. Travis (Ed.), *Handbook of speech pathology*. New York: Appleton-Century-Crofts.

Miller, S. (2004). Voice therapy for vocal fold paralysis. *Otolaryngologic Clinics of North America, 3*, 105–119.

Milutinovic, Z. (1994). Social environment and incidence of voice disturbances in children. *Folia Phoniatrica et Logopaedica, 46*, 135–138.

Minckler, J. (1972). *Functional organization and maintenance. Introduction to neuroscience.* St. Louis, MO: Mosby.

Minifie, F. D. (1994). *Introduction to communication sciences and disorders.* San Diego, CA: Singular.

Miyamoto, R. C., Cotton, R. T., Rope, A. F., Hopkin, R. J., Cohen, A. P., Shott, S. R., et al. (2004). Association of anterior glottic webs with velocardiofacial syndrome (chromosome 22q11.2 deletion). *Journal of Otolaryngology—Head and Neck Surgery, 130*, 415–417.

Moini, J. (2012). *Anatomy and physiology for health professionals.* New York: Jones & Bartlett Learning.

Molyneux, I. D. (2011). Airway reflux, cough and respiratory disease. *Therapeutic Advances in Chronic Disease, 2*, 237–248.

Monsen, R. B. (1976). Second formant transitions in speech of deaf and normal-hearing children. *Journal of Speech and Hearing Research, 19*, 279–289.

Moolenaar-Bijl, A. (1953). The importance of certain consonants in esophageal voice after laryngectomy. *Annals of Otology, Rhinology, and Laryngology, 62*, 979–989.

Moore, G. P., & von Leden, H. (1958). Dynamic variations of the vibratory pattern in the normal larynx. *Folia Phoniatrica et Logopaedica, 10*, 205–238.

Morgan, J. E., Zraick, R. I., Griffin, A. W., Bowen, T. L., & Johnson, F. L. (2007). Injection versus medialization laryngoplasty for the treatment of unilateral vocal fold paralysis. *Laryngoscope, 117*, 2068–2074.

Morini, F., Iacobelli, B. D., Crocoli, A., Bottero, S., Trozzi, M., Conforti, A., et al. (2011). Symptomatic vocal cord paresis/paralysis in infants operated on for esophageal atresia and/or tracheo-esophageal fistula. *Journal of Pediatrics, 158*, 973–976.

Morris, H. L., & Smith, J. K. (1962). A multiple approach evaluating velopharyngeal competency. *Journal of Speech and Hearing Disorders, 27*, 218–226.

Morrison, M., & Rammage, L. (1994). *The management of voice disorders*. San Diego, CA: Singular.

Morrison, M. D., Rammage, L. A., Belisle, G. M., Pullan, C. B., & Nichol, H. (1983). Muscular tension dysphonia. *Journal of Otolaryngology, 12*, 302–306.

Mueller, A. H. (2011). Laryngeal pacing for bilateral vocal fold immobility. *Current Opinion in Otolaryngology & Head and Neck Surgery, 19*, 439–443.

Mulrow, C. D., & Lichtenstein, M. J. (1991). Screening for hearing impairment in the elderly: Rationale and strategy. *Journal of General Internal Medicine, 6*, 249–258.

Munier, C., & Kinsella, R. (2008). The prevalence and impact of voice problems in primary school teachers. *Occupational Medicine, 58*, 74–76.

Munin, M. C., Rosen, C. A., & Zullo, T. (2003). Utility of laryngeal electromyography in predicting recovery after vocal fold paralysis. *Archives of Physical Medicine and Rehabilitation, 84*, 1150–1153.

Murdoch, B. E., Thompson, E. C., & Stokes, P. D. (1994). Phonatory and laryngeal dysfunction following upper motor neuron vascular lesions. *Journal of Medical Speech-Language Pathology, 2*, 177–190.

Murry, T., Branski, R., Yu, K., Cukier-Blaj, S., Duflo, S., & Aviv, J. E. (2010). Laryngeal sensory deficits in patients with chronic cough and paradoxical vocal fold movement disorder. *Laryngoscope, 120*, 1576–1581.

Murry, T., Tabaee, A., & Aviv, J. E. (2004). Respiratory retraining of refractory cough and laryngopharyngeal reflux in patients with paradoxical vocal fold movement disorder. *Laryngoscope, 114*, 1341–1345.

Murry, T., & Woodson, G. E. (1995). Combined-modality treatment of adductor spasmodic dysphonia with botulinum toxin and voice therapy. *Journal of Voice, 9*, 460–465.

Nagata, K., Kurita, S., Yasumoto, S., Maeda, T., Kawaski, H., & Hirano, M. (1983). Vocal fold polyps and nodules: A 10-year review of 1,156 patients. *Auris Nasus Larynx, 10*(Suppl.), S27–S35.

Nakagawa, H., Miyamoto, M., Kusuyama, T., Mori, Y., &, Fukuda, H. (2012). Resolution of vocal fold polyps with conservative treatment. *Journal of Voice, 26*, e107–e110.

National Academy on an Aging Society. (1999). *Hearing loss: A growing problem that affects quality of life*. Washington, DC: Author. Retrieved from www.agingsociety.org

National Emphysema Foundation (NEF). (2007). Archives. Retrieved from www.emphysema-foundation.org

National Institute for Deafness and Other Communication Disorders (NIDCD). (2007). *Strategic plan*. Bethesda, MD: Author.

Nemetz, M. A., Pontes, P. A., & Vieira, V. P. (2005). Vestibular fold configuration during phonation in adults with and without dysphonia. *Revista Brasileira Otorrinolaringologia, 71*, 6–12.

Netsell, R., & Hixon, T. (1981). A noninvasive method for clinically estimating subglottal air pressure. *Journal of Speech and Hearing Disorders, 43*, 326–330.

Newby, H. A. (1972). *Audiology*. New York: Appleton-Century-Crofts.

Newman, K. B., Mason, U. G., & Schmaling, K. B. (1995). Clinical features of vocal cord dysfunction. *American Journal of Respiratory Critical Care Medicine, 152*, 1382–1386.

Novakovic, D., Waters, H. H., D'Elia, J. B., & Blitzer, A. (2011). Botulinum toxin treatment of adductor spasmodic dysphonia: Longitudinal functional outcomes. *Laryngoscope, 121*, 606–612.

Nuss, R. C., Ward, J., Recko, T., Huang, L., & Woodnorth, G. H. (2012). Validation of a pediatric vocal fold nodule rating scale based on digital video images. *Annals of Otology, Rhinology, and Laryngology, 121*, 1–6.

Oates, J. (2006). Evidence based practice. In R. K. Adler, S. Hirsch, & M. Mordaunt (Eds.), *Voice and communication therapy for the transgender/transsexual client* (pp. 23–44). San Diego, CA: Plural.

Oates, J. M., & Dacakis, G. (1983). Speech pathology considerations in the management of transsexualism. *British Journal of Disorders of Communication, 18*, 139–151.

O'Connor, R. (2004). *Measuring quality of life in health*. New York: Elsevier.

Oestreicher-Kedem, Y., DeRowe, A., Nagar, H., Fishman, G., & Ben-Ari, J. (2008). Vocal fold paralysis in infants with tracheoesophageal fistula. *Annals of Otology, Rhinology, and Laryngology, 117,* 896–901.

Offer, D. (1980). Normal adolescent development. In H. I. Kaplan, A. M. Freedman, & B. J. Sadock (Eds.), *Comprehensive textbook of psychiatry* (3rd ed.). Baltimore, MD: Lippincott.

O'Hollaren, M. T. (1995). Dysphea and the larynx. *Annals of Allergy, Asthma, and Immunology, 75,* 1–4.

O'Hollaren, M. T., & Everts, E. C. (1991). Evaluating the patient with stridor. *Annals of Allergy, Asthma, and Immunology, 67,* 301–306.

Ongkasuwana, J., & Courey, M. (2011). The role of botulinum toxin in the management of airway compromise due to bilateral vocal fold paralysis. *Current Opinion in Otolaryngology & Head and Neck Surgery, 19,* 444–448.

Orlikoff, R. (1990). The relationship of age and cardiovascular health to certain acoustic characteristics of male voices. *Journal of Speech and Hearing Research, 33,* 450–457.

Pack, M. A. (2008). *The effect of voice disorders on adolescents' physical/social concerns and career decisions.* Unpublished thesis. Miami University.

Paniello, R. C., Edgar, J. D., Kallogeri, D., & Piccirillo, J. F. (2011). Medialization versus reinnervation for unilateral vocal fold paralysis: A multicenter randomized clinical trial. *Laryngoscope, 121,* 2172–2179.

Park, J-O., Shim, M-R., Hwang, Y-S., Cho, K-J., Joo, Y-H., Cho, J-H., et al. (2012). Combination of voice therapy and anti-reflux therapy rapidly recovers voice-related symptoms in laryngopharyngeal reflux patients. *Journal of Otolaryngology—Head and Neck Surgery, 146,* 92–97.

Park, W., Hicks, D. M., Khandwala, F., Richter, J. E., Abelson, T. I., Milstein, C., et al. (2005). Laryngopharyngeal reflux: Prospective cohort study evaluating optimal dose of proton-pump inhibitor therapy and pretherapy predictors of response. *Laryngoscope, 115,* 1230–1238.

Parkin, D. M., Whelan, S. L., Ferlay, J., Teppo, L., & Thomas, D. B. (Eds.) (2002). Cancer Incidence in Five Continents, Vol VIII. IARC Scientific Publications No. 155. Lyon, France: IARC.

Parkinson, A., Flagmeiera, S. G., Manesa, J. L., Larson, C. R., Rogers, B., & Robin, D. A. (2012).

Understanding the neural mechanisms involved in sensory control of voice production. *NeuroImage, 61,* 314–322.

Patel, R., Dailey, S., & Bless, D. M. (2008). Comparison of high-speed digital imaging with stroboscopy for laryngeal imaging of glottal disorders. *Annals of Otology, Rhinology and Laryngology, 117*(6), 413–424.

Patel, R., Dixon, A., Richmond, A., & Donohue, K. D. (2012). Pediatric high-speed digital imaging of vocal fold vibration: A normative pilot study of glottal closure and phase closure characteristics. *International Journal of Pediatric Otorhinolaryngology, 76,* 954–959.

Patel, S., Shrivastav, R., & Eddins, D. A. (2010). Perceptual distances of breathy voice quality: A comparison of psychophysical methods. *Journal of Voice, 24,* 168–177.

Paul, R. (2002). *Introduction to clinical methods in communication disorders.* Baltimore, MD: Brookes.

Pauloski, B. R., Fisher, H. B., Kempster, G. B., & Blom, E. D. (1989). Statistical differentiation of tracheoesophageal speech produced under four prosthetic/occlusion speaking conditions. *Journal of Speech and Hearing Research, 32,* 591–599.

Pawar, S., Lim, H. J., Gill, M., Smith, T. L., Merati, A., Toohill, R. J., et al. (2007). Treatment of postnasal drip with proton pump inhibitors: A prospective, randomized, placebo-controlled study. *American Journal of Rhinology, 21,* 695–701.

Pearl, N. B., & McCall, G. N. (1986). *Laryngeal function during two types of whisper: A fiberoptic study.* Paper presented at ASHA Convention, Detroit, MI.

Pedersen, M., Beranova, A., & Moller, S. (2004). Dysphonia: Medical treatment and a medical voice hygiene advice approach. A prospective randomised pilot study. *European Archives of Otorhinolaryngology, 261,* 312–315.

Pedersen, M., & McGlashan, J. (2001). Surgical versus non-surgical interventions for vocal cord nodules. *Cochrane Database of Systematic Reviews, 2. Art. No.: CD001934.* doi:10.1002/14651858. CD001934.

Peggy, E. K. (2005). Surgical treatment of laryngomalacia. *Operative Techniques in Otolaryngology—Head and Neck Surgery, 16,* 198–202.

Perkins, W. H. (1983). Optimal use of voice: Prevention of chronic vocal abuse. *Seminars in Speech and Language, 4,* 273–286.

Pershall, K. E., & Boone, D. R. (1987). Supraglottic contribution to voice quality. *Journal of Voice, 1,* 186–190.

Peterson, G. E., & Barney, H. L. (1952). Control methods used in a study of the vowels. *Journal of the Acoustical Society, 24,* 175–184.

Peterson-Falzone, S. J., Hardin-Jones, M. A., & Karnell, M. P. (2001). *Cleft palate speech* (3rd ed.). St. Louis, MO: Mosby.

Petrovic-Lazic, M., Babac, S., Vukovic, M., Kosanovic, R., & Ivankovic, Z. (2009). Acoustic voice analysis of patients with vocal polyp. *Journal of Voice, 23,* 672–679.

Plassman, B. L., & Lansing, R. W. (1990). Perceptual cues used to reproduce an inspired lung volume. *Journal of Applied Physiology, 69,* 1123–1130.

Poburka, B. J. (1999). A new stroboscopy rating form. *Journal of Voice, 13,* 403–413.

Pontes, P., & Behlau, M. (1993). Treatment of sulcus vocalis: Auditory perceptual and acoustic analysis of the slicing mucosa surgical technique. *Journal of Voice, 7,* 365–376.

Pontes, P., Brasolotto, A., & Behlau, M. (2005). Glottic characteristics and voice complaints in the elderly. *Journal of Voice, 19,* 84–94.

Pontes, P., Yamasaki, R., & Behlau, M. (2006). Morphological and functional aspects of the senile larynx. *Folia Phoniatrica et Logopaedica, 58,* 151–158.

Popolo, P. S., Švec, J. G., & Titze, R. I. (2005). Adaptation of a pocket PC for use as a wearable voice dosimeter. *Journal of Speech, Language, and Hearing Research, 48*(4), 780–791.

Porges, S. W. (2003). The Polyvagal theory: Phylogenetic contributions to social behavior. *Physiology and Behavior, 79,* 503–513.

Portone, C. R., Hapner, E. R., McGregor, L., Otto, K., & Johns, M. M. (2007). Correlation of the Voice Handicap Index (VHI) and the Voice-Related Quality of Life Measure (V-RQOL). *Journal of Voice, 21,* 723–734.

Prater, R. J., Swift, R. W., Miller, L., & Deem, J. L. (1999). *Manual of voice therapy* (2nd ed.). Austin, TX: Pro-Ed.

Pribusiene, R., Uloza, V., & Kardisiene, V. (2011). Voice characteristics of children aged between 6 and13 years: Impact of age, gender, and vocal training. *Logopedics, Phoniatrics, and Vocology, 36,* 150–155.

Ptacek, P. H., & Sander, E. K. (1966). Age recognition from voice. *Journal of Speech and Hearing Research, 9,* 273–277.

Putzer, M., Barry, W. J., & Moringlane, J. R. (2008). Effect of bilateral stimulation of the subthalamic nucleus on different speech systems in patients with Parkinson's disease. *Clinical Linguistics and Phonetics, 22,* 957–973.

Raj, A., Gupta, B., Chowdhury, A., & Chadha, S. (2010). A study of voice changes in various phases of menstrual cycle and in postmenopausal women. *Journal of Voice, 24,* 363–368.

Ramig, L. O., Bonitati, C. M., Lemke, J. H., & Horii, Y. (1994). Voice treatment for patients with Parkinson disease: Development of an approach and preliminary efficacy data. *Journal of Medical Speech-Language Pathology, 2,* 191–209.

Ramig, L. O., & Ringel, R. (1983). Effects on physiologic aging on selected acoustic characteristics of voice. *Journal of Speech and Hearing Research, 26,* 22–30.

Ramig, L. O., Sapir, S., Fox, S., & Countryman, S. (2001). Changes in vocal loudness following intensive voice treatment (LSVT®) in individuals with Parkinson's disease: A comparison with untreated patients and normal age-matched controls. *Movement Disorders, 16,* 79–83.

Ramig, L. O., & Verdolini, K. (1998). Treatment efficacy: Voice disorders. *Journal of Speech, Language, and Hearing Research, 41,* 101–116.

Rastatter, M. P., & Hyman, M. (1982). Maximum phoneme duration of /s/ and /z/ by children with vocal nodules. *Language, Speech, and Hearing Services in Schools, 13,* 197–199.

Raza, S. A., Mahendran, S., Rahman, N., & Williams, R. G. (2002). Familial vocal fold paralysis. *Journal of Laryngology and Otology, 116,* 1047–1049.

Remacle, M., Matar, N., Verduyckt, I., & Lawson, G. (2010). Relaxation thyroplasty for mutational falsetto treatment. *Annals of Otology, Rhinology, and Laryngology, 119,* 105–109.

Rigueiro-Veloso, M. T., Pego-Reigosa, R., & Branas-Fernandez, F. (1997). Wallenberg syndrome: A review of 25 cases. *Revista de Neurologia, 25,* 1561–1564.

Ringel, R. L., & Chodzko-Zajko, W. J. (1987). Vocal indices of biological age. *Journal of Voice, 1,* 31–37.

Rizzo, A., & Kim, G. (2005). A SWOT analysis of the field of virtual reality rehabilitation and therapy. *Presence: Teleoperators & Virtual Environments, 14*(2), 119–146.

Robb, M. P., Chen, Y., Gilbert, H. R., & Lerman, J. W. (2001). Acoustic comparison of vowel articulation in normal and reverse phonation. *Journal of Speech, Language and Hearing Research, 44,* 118–127.

Rochet, A. (1991). Aging and the respiratory system. In D. Ripich (Ed.), *Handbook of geriatric communication disorders* (pp. 145–163). Austin, TX: Pro-Ed.

Rohde, S. L, Wright, C. T., Muckala, J. C., Wiggleton, J., Rousseau, B., & Netterville, J. L. (2012). Voice quality after recurrent laryngeal nerve resection and immediate reconstruction. *Journal of Otolaryngology—Head and Neck Surgery, 147,* 733–736.

Rosen, C. A. (2005). Stroboscopy as a research instrument: Development of a perceptual evaluation tool. *Laryngoscope, 115,* 423–428.

Rosen, C. A., Gartner-Schmidt, J., Casiano, R., Anderson, T. D., Johnson, F. L., Remacle, M., Sataloff, R., Abitbol, J., Shaw, G., Archer, S., & Zraick, R. I. (2009). Vocal fold augmentation with calcium hydroxylapatite (CaHA): Twelve month report. *Laryngoscope, 119,* 1033–1041.

Rosen, C. A., Gartner-Schmidt, J., Hathaway, B., Simpson, B., Postma, G. N., Courey, M., & Sataloff, R. T. (2012). A nomenclature paradigm for benign mid-membranous vocal fold lesions. *Laryngoscope, 122,* 1335–1341.

Rosen, C. A., Lee, A. S., Osborne, J., Zullo, T., & Murry, T. (2004). Development and validation of the Voice Handicap Index–10. *Laryngoscope, 114,* 1549–1556.

Rosen, C. A., & Murry, T. (2000a). Nomenclature of voice disorders and vocal pathology. *Otolaryngology Clinics of North America, 33,* 1035–1045.

Rosen, C. A., Woodson, G. E., Thompson, J. W., Hengesteg, A. P., & Bradlow, H. L. (1998). Preliminary results of the use of indole-3-carginol for recurrent respiratory papillomatosis. *Current Opinion in Otolaryngology & Head and Neck Surgery, 118,* 810–815.

Rothberg, M. B., Haessler, S. D., & Brown, R. B. (2008). Complications of viral influenza. *American Journal of Medicine, 121,* 258–264.

Roy, N. (2010). Differential diagnosis of muscle tension dysphonia and spasmodic dysphonia. *Current Opinion in Otolaryngology and Head and Neck Surgery, 18,* 165–170.

Roy, N., Ford, C. N., & Bless, D. M. (1996). Muscle tension dysphonia and spasmodic dysphonia: The role of manual laryngeal tension reduction in diagnosis and management. *Annals of Otology, Rhinology and Laryngology, 105,* 851–856.

Roy, N., Gouse, M., Mauszycki, S. C., Merrill, R. M., & Smith, M. (2005). Task specificity in adductor spasmodic dysphonia versus muscle tension dysphonia. *Laryngoscope, 115,* 311–316.

Roy, N., Gray, S., Simon, M., Dove, H., Corbin-Lewis, K., & Stemple, J. (2001). An evaluation of the effects of two treatment approaches for teachers with voice disorders: A prospective randomized clinical trial. *Journal of Speech, Language, and Hearing Research, 44,* 286–296.

Roy, N., Holt, K. I., Redmond, S., & Muntz, H. (2007). Behavioral characteristics of children with vocal fold nodules. *Journal of Voice, 21,* 157–168.

Roy, N., & Leeper, H. A. (1993). Effects of the manual laryngeal musculoskeletal tension reduction technique as a treatment for functional voice disorders: Perceptual and acoustic measures. *Journal of Voice, 7,* 242–249.

Roy, N., Mauszycki, S. C., Merrill, R. M., Gouse, M., & Smith, E. M. (2007). Toward improved differential diagnosis of adductor spasmodic dysphonia and muscle tension dysphonia. *Folia Phoniatrica et Logopaedica, 59,* 83–90.

Roy, N., Merrill, R. M., Gray, S. D., & Smith, E. M. (2005). Voice disorders in the general population: Prevalence, risk factors, and occupational impact. *Laryngoscope, 115,* 1988–1995.

Roy, N., Merrill, R. M., Thibeault, S., Gray, S. D., & Smith, E. M. (2004). Voice disorders in teachers and the general population: Effects on work performance, attendance, and future career choices. *Journal of Speech, Language, and Hearing Research, 47,* 542–551.

Roy, N., Stemple, J. C., Merrill, R. M., & Thomas, L. (2007). Epidemiology of voice disorders in the elderly: Preliminary findings. *Laryngoscope, 117,* 628–633.

Roy, N., Weinrich, B., Gray, S. D., Tanner, K., Stemple, J. C., & A Sapienza, C. M. (2003). Three treatments for teachers with voice disorders: A randomized clinical trial. *Journal of Speech-Language Hearing Research, 46,* 670–688.

Roy, N., Weinrich, B., Gray, S. D., Tanner, K., Toledo, S. W., Dove, H., et al. (2002). Voice amplification versus vocal hygiene instruction for teachers with voice disorders: A treatment outcomes study. *Journal of Speech, Language, and Hearing Research, 45,* 625–638.

Roy, N., Whitchurch, M., Merrill, R. M., Houtz, D., & Smith, M. E. (2008). Differential diagnosis of adductor spasmodic dysphonia and muscle tension dysphonia using phonatory break analysis. *Laryngoscope, 118,* 2245–2253.

Roy, S., & Vivero, R. J. (2008). Recurrent respiratory papillomatosis. *Ear, Nose & Throat Journal, 87,* 18–19.

Ruben, R. J. (2000). Redefining the survival of the fittest: Communication disorders in the 21st century. *Laryngoscope, 110,* 241–245.

Rubin, A., & Sataloff, R. (2007). Vocal fold paresis and paralysis. *Otolaryngologic Clinics of North America, 40,* 1109–1131.

Rubin, J. S., & Yanagisawa, E. (2003). Benign vocal fold pathology through the eyes of the laryngologist. In J. S. Rubin, R. T. Sataloff, & G. S. Korovin (Eds.), *Diagnosis and treatment of voice disorders* (2nd ed.). New York: Delmar Learning.

Rudolf, R., & Sibylle, B. (2012). Laryngoplasty with hyaluronic acid in patients with unilateral vocal fold paralysis. *Journal of Voice, 26,* 785–791.

Rundell, K. W., & Spiering, B. A. (2003). Inspiratory stridor in elite athletes. *Chest, 123,* 468–474.

Ruotsalainen, J. H., Sellman, J., Lehto, L., Jauhiainen, M., & Verbeek, J. H. (2007). Interventions for treating functional dysphonia in adults. *Cochrane Database of Systematic Reviews, 3.* Art. No.: CD00-6373. doi:10.1002/14651858.CD006373.pub2

Ruscello, D. M. (2008). An examination of non-speech oral motor exercises for children with velopharyngeal inadequacy. *Seminars in Speech and Language, 29,* 294–303.

Ruscello, D. M., Lass, N. J., & Podbesek, J. (1988). Listeners' perceptions of normal and voice-disordered children. *Folia Phoniatrica et Logopaedica, 40,* 290–296.

Russell, J. A., Ciucci, M. R., Connor, N. P., & Schallert, T. (2010). Targeted exercise therapy for voice and swallow in persons with Parkinson's disease. *Brain Research, 1341,* 3–11.

Ryan, W., & Burk, K. (1974). Perceptual and acoustic correlates in the speech of males. *Journal of Communication Disorders, 7,* 181–192.

Ryan, E. B., & Capadano, H. L. (1978). Age perceptions and evaluative reactions toward adult speakers. *Journal of Gerontology, 33,* 98–102.

Sakae, F. A., Imamura, R., Sennes, L. U., Mauad, T., Saldiva, P. H., & Tsuji, D. H. (2008). Disarrangement of collagen fibers in Reinke's edema. *Laryngoscope, 118,* 1500–1503.

Sano, D., & Myers, J. N. (2009). Xenograft models of head and neck cancers. *Head and Neck Oncology, 1,* 32.

Sapienza, C. M., & Ruddy, B. H. (2009). *Voice disorders.* San Diego, CA: Plural.

Sapienza, C. M., Ruddy, B. H., & Baker, S. (2004). Laryngeal structure and function in the pediatric larynx. *Language, Speech, and Hearing Services in Schools, 35,* 299–307.

Sapir, S., Ramig, L. O., Hoyt, P., Countryman, S., O'Brien, C., & Hoehn, M. (2002). Speech loudness and quality 12 months after intensive voice treatment (LSVT) for Parkinson's disease: A comparison with an alternative speech treatment. *Folia Phoniatrica et Logopaedica, 54,* 296–303.

Sasaki, C. T., & Toolhill, R. J. (2000). Ambulatory pH monitoring for extraesophageal reflux: Introduction. *Annals of Otology, Rhinology and Laryngology, 109*(Suppl.), 2–3.

Sataloff, R. T. (1981). Professional singers: The science and art of clinical care. *American Journal of Otolaryngology, 2,* 251–266.

Sataloff, R. T. (Ed.). (1997). *Professional voice: The science and art of clinical care* (2nd ed.). San Diego, CA: Singular.

Sataloff, R. T. (2005). *Voice science*. San Diego, CA: Plural.

Sataloff, R. T., Spiegel, J. R., & Hawkshaw, M. J. (2003). History and physical examination of patients with voice disorders. In J. S. Rubin, R. T. Sataloff, & G. S. Korovin (Eds.), *Diagnosis and treatment of voice disorders* (2nd ed.). New York: Delmar Learning.

Sataloff, R. T., Spiegel, J. R., Hawkshaw, M., & Caputo Rosen, D. (1996). Severe hyperkeratosis mimicking carcinoma. *Ear, Nose & Throat Journal, 75*, 647.

Saunders, W. H. (1956). Dysphonia plica ventricularis: An overlooked condition causing chronic hoarseness. *Annals of Otology, Rhinology, and Laryngoscopy, l65*, 665–673.

Scarsellone, J. M., Rochet, A. P., & Wolfaardt, J. F. (1999). The influence of dentures on nasalance values in speech. *Cleft Palate–Craniofacial Journal, 36*, 51–56.

Schalen, L., & Rydell, R. (1995). Dysphonia in children. Not necessarily due to vocal abuse. *Voice, 4*, 44–56.

Schindler, A., Bottero, A., Capaccio, P., Ginocchio, D., Adorni, F., & Ottaviani, F. (2008). Vocal improvement after voice therapy in unilateral vocal fold paralysis. *Journal of Voice, 22*, 113–118.

Schneider, B., Zumtobel, M., Prettenhofer, W., Aichstill, B., & Jocher W. (2010). Normative voice range profiles in vocally trained and untrained children aged between 7 and 10 years. *Journal of Voice, 24*, 153–160.

Schneider-Stickler, B., Knell, C., Aichstill, B., & Jocher, W. (2012). Biofeedback on voice use in call center agents in order to prevent occupational voice disorders. *Journal of Voice, 26*, 51–62.

Schweinfurth, J. M., Billante, M., & Courey, M. S. (2002). Risk factors and demographics in patients with spasmodic dysphonia. *Laryngoscope, 112*, 220–223.

Seifert, E., & Kollbrunner, J. (2005). Stress and distress in non-organic voice disorders. *Swiss Medical Weekly, 135*, 387–397.

Seifert, E., & Kollbrunner, J. (2006). An update in thinking about nonorganic voice disorders. *Head and Neck Surgery, 132*, 1128–1132.

Seifert, E., Oswald, M., Bruns, U., Vischer, M., Kompis, M., & Haeusler, R. (2002). Changes of voice and articulation in children with cochlear implants. *International Journal of Pediatric Otorhinolaryngology, 66*, 115–123.

Seikel, J. A., King, D. W., & Drumright, D. G. (2010). *Anatomy and physiology for speech, language and hearing* (3rd ed.). Clifton Park, NJ: Thomson Learning.

Shah, R. K., Engel, S. H., & Choi, S. S. (2008). Relationship between voice quality and vocal nodule size. *Journal of Otolaryngology—Head and Neck Surgery, 139*, 723–726.

Shah, R. K., Feldman, H. A., & Nuss, R. C. (2007). A grading scale for pediatric vocal fold nodules. *Journal of Otolaryngology—Head and Neck Surgery, 136*, 193–197.

Shah, R. K., Woodnorth, G. H., Glynn, A., & Nuss, R. C. (2005). Pediatric vocal nodules: Correlation with perceptual voice analysis. *International Journal of Pediatric Otorhinolaryngology, 69*, 903–909.

Shelton, R. L., Hahn, E., & Morris, H. L. (1968). Diagnosis and therapy. In D. C. Spriestersbach & D. Sherman (Eds.), *Cleft palate and communication*. New York: Academic Press.

Shelton, R. L., & Trier, W. C. (1976). Issues involved in the evaluation of velopharyngeal closure. *Cleft Palate Journal, 13*, 127–137.

Shipp, T., & Hollien, H. (1969). Perception of the aging male voice. *Journal of Speech and Hearing Research, 12*, 703–712.

Shively, S. B., & Perl, D. P. (2012). Traumatic brain injury, shell shock, and post-traumatic stress disorder in the military: Past, present, and future. *Journal of Head Trauma Rehabilitation, 27*, 234–239.

Shrivastav, R., Sapienza, C., & Nandur, V. (2005). Application of psychometric theory to the measurement of voice quality using rating scales. *Journal of Speech, Language, and Hearing Research, 48*, 323–335.

Siegel, R., Ward, E., Brawley, O., & Jemal, A. (2011), Cancer statistics, 2011. *CA: A Cancer Journal for Clinicians, 61*, 212–236.

Sieron, A., Namysloski, G., Misiolek, M., Adamek, M., & Kawczyk-Krupka, A. (2001).

Photodynamic therapy of premalignant lesions and local recurrence of laryngeal and hypopharyngeal cancers. *European Archives of Otorhinolaryngology, 258,* 349–352.

Signorelli, M. E., Madill, C. J., & McCable, P. (2011). The management of vocal fold nodules in children: A national survey of speech-language pathologists. *International Journal of Speech-Language Pathology, 13,* 227–238.

Silverman, E. M., & Zimmer, Z. H. (1975). Incidence of chronic hoarseness amongst school age children. *Journal of Speech and Hearing Disorders, 40,* 211–215.

Silverman, E. P., Sapienza, C. M., Saleem, A., Carmichael, C., Davenport, P. W., Hoffman-Ruddy, B., et al. (2006). Tutorial on maximum inspiratory and expiratory mouth pressures in individuals with idiopathic Parkinson disease (IPD) and the preliminary results of an expiratory muscle strength training program. *Neurorehabilitation, 21,* 71–79.

Simberg, S., Sala, E., Tuomainen, J., Sellman, J., & Ronnemaa, A-M. (2006). The effectiveness of group therapy for students with mild voice disorders: A controlled clinical trial. *Journal of Voice, 20,* 97–109.

Simonyan, K., & Horwitz, B. (2011). Laryngeal motor cortex and control of speech in humans. *Neuroscientist, 17,* 197–208.

Sipp, J. A., Kerschner, J. E., Braune, N., & Hartnick, C. J. (2007). Vocal fold medicalization in children: Injection laryngoplasty, thyroplasty, or nerve reinnervation? *Archives of Otolaryngology, Head and Neck Surgery, 133,* 767–771.

Siupsinskiene, N., & Lycke, H. (2011). Effects of vocal training on singing and speaking voice characteristics in vocally healthy adults and children based on choral and nonchoral data. *Journal of Voice, 25,* e177–e189.

Slater, S. C. (1992). Omnibus survey: Portrait of the professions. *ASHA Leader, 3,* 61–65.

Smith, B. E., & Guyette, T. W. (1996). Observation: Pressure-flow differences in performance during production of the CV syllables /pi/ and /pa/. *The Cleft Palate–Craniofacial Journal, 33,* 74–76.

Smith, B. E., Guyette, T. W., Patil, Y., & Brannan, T. (2003). Pressure-flow measurements for selected nasal sound segments produced by normal children and adolescents: A preliminary study. *The Cleft Palate–Craniofacial Journal, 40,* 158–164.

Smith, B. E., Kempster, G. B., & Sims, H. S. (2009). Patient factors related to voice therapy attendance and outcomes. *Journal of Voice, 24,* 694–701.

Smith, M. E., Roy, N., & Stoddard, K. (2008). ANSA-RLN innervation for unilateral vocal fold paralysis in adolescents and young children. *International Journal of Pediatric Otorhinolaryngology, 72,* 1311–1316.

Smith, M. E., Roy, N., & Wilson, C. (2006). Lidocaine block of the recurrent laryngeal nerve in adductor spasmodic dysphonia: A multidimensional assessment. *The Laryngoscope, 116,* 591–595.

Smith, M. E., & Sauder, C. (2009). Pediatric vocal fold paralysis/immobility. *ASHA Special Interest Group 3: Perspectives on Voice and Voice Disorders, 19,* 113–121.

Smitheran, J., & Hixon, T. (1981). A clinical method for estimating laryngeal airway resistance during vowel production. *Journal of Speech and Hearing Disorders, 46,* 138–146.

Solomon, N. P., & Charron, S. (1998). Speech breathing in able-bodied children and children with cerebral palsy: A review of the literature and implications for clinical intervention. *American Journal of Speech-Language Pathology, 7,* 61–78.

Solomon, N. P., Helou, L. B., & Stojadinovic, A. (2011). Clinical versus laboratory ratings of voice using the CAPE-V. *Journal of Voice, 25,* e7–e14.

Soman, B. (1997). The effect of variations in method of elicitation on maximum sustained phoneme duration. *Journal of Voice, 11,* 285–294.

Sorenson, D. (1984). Frequency characteristics of male and female speakers in the pulse register. *Journal of Communication Disorders, 17,* 65–73.

Sorenson, D. N., & Parker, P. A. (1992). The voiced/voiceless phonation time in children with and without laryneal pathology. *Language, Speech and Hearing Service in Schools, 23,* 163–168.

Speyer, R., Bogaardt, H. A. C., Passos, V. L., Roodenburg, N. P. H. D., Zumach, A., Heijnen, M. A. M., et al. (2010). Maximum phonation time: Variability and reliability. *Journal of Voice, 24,* 261–284.

Speyer, R., Speyer, I., & Heijnen, M. A. M. (2008). Prevalence and relative risk of dysphonia in rheumatoid arthritis. *Journal of Voice, 22,* 232–237.

Spielman, J., Mahler, L., Halpern, A., Gilley, P., Klepitskay, O., & Ramig, L. (2011). Intensive voice treatment (LSVT®LOUD) for Parkinson's disease following deep brain stimulation of the subthalamic nucleus. *Journal of Communication Disorders, 44,* 688–700.

Spielman, J., Starr, A. C., Popolo, P. S., & Hunter, E. J. (2007). Recommendations for the creation of a voice acoustics laboratory. *The National Center for Voice and Speech Online Technical Memo, 7, Version 1.4.* Retrieved from www.ncvs.org.

Stanton, A. E., Sellars, C., Mackenzie, K., McConnachie, A., & Bucknall, C. E. (2009). Perceived vocal morbidity in a problem asthma clinic. *Journal of Laryngology & Otology, 123,* 96–102.

Stathopoulos, E. T., & Sapienza, C. M. (1993). Respiratory and laryngeal function of women and men during vocal intensity variation. *Journal of Speech-Language and Hearing Research, 36,* 64–75.

Stathopoulos, E. T., & Sapienza, C. M. (1997). Developmental changes in laryngeal and respiratory function with variations in sound pressure level. *Journal of Speech, Language, and Hearing Research 40,* 595–614.

Stathopoulos, E. T., & Weismer, G. (1985). Oral airflow and air pressure during speech production: A comparative study of children, youths and adults. *Folia Phoniatrica et Logopaedica, 37,* 152–159.

Stavroulaki, P. (2006). Diagnostic and management problems of laryngopharyngeal reflux disease in children. *International Journal of Pediatric Otorhinolaryngology, 70,* 579–590.

Stemple, J. C. (2000). *Voice therapy: Clinical studies* (2nd ed.). San Diego, CA: Singular.

Stemple, J. C. (2005). A holistic approach to voice therapy. *Seminars in Speech and Language, 26,* 131–137.

Stemple, J. C. (2007). *Principles of physiologic voice therapy. Short course.* Tempe: Arizona State University.

Stemple, J. C., Gerdeman, B. K., & Glaze, L. E. (1994). *Clinical voice management.* San Diego, CA: Singular.

Stemple, J. C., Glaze, L. E., & Klaben, B. G. (2000). *Clinical voice pathology: Theory and management* (3rd ed.). San Diego, CA: Thomson Learning.

Stemple, J. C., Glaze, L. E., & Klaben, B. G. (2010). *Clinical voice pathology: Theory and management* (4th ed.). San Diego, CA: Thomson Learning.

Stemple, J. C., & Holcomb, B. (1988). *Effective voice and articulation.* Columbus, OH: Merrill.

Stemple, J. C., & Thomas, L. (2007). Voice therapy: Does science support the art? *Communicative Disorders Review, 1,* 49–77.

Stewart, C. F., Allen, E. L., Tureen, P., Diamond, B. E., Blitzer, A., & Brin, M. F. (1997). Adductor spasmodic dysphonia: Standard evaluation of symptoms and severity. *Journal of Voice, 11,* 95–103.

Stoll, C., Hochmuth, M., Meister, P., & Soost, F. (2001). Refinement of velopharyngoplasty in patients with cleft palate by covering the pharyngeal flap with nasal mucosa of the velum. *Journal of Craniomaxillofacial Surgery, 29,* 185–186.

Strauss, L., Hejal, R., Galan, G., Dixon, L., & McFadden, E. R., Jr. (1997). Observations on the effects of aerosolized albuterol in acute asthma. *American Journal of Respiratory Critical Care Medicine, 155,* 826–832.

Stroh, B. C., Faust, R. A., & Rimell, F. L. (1998). Results of esophageal biopsies performed during triple endoscopy in the pediatric patient. *Archives of Otolaryngology—Head and Neck Surgery, 124,* 545–549.

Strome, M. (1982). Common laryngeal disorders in children. In M. D. Filter (Ed.), *Phonatory voice disorders in children.* Springfield, IL: Charles C. Thomas.

Su, C. Y., Tsai, S. S., Chiu, J. F., & Cheng, C. A. (2004). Medialization laryngoplasty with strap muscle transposition for vocal fold atrophy with or without sulcus vocalis. *Laryngoscope, 114,* 1106–1112.

Su, C. Y., Tsai, S. S., Chuang, H. C., & Chiu, J. F. (2005). Functional significance of arytenoid adduction with the suture attaching to cricoid cartilage versus to thyroid cartilage for unilateral paralytic dysphonia. *Laryngoscope, 115,* 1752–1759.

Su, W-F., Hsu, Y-D., Chen, H-C., & Sheng, H. (2007). Laryngeal reinnervation by ansa cervicalis nerve implantation for unilateral vocal cord paralysis in humans. *Journal of the American College of Surgeons, 204,* 64–72.

Sugumaran, M., Sulica, L., & Branski, R. C. (2011). Reinke edema finding on positron emission tomography. *Archives of Otolaryngology—Head and Neck Surgery, 137,* 620–621.

Sulica, L., Rosen, C. A., Postma, G. N., Simpson, B., Amin, M., Courey, M., et al. (2010). Current practice in injection augmentation of the vocal folds: Indications, treatment principles, techniques, and complications. *Laryngoscope, 120,* 319–325.

Sullivan, M. D., Heywood, B. M., & Beukelman, D. R. (2001). A treatment for vocal cord dysfunction in female athletes: An outcome study. *Laryngoscope, 111,* 1751–1755.

Svirsky, M. A., Lane, H., Perkell, J. S., & Wozniak, J. (1992). Effects of short-term auditory deprivation on speech production in adult cochlear implant users. *Journal of the Acoustical Society of America, 92,* 1284–1300.

Tachimura, T., Nohara, K., & Wada, T. (2000). Effect of placement of speech appliance on levator veli palatini muscle activity during speech. *Cleft Palate–Craniofacial Journal, 37,* 478–482.

Tait, N. A., Michel, J. F., & Carpenter, M. A. (1980). Maximum duration of sustained /s/ and /z/ in children. *Journal of Speech and Hearing Disorders, 45,* 239–246.

Tanner, K., Roy, N., Merrill, R. M., Sauder, C., Houtz, D. R., & Smith, M. E. (2012). Case-control study of risk factors for spasmodic dysphonia: A comparison with other voice disorders. *Laryngoscope, 122,* 1082–1092.

Tasker, A., Dettmar, P. W., Penetti, M., Koufman, J. A., Birchall, J. P., & Pearson, J. P. (2002). Is gastric reflux a cause of otitis media with effusion in children? *Laryngoscope, 112,* 1930–1934.

Tavares, E., Brasolotto, A. G., Rodrigues, S. A., Pessin, A., & Martins, R. (2012). Maximum phonation time and s/z ratio in a large child cohort. *Journal of Voice* [epub ahead of print]. doi:10.1016/j.jvoice.2012.03.001

Templin, M. C., & Darley, F. L. (1980). *The Templin-Darley Tests of Articulation.* Iowa City, IA: Bureau of Education Research and Service.

Theis, S. M. (2011). Reflux in children and its effects on assessment and management of voice disorders from a speech-language pathologist's perspective. *ASHA Special Interest Group 3: Perspectives on Voice and Voice Disorders, 21,* 106–111.

Theis, S. M., & Heatley, D. G. (2009). Evaluation and treatment of pediatric gastroesophageal reflux and its effects on voice. *ASHA Special Interest Group 3: Perspectives on Voice and Voice Disorders, 19,* 90–95.

Theodoros, D., Scudamore, S., Baldock, P., Coman, S. & Hancock, K. (2007). The effects of Botox and voice therapy in the management of severe muscle tension dysphonia: A case study. *Journal of Medical Speech-Language Pathology, 15,* 293–304.

Thibeault, S. L. (2005). Advances in our understanding of the Reinke space. *Current Opinion in Otolaryngology & Head and Neck Surgery, 13,* 148–151.

Thibeault, S. L. (2007). What are the roles of the laryngologist and speech language pathologist in management of patients with dysphonia? *ASHA Special Interest Group 3: Perspectives on Voice and Voice Disorders, 17,* 4–8.

Thomas, L. B., & Stemple, J. C. (2007). Voice therapy: Does science support the art? *Communication Disorders Review, 1,* 49–77.

Timmermans, B., de Bodt, M. S., Wuyts, F. L., & Van de Heyning, P. H. (2005). Analysis and evaluation of a voice-training program in future professional voice users. *Journal of Voice, 19,* 201–210.

Tindall, L. R., Huebner, R. A., Stemple, J. C., & Kleinert, H. L. (2008). Videophone-delivered voice therapy: A comparative analysis of outcomes to traditional delivery for adults with Parkinson's disease. *Telemedicine and e-Health, 14*(10), 1070–1077.

Ting, J. Y., Patel, R., & Halum, S. L. (2012). Managing voice impairment after injection laryngoplasty. *Journal of Voice, 26,* 797–800.

Titze, I. R. (1994). *Principles of voice production.* New York: Prentice Hall.

Titze, I. R. (2006). Voice training and therapy with a semi-occluded vocal tract: Rationale and scientific underpinnings. *Journal of Speech, Language and Hearing Research, 49,* 448–454.

Titze, I. R., Lemke, J., & Montequin, D. (1997). Populations in the U.S. workforce who rely on voice as a primary tool of trade: A preliminary report. *Journal of Voice, 11,* 254–259.

Treole, K., & Trudeau, M. D. (1997). Changes in sustained production tasks among women with bilateral vocal nodules before and after voice therapy. *Journal of Voice, 11*, 462–469.

Trost-Cardamone, J. E. (1990). The development of speech: Cleft palate misarticulations. In D. E. Kernahan & S. W. Rosenstein (Eds.), *Cleft lip and palate: A system of management.* Baltimore, MD: Lippincott.

Trudeau, M. D. (1998). Paradoxical vocal cord dysfunction among juveniles. *Voice and Voice Disorders, 8*, 11–13.

Trudeau, M. D., & Forrest, L. A. (1997). The contributions of phonatory volume and transglottal airflow to the s/z ratio. *American Journal of Speech-Language Pathology, 6*, 65–69.

Tsukahara, K., Tokashiki, R., Hiramatsu, H., & Suzuki, M. (2005). A case of high-pitched diplophonia that resolved after a direct pull of the lateral cricoarytenoid muscle. *Acta Otolaryngologica, 125*, 331–333.

Tucker, H. M. (1980). Vocal cord paralysis—etiology and management. *Laryngoscope, 90*, 585–590.

Tulunay, O. E. (2008). Laryngitis—diagnosis and management. *Otolaryngologic Clinics of North America, 41*, 437–451.

Tunkel, D. E., Hotchkiss, K. S., Ishman, S., & Brown, D. (2008). Supraglottoplasty in infants using sinus instruments. *Medscape Journal of Medicine, 10*(11), 269.

Ubrig, M. T., Goffi-Gomez, M. V. S., Weber, R., Menezes, M. H. M., Nemr, N. K., Tsuji, D. H., et al. (2011). Voice analysis of postlingually deaf adults pre- and post-cochlear implantation. *Journal of Voice, 6*, 692–699.

Umeno, H., Chitose, S., Sato, K., Ueda, Y., & Nakashima, T. (2012). Long-term postoperative vocal function after thyroplasty type I and fat injection laryngoplasty. *Annals of Otology, Rhinology, and Laryngology, 121*, 185–191.

United States Administration on Aging. (2004). Retrieved May 16, 2012, from www.aoa.gov

United States Bureau of the Census. (2010). Retrieved May 15, 2012, from www.census.gov

United States Department of Labor, Bureau of Labor Statistics. (2006). Occupational employment and wages, 2006 [data file]. Retrieved May 15, 2012, from www.bls.gov/oes

Vaezi, M. F., Hicks, D. M., Abelson, T. I., & Richter, J. E. (2003). Laryngeal signs and symptoms and gastroesophageal reflux disease (GERD): A critical assessment of cause and effect association. *Clinical Gastroenterology and Hepatology, 1*, 333–344.

Van Borsel, J., & De Maesschalek, D. (2008). Speech rate in males, females, and male-to-female transsexuals. *Clinical Linguistics & Phonetics, 22*, 679–685.

Van Borsel, J., Janssens, J., & De Bodt, M. (2009). Breathiness as a feminine voice characteristic: A perceptual approach. *Journal of Voice, 23*, 291–294.

van den Berg, J. (1958). Myoelasatic-aerodynamic theory of voice production. *Journal of Speech and Hearing Research, 1*, 227–243.

Van der Meer, G., Ferreira, Y., & Loock, J. W. (2010). The s/z ratio: A simple and reliable clinical method of evaluating laryngeal function in patients after intubation. *Journal of Critical Care, 25*, 489–492.

van der Merwe, A. (2004). The voice use reduction program. *American Journal of Speech-Language Pathology, 13*, 208–218.

Vanhoudt, I., Thomas, G., Wellens, W. A. R., Vertommen, H., & de Jong, F. I. C. R. S. (2008). The background biopsychosocial status of teachers with voice problems. *Journal of Psychosomatic Research, 65*, 371–380.

Van Houtte, E., Van Lierde, K., & Claeys, S. (2011). Pathophysiology and treatment of muscle tension dysphonia: A review of the current knowledge. *Journal of Voice, 25*, 202–207.

Van Houtte, E., Van Lierde, K. M., d'Haeseleer, D., & Claeys, S. (2010). The prevalence of laryngeal pathology in a treatment-seeking population with dysphonia. *Laryngoscope, 120*, 306–313.

van Leer, E., & Conner, N. P. (2012). Use of portable digital media players increases patient motivation and practice in voice therapy. *Journal of Voice, 26*, 447–453.

van Leer, E., Hapner, E., & Connor, N. P. (2008). Transtheoretical model of health behavior change applied to voice therapy. *Journal of Voice, 22*, 688–698.

Van Lierde, K. M., De Ley, S., Clement, G., De Bodt, M., & Cauwenberge, P. (2004). Outcome of laryngeal manual therapy in four Dutch adults with persistent moderate to severe vocal hyperfunction: A pilot study. *Journal of Voice, 18*, 467–474.

Van Lierde, K. M., d'Haeseleer, E., Baudonck, N., Claeys, S., De Bodt, M., & Behlau, M. (2011). The impact of vocal warm-up exercises on the objective vocal quality in female students training to be speech-language pathologists. *Journal of Voice, 25*, e115–e121.

Van Lierde, K. M., d'Haeseleer, E., De Ley, S., Luyten, A., Baudonck, N., Claeys, S., et al. (2012). The impact of a voice counseling procedure to select students with normal vocal characteristics for starting a master program in speech-language pathology: A pilot study. *Journal of Voice, 26*, 623–628.

Van Riper, C., & Irwin, J. V. (1958). *Voice and articulation.* Englewood Cliffs, NJ: Prentice Hall.

Verdolini, K. (2000). Resonant voice therapy. In J. C. Stemple (Ed.), *Voice therapy: Clinical studies* (2nd ed.). San Diego, CA: Singular.

Verdolini, K., & Ramig, L. (2001). Review: Occupational risks for voice problems. *Logopedics, Phoniatrics, and Vocology, 26*, 37–46.

Verdolini, K., Rosen, C. A., & Branski, R. C. (2006). *Classification manual for voice disorders—I.* Mahwah, NJ: Lawrence Erlbaum Associates.

Verdolini-Marston, K., Burke, M. K., Lessac, A., Glaze, L., & Caldwell, E. (1995). Preliminary study of two methods of treatment for laryngeal nodules. *Journal of Voice, 9*, 74–85.

Verdonck-de Leeuw, I. M., & Mahieu, H. F. (2004). Vocal aging and the impact on daily life: A longitudinal study. *Journal of Voice, 18*, 193–202.

Verduyckt, I., Remacle, M., Jamart, J., Benderitter, C., & Morsomme, D. (2011). Voice-related complaints in the pediatric population. *Journal of Voice, 25*, 373–380.

Vertigan, A. E., & Gibson, P. G. (2012). The role of speech pathology in the management of patients with chronic refractory cough. *Lung, 190*, 35–40.

Vertigan, A. E., Theodoros, D. G., Gibson, P. G., & Winkworth, A. L. (2006). The relationship between chronic cough and paradoxical vocal fold movement: A review of the literature. *Journal of Voice, 20*, 466–480.

Vertigan, A. E., Theodoros, D. G., Winkworth, A. L., & Gibson, P. G. (2007). Perceptual voice characteristics in chronic cough and paradoxical vocal fold movement. *Folia Phoniatrica et Logopaedica, 59*, 256–267.

Vinson, K. N., Zraick, R. I., & Ragland, F. J. (2010). Injection versus medialization laryngoplasty for the treatment of unilateral vocal fold paralysis: Follow-up at 6 months. *Laryngoscope, 120*, 1802–1807.

Von Berg, S., & McFarlane, S. C. (2002a). A collaborative approach to the diagnosis and treatment of child voice disorders. *ASHA Special Interest Group 3, Perspectives on Voice and Voice Disorders, 12*, 19–22.

Von Berg, S., & McFarlane, S. C. (2002b). *Differential diagnosis of dysphonia in an adolescent with complex medical history.* Paper presented at the annual convention of the American Speech-Language-Hearing Association, Atlanta, GA.

Von Berg, S., Watterson, T. L., & Fudge, L. A. (1999). Behavioral management of paradoxical vocal fold movement. *Phonoscope, 2*(3), 145–149.

Walner, D. L., & Cotton, R. T. (1999). Acquired anomalies of the larynx and trachea. In R. T. Cotton & C. M. Meyer (Eds.), *Practical pediatric otolaryngology* (3rd ed., pp. 515–538). Philadelphia, PA: Lippincott-Raven.

Ward, E. C., Koh, S. K., Frisby, J., & Hodge, R. (2003). Differential modes of alaryngeal communication and long-term voice outcomes following pharyngolaryngectomy and laryngectomy. *Folia Phoniatrica et Logopaedica, 55*(1), 39–49.

Warren, D. W. (1979). PERCI: A method for rating palatal efficiency. *Cleft Palate Journal, 16*, 279–285.

Watterson, T. L., Hansen-Magorian, H., & McFarlane, S. C. (1990). A demographic description of laryngeal contact ulcer patients. *Journal of Voice, 4*, 71–75.

Watterson, T. L., Hinton, J., & McFarlane, S. C. (1996). Novel stimuli for obtaining nasalance measures from young children. *Cleft Palate–Craniofacial Journal, 33*, 67–73.

Watterson, T. L., Lewis, K. E., & Deutsch, C. (1998). Nasalance and nasality in low pressure and high pressure speech. *Cleft Palate–Craniofacial Journal, 35*, 293–298.

Watterson, T. L., & McFarlane, S. C. (1990). Transnasal videoendoscopy of the velopharyngeal port mechanism. *Seminars in Speech and Language, 11*, 27–37.

Watterson, T. L., York, S. L., & McFarlane, S. C. (1994). Effect of vocal loudness on nasalance measures. *Journal of Communication Disorders, 27*, 257–262.

Watts, C., Murphy, J., & Barnes-Burroughs, K. (2003). Pitch matching accuracy of trained singers, untrained subjects with talented singing voices, and untrained subjects with nontalented singing voices in conditions of varying feedback. *Journal of Voice, 17,* 185–194.

Watts, C. R., & Awan, S. N. (2011). Use of spectral/cepstral analyses for differentiating normal from hypofunctional voices in sustained vowel and continuous speech contexts. *Journal of Speech, Language and Hearing Research, 54,* 1525–1537.

Weed, D. T., Jewett, B. S., Rainey, C., Zealear, D. L., Stone, R. E., Ossoff, R. H., et al. (1996). Long-term follow-up of recurrent laryngeal nerve avulsion for the treatment of spastic dysphonia. *Annals of Otology, Rhinology and Laryngology, 105,* 592–601.

Wei, J., & Bond, J. (2011). Management and prevention of endotracheal intubation injury in neonates. *Current Opinion in Otolaryngology & Head & Neck Surgery, 19,* 474–477.

Weinrich, B. (2002). Common voice disorders in children. *ASHA Special Interest Group 3: Perspectives on Voice and Voice Disorders, 12*(1), 13–16.

Weismer, G., & Liss, J. M. (1991). Speech motor control and aging. In D. Ripich (Ed.), *Handbook of geriatric communication disorders* (pp. 205–225). Austin, TX: Pro-Ed.

Wetmore, S. I., Key, J. M., & Suen, J. Y. (1985). Complications of laser surgery for laryngeal papillomatosis. *Laryngoscope, 95,* 798–803.

Wheeler, K. M., Collins, S. P., & Sapienza, C. M. (2006). The relationship between VHI scores and specific acoustic measures of mildy disordered voice production. *Journal of Voice, 20,* 308–317.

Whymark, A. D., Clement, W. A., Kubba, H., & Geddes, N. K. (2006). Laser epiglottopexy for laryngomalacia: 10 years' experience in the west of Scotland. *Archives of Otolaryngology, Head and Neck Surgery, 132,* 978–982.

Wilson, D. K. (1987). *Voice problems of children* (3rd ed.). Baltimore, MD: Lippincott.

Wilson, F. B., Oldring, D. J., & Mueller, J. (1980). Recurrent laryngeal nerve dissection: A case report involving return of spastic dysphonia after initial surgery. *Journal of Speech and Hearing Disorders, 45,* 112–118.

Wilson, J. J., Theis, S. M., & Wilson, E. M. (2009). Evaluation and management of vocal cord dysfunction in the athlete. *Current Sports Medicine Reports, 8,* 65–70.

Wingate, J., Brown, W., Shrivastav, R., Davenport, P., & Sapienza, C. (2007). Treatment outcomes for professional voice users. *Journal of Voice, 21,* 433–449.

Wingate, J., & Collins, S. (2005, November). *Consistency of voice range profiles in normal speakers.* Paper presented at the annual ASHA Convention, San Diego, CA.

Wingfield, W. L., Pollock, D., & Gunert, R. R. (1969). Therapeutic efficacy of amantadine-HCL and rumantidine-HCL in naturally occurring influence A2 respiratory illness in many. *New England Journal of Medicine, 281,* 579–584.

Winkler, R., & Sendlmeier, W. (2006). EGG open quotient in aging voices—Changes with increasing chronological age and its perception. *Logopedics Phoniatrics Vocology, 31,* 51–56.

Wirz, S. (1986). The voice of the deaf. In M. Fawcus (Ed.), *Voice disorders and their management.* London: Croom Helm.

Witt, P., Cohen, D., Grames, L. M., & Marsh, J. (1999). Sphincter pharyngoplasty for the surgical management of speech dysfunction associated with velocardiofacial syndrome. *British Journal of Plastic Surgery, 52,* 613–618.

Wolfe, V. I., Ratusnik, D. I., Smith, F. H., & Northrop, G. (1990). Intonation and fundamental frequency in male-to-female transsexuals, *Journal of Speech and Hearing Disorders, 5,* 43–50.

Wolpe, J. (1987). *Essential principles and practices of behavior therapy.* Phoenix, AZ: Milton H. Erickson Foundation.

Woo, P. (2006). Office-based laryngeal procedures. *Otolaryngologic Clinics of North America, 39,* 111–133.

Woodson, G. E. (2011). Arytenoid abduction for bilateral vocal fold immobility. *Current Opinion in Otolaryngology & Head and Neck Surgery, 19,* 428–438.

Woodson, G. E., & Murry, T. (1994). Botulinum toxin in the treatment of recalcitrant mutational dysphonia. *Journal of Voice, 8,* 347–351.

Xu, J., & Fung, K. (2012). Laryngectomy-concepts and shifting paradigms. *ASHA Special Interest*

Group 3: Perspectives on Voice and Voice Disorders, 22, 25–32.

Xu, J. H., Ikeda, Y., & Komiyama, S. (1991). Biofeedback and the yawning breath pattern in voice therapy: A clinical trial. *Auris Nasus Larynx, 18*(1), 67–77.

Xu, Z., Xia, Z., Wang, Z., & Jiang, F. (2007). Pediatric sulcus vocalis. *Lin Chung Er Bi Yan Hou Tou Jing Wai Ke Za Zh, 21,* 550–551.

Yan, Y., Olszewski, A. E., Hoffman, A. E., Zhuang, P., Ford, C. N., Dailey, S. H., et al. (2010). Use of lasers in laryngeal surgery. *Journal of Voice, 24,* 102–109.

Yorkston, K. M., Beukelman, D. R., Strand, E. A., & Hakel, M. (2010). *Management of motor speech disorders in children and adults* (3rd ed.). Austin, TX: Pro-Ed.

Yorkston, K. M., Miller, R. M., & Strand, E. A. (2004). *Management of speech and swallowing in degenerative diseases.* Tuscon, AZ: Communication Skill Builders.

Young, V., & Smith, L. J. (2012). Saccular cysts: A current review of characteristics and management. *Laryngoscope, 122*(3), 595–599.

Zealer, D. L., Billante, C. R., Courey, M. S., Netterville, J. L., Paniello, R. C., Sanders, I., et al. (2003). Reanimation of the paralyzed human larynx with an implantable electrical stimulation device. *Laryngoscope, 113,* 1149–1156.

Zeine, L., & Walter, K. L. (2002). The voice and its care: Survey findings from actors' perspectives. *Journal of Voice, 16,* 229–243.

Zeitels, S. M., Hillman, R. E., Desloge, R., Mauri, M., & Doyle, P. B. (2002). Phonomicrosurgery in singers and performing artists: Treatment outcomes, management theories, and future directions. *Annals of Otology, Rhinology and Laryngology, Supplement 190,* 21–40.

Zemlin, W. R. (1998). *Speech and hearing science: Anatomy and physiology* (4th ed.). Englewood Cliffs, NJ: Prentice Hall.

Zhang, Y., Beiging, E., Tsui, H., & Jiang, J. J. (2010). Efficient and effective extraction of vocal fold vibratory patterns from high-speed digital imaging. *Journal of Voice, 24,* 21–29.

Zraick, R. I. (2009). Voice use reduction for the treatment of chronic dysphonia. In J. C. Stemple & L. B. Thomas (Eds.), *Voice therapy: Clinical studies* (pp. 93–98). San Diego, CA: Plural.

Zraick, R. I., & Atcherson, S. R. (2012). Readability of patient-reported outcome questionnaires for use with persons with dysphonia. *Journal of Voice, 26,* 635–641.

Zraick, R. I., Atcherson, S. R., & Brown, A. M. (2012). Readability of patient-reported outcome questionnaires for use with persons who stutter. *Journal of Fluency Disorders, 37,* 20–24.

Zraick, R. I., Atcherson, S. R., & Ham, B. K. (2012). Readability of patient-reported outcome questionnaires for use with persons with swallowing disorders. *Dysphagia, 27,* 3, 346–352.

Zraick, R. I., Birdwell, K. Y., & Smith-Olinde, L. K. (2005). The effect of speaking sample duration on determination of habitual pitch. *Journal of Voice, 19,* 197–201.

Zraick, R. I., Davenport, D. J., Tabbal, S. D., Hicks, G. S., Hutton, T. J., & Patterson, J. (2004). Reliability of speech intelligibility ratings using the Unified Huntington's Disease Rating Scale. *Journal of Medical Speech-Language Pathology, 12,* 31–40.

Zraick, R. I., Dennie, T. M., Tabbal, S. D., Hutton, T. J., Hicks, G. S., & O'Sullivan, P. (2003). Reliability of speech intelligibility ratings using the Unified Parkinson's Disease Rating Scale. *Journal of Medical Speech-Language Pathology, 11,* 227–240.

Zraick, R. I., Gentry, M. A., Smith-Olinde, L., & Gregg, B. A. (2006). The effect of speaking context on determination of habitual pitch. *Journal of Voice, 20,* 545–554.

Zraick, R. I., Gregg, B. A., & Whitehouse, E. L. (2006). Speech and voice characteristics of geriatric speakers: A review of the literature and a call for research and training. *Journal of Medical Speech-Language Pathology, 14,* 133–142.

Zraick, R. I., Kempster, G. B., Connor, N. P., Thibault, S., Klaben, B. K., Bursac, Z., et al. (2011). Establishing validity of the Consensus Auditory Perceptual Evaluation of Voice. *American Journal of Speech-Language Pathology, 20,* 14–22.

Zraick, R. I., Keyes, M., Montague, J., & Keiser, J. (2002). Mid-basal-to-ceiling versus mid-ceiling-to-basal elicitation of maximum phonational frequency range. *Journal of Voice, 16,* 317–322.

Zraick, R. I., Klaben, B., Connor, N., Thiebault, S., Kempster, G., Glaze, L., et al. (2007, November). *Results of the CAPE-V validation study.* Seminar at the Annual Convention of the American Speech-Language-Hearing Association, Boston, MA.

Zraick, R. I., & LaPointe, L. L. (2008). Hyperkinetic dysarthria. In M. R. McNeil (Ed.), *Clinical management of sensorimotor speech disorders* (2nd ed., pp. 152–165). New York: Thieme Medical Publishers.

Zraick, R. I., & Liss, J. M. (2000). A comparison of equal-appearing interval scaling and direct magnitude estimation of nasal voice quality. *Journal of Speech and Hearing Research, 43,* 979–988.

Zraick, R. I., Liss, J. M., Dorman, M. F., Case, J. L., LaPointe, L. L., & Beals, S. P. (2000). Multidimensional scaling of nasal voice quality. *Journal of Speech and Hearing Research, 43,* 989–996.

Zraick, R. I., Marshall, W. C., Smith-Olinde, L., & Montague, J. C. (2004). The effect of speaking task on determination of habitual loudness. *Journal of Voice, 18,* 176–182.

Zraick, R. I., Nelson, J. C., Montague, J. C., & Monoson, P. K. (2000). The effect of task on determination of maximum phonational frequency range. *Journal of Voice, 14,* 154–160.

Zraick, R. I., Pickett, H., Guyette, T. W., Gregg, B. A., & McWeeny, E. (June 2009). *Voice use reduction as a treatment for chronic dysphonia: A case study.* Poster at the Voice Foundation's 38th Annual Symposium: Care of the Professional Voice, Philadelphia, PA.

Zraick, R. I., & Risner, B. Y. (2008). Assessment of quality of life in persons with voice disorders. *Current Opinion in Otolaryngology—Head and Neck Surgery, 16,* 188–193.

Zraick, R. I., Risner, B. Y., Smith-Olinde, L., Gregg, B. A., Johnson, F. L., & McWeeny, E. K. (2006). Patient versus partner perception of voice handicap. *Journal of Voice, 21,* 485–494.

Zraick, R. I., Skaggs, S. D., & Montague, J. C. (2000). The effect of task on determination of habitual pitch. *Journal of Voice, 14,* 484–489.

Zraick, R. I., Smith-Olinde, L. S., & Shotts, L. (2012). Adult normative data for the KayPentax Phonatory Aerodynamic System Model 6600. *Journal of Voice, 26,* 164–176.

Zraick, R. I., Wendel, K. W., & Smith-Olinde, L. (2005). The effect of speaking task on perceptual judgment of the severity of dysphonic voice. *Journal of Voice, 19,* 574–581.

Zur, K., Cotton, S., Kelchner, L., Baker, S., Weinrich, B., & Lee, L. (2007). Pediatric Voice Handicap Index (pVHI): A new tool for evaluating pediatric dysphonia. *International Journal of Pediatric Otorhinolaryngology, 71,* 77–82.

Zwitman, D. H. (1990). Utilization of transoral endoscopy to assess velopharyngeal closure. *Seminars in Speech and Language, 11,* 38–46.

Zwitman, D. H., & Calcaterra, T. C. (1973). The "silent cough" method for vocal hyperfunction. *Journal of Speech and Hearing Disorders, 38,* 119–125.

Zwitman, D. H., Gyepes, M. T., & Ward, P. H. (1976). Assessment of velar and lateral wall movement by oral telescope and radiographic examination in patients with velopharyngeal inadequacy and in normal subjects. *Journal of Speech and Hearing Disorders, 41,* 381–389.

COMPANIES AND ORGANIZATIONS

Blue Tree Publishing, www.bluetreepublishing.com/iEducate.cfm

Casa Futura Technologies (Boulder, CO), www.casafuturatech.com/index.php/

CTS Informatica (Paraná, Brazil), www.ctsinf.com/english/#produtos.html

Griffin Laboratories (Temecula, CA), http://www.griffinlab.com/

International Association of Laryngectomees (Atlanta, GA), www.theial.com/ial/

KayPENTAX® Corp. (Montvale, NJ), www.kaypentax.com

National Association of Teachers of Singing (NATS) (Jacksonville, FL), www.NATS.org

Pro-Ed Inc. (Austin, TX), www.proedinc.com

Tiger DRS, Inc. (Seattle, WA), tiger-electronics@att.net

Voice and Speech Trainers Association (VASTA) (City, ST), www.VASTA.org

WebWhispers (Gold Hill, OR), www.webwhispers.org/

World Professional Association for Transgender Health (City, ST), www.WPATH.org

Index